Questions & Answers

Exam-Oriented
ANATOMY
Below Diaphragm

Questions & Answers

Exam-Oriented

ANATOMY

Below Diaphragm

**(Gross Anatomy, Systemic Histology, Systemic Embryology
of Abdomen, Infex, General Anatomy, General Histology,
General Embryology and Genetics)**

(With Colour Diagrams)

Shoukat N. Kazi

M.S. (Anatomy), D.T.C.D., B.Sc., L.L.B., M.B.A. (Hospital Admin.)

Professor, Dr. D.Y. Patil Medical College
(Dr. D.Y. Patil Vidhyapeeth—deemed university),
Pune - 411 018 (India)

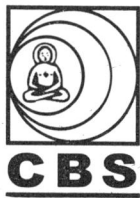

CBS

CBS Publishers & Distributors Pvt. Ltd.

New Delhi • Bengaluru • Chennai • Kochi • Kolkata • Mumbai
Hyderabad • Uttarakhand • Nagpur • Patna • Pune • Jharkhand

ISBN: 81-239-1121-1

First Edition: 2004
Reprint: 2006, 2008, 2009, 2010, 2012, 2013,
          2014, 2015, 2017, 2018, 2019, 2020

Published by **Satish Kumar Jain** and produced by **Varun Jain** for
CBS Publishers & Distributors Pvt. Ltd.,
4819/XI Prahlad Street, 24 Ansari Road, Daryaganj, New Delhi - 110002
delhi@cbspd.com, cbspubs@airtelmail.in • www.cbspd.com
Ph.: 23289259, 23266861, 23266867 • Fax: 011-23243014

Corporate Office: 204 FIE, Industrial Area, Patparganj, Delhi - 110 092
Ph: 49344934 • Fax: 011-49344935
E-mail: publishing@cbspd.com • publicity@cbspd.com

Branches:
• *Bengaluru:* 2975, 17th Cross, K.R. Road, Bansankari 2nd Stage,
  Bengaluru - 70 • Ph: +91-80-26771678/79 • Fax: +91-80-26771680
  E-mail: cbsbng@gmail.com, bangalore@cbspd.com
• *Chennai:* No. 7, Subbaraya Street, Shenoy Nagar, Chennai - 600030
  Ph: +91-44-26681266, 26680620 • Fax: +91-44-42032115
  E-mail: chennai@cbspd.com
• *Kochi:* Ashana House, 39/1904, A.M. Thomas Road, Valanjambalam,
  Ernakulum, Kochi • Ph: +91-484-4059061-65
  Fax: +91-484-4059065 • E-mail: cochin@cbspd.com
• *Kolkata:* 6-B, Ground Floor, Rameshwar Shaw Road, Kolkata - 700014
  Ph: +91-33-22891126/7/8 • E-mail: kolkata@cbspd.com
• *Mumbai:* 83-C, Dr. E. Moses Road, Worli, Mumbai - 400018
  Ph: +91-9833017933, 022-24902340/41 • E-mail: mumbai@cbspd.com

Representatives:

• Hyderabad: 0-9885175004	• Nagpur: 0-9021734563
• Patna: 0-9334159340	• Pune: 0-9623451994
• Jharkhand: 0-9811541605	• Uttarakhand: 0-9716462459

Printed at:
SDR Printers Pvt. Ltd., Delhi (India)

DEDICATED

TO

MY PARENTS

Haji Nizamsaheb K. Kazi
Mrs. Jainnabbi N. Kazi

&

STUDENTS

ABOUT THE BOOK

Medical Council of India has reduced the duration of first year M.B.B.S. by 6 months and introduced new pattern of questions which include long answer question, short notes, short answer question, clinical problems and multiple choice question. The students are expected to know all the topics as well as specific information and minute, relevant details having clinical importance.

There is no source for the definition and the extent of the contents of the various terms used in the theory questions. The author has extensively discussed these terms with eminent anatomist in India and attempted to define these terms. He is aware of the limitations and has high regard about others views.

To all above problems the author has given a solution by a book **'Exam Oriented Anatomy'**.

The salient features of the book are
- The book is written using short and simple sentences.
- Three types of questions are discussed 47 LAQs (Long Answer Questions), 125 SN (Short Notes) & 38 SAQs (Short Answer Questions).
- The information given in italic is the information required to answer the MCQs.
- The answers are written in the form of points by using indentation.
  1.
     A.
        a.
           I.
              i.
              -
  2.
- Tables are used to save the time and display the information for immediate references for the students and examiners.
- The relevant, simple, linear, informative diagrams are drawn with the respective colours.
- Histology diagrams are drawn by pink and violet colour.
- The question of the development of organ is discussed by applying rule of five wives and one husband by using key word NORTHY (Whe**n**, Wh**o**, Whe**re**, Wha**t**, **H**ow & **W**hy).
  o Chronological age: When.
  o Germ layer: Who.
  o Site: Where.
  o Source: What and how.
  o Anomalies: Deviation from normal. Anomalies are described depending upon the incidence.
- Important key words, which help to memorize the subject without taxation to the memory.
- **'Key to memory'** is displayed at the end of the book, which help the student to revise important points.

The author humbly request all the students, teachers and well wishers to point out any corrections, which will be rectified in the next edition. He is very much free for correction and welcomes all sorts of criticism.

FOREWORD

Prof. S. N. Kazi's Book is intended to help medical Students rapidly master complex intricacies of human anatomy that is essential to clinical care.

This book was written to fulfill the need for a brief, but readable, summary of the relevant anatomy, with succinct notes on applied anatomy wherever indicated. It addresses the diverse and mounting need of medical students preparing for professional examinations. The text will not only enhance the knowledge to an extent sufficient to satisfy the examiners but will equip the readers with the necessary understanding of applied anatomy for future practice. A recurring problem in medical education is the common inability of the students to relate the large body of factual knowledge to practical application in their future clinical training. A commendable endeavour has been made by Pro. Kazi to bridge the gap between rote anatomy and clinical relevance. The mnemonics and humour in this book do not intend any disrespect for anyone, rather they are employed as an educational device, as it is well known that the best memory techniques involve the use of ridiculous association. Stephen Goldberg in his unique book titled. " Clinical Neuroanatomy made ridiculous simple", has already demonstrated their efficacy superbly. **Further more, this book is very well-illustrated with 47 LAQs, 38 SAQs & 125 SNs, 49 key words, 254 line diagrams and elegantly constructed 47 tables.**

This book is not designed to replace standard reference texts, but rather is to be read as a companion text before appearing in an examination. This will enable the student to gain an overall perspective of essential anatomy.

My best wishes for the success of this endeavor which merits appreciation.

Formerly:-
Professor & Chairman
Department of Anatomy &
Founder Director,
Inter Disciplinary Brain Research Center,
Dean, Principal & Chief medical Suptdt.
Jawaharlal Nehru Medical College,
Aligarh Muslim University
Aligarh 202 002 U. P. (India)

Prof. Dr. Mahdi Hasan
M.B.B.S., (Hons.) FICS, FAMS. Ph. D.,D.Sc.,
FNA
Professor Emeritus
INSA Senior Scientist
Department of Anatomy
Chhatrapati Shahuji Maharaj Medical University,
(Upgrapati King George's Medical College)
Lucknow-226 003
U. P. India.

FOREWORD

All the Medical Colleges in the state of Maharashtra were affiliated to eight different conventional universities in the state up to 1997. After the establishment of Maharashtra University of health sciences in the state in 1998, all of them were affiliated to this single state level university. Previously syllabi and pattern of examination were different but new pattern (1+1½ + 2 yrs.) of curriculum recommended by the Medical Council of India while the conventional universities were following the old (1½ + 1½ + 1½ yrs.) pattern. First time in the examination LAQ, SAQ and MCQ patterns were introduced by MUHS. On the background of the reduced duration for both students (for learning) and teachers (for teaching) of I MBBS there was a need for examination oriented revision book.

It is really a great pleasure for me to introduce this book on Human Anatomy written by one of my ex-colleague Dr. S. N. Kazi. I have gone through the manuscript of this book which adequately covers the subject. Usually students have to purchase separate books for Anatomy, Histology, Embryology, Gen. Anatomy, Genetics etc. Dr. Kazi has tried to cover all these branches in simple language with the help of computerized line diagrams. It is designed to meet the need of the undergraduate exam going students. Most of the information is given in tabular forms, easy to compare and remember and clinical applications of the subject have been touched adequately.

The book speaks the long experience of the author in the subject and will minimize the stress and strain of a medical student during pre-examination period. I congratulate the author for this venture and wish the book great success.

Dr. Shingare P. H.
Prof. & Head,
Dept. of Anatomy
Grant Medical College &
Sir J.J. Group of Hospitals
Byculla, Mumbai 400 008.

- Ex. Dean, Faculty of Medicine - North Maharashtra University.
- Ex. Controller of Exam - MUHS, Nashik.
- Ex. Chairman BOS Preclinical - MUHS, Nashik.
- Member of BOS Preclinical Faculty of Medicine & Faculty of Dentistry - MUHS.
- Ex. Vice Dean U. G. - Grant Medical College, Mumbai.
- Ex. Vice Dean P. G. - Grant Medical College, Mumbai.

ACKNOWLEDGMENT

Writing acknowledgment is a sign of sigh of relief. It is the last leaf of the process of book writing. Though there is a feeling that the phenomenon of book writing has ended, in reality it is the beginning of shouldering the responsibility of the contents. Though I have authored the contents, it was indeed a teamwork. Many of my friends, colleagues and students have contributed immensely .It is great pleasure to acknowledge them.

When I proposed the idea of writing an 'Exam Oriented Anatomy' book to late Dr. Indra Bhargava, he patted on my back and gave an encouragement to take the first step in this direction. My sincere and humble salutations to the great soul.

Prof. Dr. Mahdi Hasan (Professor & Chairman, Department of Anatomy & Founder Director, Inter Disciplinary Brain Research Center, Dean, Principal & Chief Medical Superintendent, Jawaharlal Nehru Medical College, Aligarh Muslim University) has agreed to write a preface without any hesitation and guided me regarding the approach to the subject. I think myself fortunate to have the preface of such eminent professor in Anatomy. I salute to him from the bottom of my heart.

Dr. Inderbir Singh (Professor Emeritus, Rohtak) has thrown light upon the definition of each term used in the examination and warned to use the original diagrams. I am really thankful for cautioning me about the consequences. I am indebted to his valuable guidance. Dr. V. Balasubramanyam, (Professor and head department of anatomy St. John's Medical College, Bangalore) thoroughly went through the general lay out of the book and gave me very valuable suggestions regarding alteration of diagrams and copy right regulations.

My sincere and heartfelt thanks to following colleagues.

Dr. P. H. Shingare (Professor & Head, Department of Anatomy, Grant Medical College, Mumbai) for preparing the preface and guidance in all respects.

Dr. Kadasne (Civil Surgeon & Professor of Anatomy at Government Medical College, Nagpur), Dr. Mrs. S. L. Pathak (Associate Professor at Government Medical College, Nagpur) and Dr. Mrs. Palikundwar (Professor at Government Medical College, Nagpur) have given their invaluable guidance in drawing diagrams.

My sincere thanks are to Dr. P. L. Jahagirdar (Professor at Al-Amin Medical College, Bijapur) for encouragement in the initial stage of writing the book.

I am very much thankful to Dr. Miss. A. N. Nandedkar (Professor & HOD) for understanding me and making me free from departmental activities. She has knowingly unknowingly helped me a lot in bringing up the book. I am also thankful Dr. D. L. Ingole (Dean & Pro Vice Chancellor of Dr. D. Y. Patil Vidhyapeeth - Deemed University), Mr. B. S. Mane (Registrar) & Dr. Mrs. U. P. Dubhashi (Professor) of Dr. D. Y. Patil Medical College, Pimpri, for their constant and continued encouragement.

Dr. Herekar (Professor at Government Medical College, Miraj), Dr. Mrs. Aruna Mukherji (Ex. Deputy Dean & Professor at M. G. M. Medical College, New Mumbai), Dr. Bhatnagar (Professor Emeritus) & Dr. Sadhna Roy Chaudhary for inspiring me to write the book.

I must thank my core group who were associated with the metamorphosis of the book since inception. I thank Dr. Manvikar Purushottam Rao, Dr. R. J. Patil (Professor at Dr. D. Y. Patil Medical College) for their contribution to every section of the book in each stage of the process of writing.

My heartfelt thanks are to Ms. Benazeer Mujawar who had worked odd hours tirelessly for secretarial help. Her contribution has been indispensable. Mr. Sanjay Raut, our artist who has drawn the diagrams and patiently done numerous corrections as suggested. I must thank Mrs. Geeta Pomaji and Mr. Dinesh Kelji for immense help.

I should not fail to mention the name of my better half Mrs. Kamartaj S. Kazi who is my silent and constant inspiration. She has kept me free from all our domestic and family problems. I express my grateful appreciation for her love, patience and understanding. I also appreciate my daughter Ms. Sadiya for tolerating my absence from home. I am indebted for the support and blessings of my parents. I constantly get charged by the moral boosting by my brothers Shikandar, Kabir, Allabax and Nazir. I extend my thanks to my elder brother Mr. Akbar Kazi who has constantly encouraged to write the book. I would like to extend my thanks to Mrs. Shama Kazi for understanding me and allowing to remain absent in real time.

Last and most important are the students, without whose feed-back the book would not have taken the shape.

It has been my pleasure to work with the staff of CBS Publication and Distributors (Delhi), Mr. Satish Kumar Jain, Mr. Vinod Jain, Mr. Wajid Khan & Mr. B. R. Sharma, for their keen interest and devotion in getting this book published.

DR. S. N. KAZI
60, Atlas colony,
Mahesh Nagar, Pimpri,
Pune - 411 018.
Mobile - 94220 27718.

Special thanks

I am extending my sincere and special thanks to following persons, without whom the book would not have been completed.

- **Dr. P. H. Shingare** (Professor & Head, Department of Anatomy, Grant Medical College, Mumbai) has meticulously corrected the text and has given solutions to diagrams. He has tolerated my disturbance at odd hours in his busy schedule.

- **Dr. Mrs. Kanaklata Iyer** (Professor of Anatomy, Somaiya Medical College, New Mumbai) has really given a breakthrough to the problems of diagrams. She has helped outrightly by sparing her valuable time through her busy schedule by taking keen interest. She has contributed diagrams of gross anatomy of abdomen, inferior extremity and general embryology.

- **Dr. Savgaonkar** (Professor of Anatomy B. J. Medical College, Pune) has drawn histology diagrams of abdomen section. He being my close friend, understood the difficulties and offered his help by completing the diagrams in very short time.

- **Dr. Anjali Dhamangaonkar** (Associate Professor of Anatomy, G. S. Medical College, Mumbai) has contributed to the general embryology diagrams. It was very difficult for her to give some time. But her desire to help me has solved the problems.

- **Dr. Manvikar Purushottam Rao** (Lecturer at Dr. D. Y. Patil Medical College, Pimrpi) has drawn some of the diagrams of general histology.

- **Dr. Kadasne D. K.** has allowed me to use some of the diagrams from his book.

- **Dr. Umarji** (Professor & Head of Department, Krishna Institute of Medical Science, Karad) has drawn few diagrams of general anatomy.

Includes gross anatomy, systemic histology, systemic embryology below the diaphragm. It also includes general embryology, general anatomy and genetics.

Pattern of Question Papers

Rajiv Gandhi University of Health Sciences

Total Marks 100

Section - I
1. Long Essays: 9 Marks
2. Long Essays: 9 Marks

Section - II
Short Essays: 10 x 5 = 50 Marks

Section - III
Short Answers: 16 x 2 = 32 Marks

Bharti Vidhyapeeth Medical College

Total Marks 100

Instruction: Answer any five from each section.

Section - I
1. Short Notes: 2 x 5 = 10 Marks
2. 4 Long questions, each of 10 marks: 40 Marks
3. Short Notes: 2 x 5 = 10 Marks

Section - II
1. Short Notes: 2 x 5 = 10 Marks
2. 4 Long questions, each of 10 marks: 40 Marks
3. Short Notes: 2 x 5 = 10 Marks

Maharashtra University of Health Sciences & Dr. D. Y. Patil Vidhyapeeth Deemed University

Total Marks 50

Section A

Q. No. 1 Multiple Choice Questions (MCQ): 15 Marks {30 Minutes}

Section B

Q. No. 2 Write in brief (five out of six): 2 Marks each = 10 Marks

Q. No. 3 On applied anatomy (two out of three): 4 marks each = 8 Marks

Section C

Q. No. 4 Long Question OR

Q. No. 4 Long Question: 9 Marks

Q. No. 5 Write Short Notes (two out of three): 4 Marks each = 8 Marks

PROTOTYPE DESCRIPTION OF THE QUESTIONS

LAQ on joint
1. **Introduction :**
2. **Classification**
   A. Structural classification
      a. Depending upon the number of bones
      b. Depending upon the presence of intra articular structure
      c. Depending upon the shape of the articular surface of the bone
      d. Depending upon the presence & absence of the features of typical synovial joint
      e. Depending upon the axis
   B. Functional classification
      a. Depending upon the mobility
3. **Bones taking part any joint**
4. **Ligament :**
   A. Fibrous capsule
      a. Attachment of the capsule to the proximal and distal bones
      b. Variation of the thickness of the capsule
      c. Areas where the capsule is deficient
      d. Muscles, ligaments strengthening (reinforcing) the capsule
   B. Other ligaments
5. **Bursae in relation to joint**
6. **Movements**
   A. Name of the movement
   B. Range
   C. Axis
   D. Limiting factors
   E. Muscles bringing movement
7. **Intra articular structures**
8. **Relations**
   A. Anterior
   B. Posterior
   C. Lateral
   D. Medial
9. **Blood supply**
10. **Nerve supply**
11. **Applied anatomy.**
    A. Function :
       a. Maintenance
       b. Common diseases of the joint
    B. Disease :
       a. Dislocation or fracture of the joint
       b. Deformity
       c. Ankylosis

LAQ on Artery
1. **Introduction :**
    Region supplied
2. **Origin**
3. **Termination**
4. **Extent**
5. **Course and relations**
6. **Distribution**
7. **Branches**
    A. Muscular branches,
    B. Cutaneous branches,
    C. Nutrient branches,
    D. Articular branches,
    E. Branches to nerve,
    F. Anastomosing branches,
    G. Terminal branches,
8. **Applied anatomy**
    A. Pressure points
    B. Ligation and exposure
    C. Vulnerable points
    D. Collateral circulation
    E. Arteriography
9. **Development :**
10. **Variation :**

LAQ on Vein
1. **Introduction :**
    Area drained
2. **Formation**
    A. How?
    B. Where?
3. **Termination**
    A. How?
    B. Where?
4. **Course and relation**
5. **Subdivision**
6. **Peculiarities**
7. **Tributaries**
8. **Applied anatomy**
    A. Obstruction and collateral circulation
    B. Vulnerable points
    C. Surgical procedure

LAQ on peripheral nerve

1. **Introduction** : Region of distribution
2. **Nature**
3. **Origin and root value**
   A. Level
   B. Mode of origin
4. **Course and relations**
5. **Branches**
   A. Sensory branches,
   B. Motor branches,
   C. Articular branches,
   D. Vascular branches &
   E. Communicating
   F. Miscellaneous.
6. **Applied anatomy**
   A. Functions and testing of the nerve
   B. In disease
      a. Sensory - loss or pain
      b. Motor - paralysis deformity
   C. Vulnerable points for injury

LAQ on space
Femoral triangle, popliteal fossa, axilla, cubital fossa, triangles of neck (anterior, posterior, suboccipital) superficial and deep perineal pouch, ischiorectal fossa.
1. **Introduction :**
   A. Location
   B. Shape
2. **Boundaries :**
   A. Lateral border / wall
   B. Medial border
   C. Superior border
   D. Inferior border
   E. Roof / anterior wall
      a. Skin,
      b. Cutaneous vein, artery, nerve
      c. Superficial fascia
      d. Deep fascia
   F. Floor
3. **Content :**
   A. Neurovascular
   B. Glands
   C. Packing material
4. **Recesses :**

5.   Space :
6.   Canals
7.   Applied anatomy
  A.   Function
      a.   Protection of the contents
      b.   Accommodate for movements
  B.   Disease
      a.   Vulnerable structures
      b.   Collection of pus
      c.   Path of spread
      d.   Incision drainage

LAQ on Gross anatomy of canal
(Femoral canal, adductor canal, anal canal, pudendal canal)
1.   **Gross anatomy**
  A.   **Introduction :**
      a.   General introduction
      b.   Situation
      c.   Extent :
      d.   Length :
      e.   Direction :
      f.   Peculiarity(ies) :
      g.   Sex predilection :
  B.   **Boundaries :**
      a.   Lateral border / wall
      b.   Medial border
      c.   Superior border
      d.   Inferior border
      e.   Roof / anterior wall
          I.   Skin,
          II.   Cutaneous vein, artery, nerve
          III. Superficial fascia
          IV.   Deep fascia
      g.   Floor
  C.   **Content and relations of content**
  D.   **Defensive mechanism of the canal :**
2.   **Development**
3.   **Applied anatomy**

SN on inguinal ring
1.   **Location,**   2.   **Formation,**   3.   **Shape,**
4.   **Axis,**   5.   **Dimension,**   6.   **Relations,**
7.   **Content.**

1. **Gross anatomy (e.g. Stomach, duodenum, intestine, appendix, caecum, transverse colon, rectum, anal canal, urinary bladder, uterus):** It includes everything about a particular organ excluding *Histology, Development and Applied anatomy*

   A. Introduction :
      a. General introduction : Brief information about the organ.
      b. Location
      c. Size
      d. Peculiarity(ies)
      e. Dimension
   B. External features :
      a. Parts : Subdivision
      b. Situation, extent &
      c. Capacity.
   C. Internal features (orifices)
   D. Relations
      a. Peritoneal &
      b. Visceral.
   E. Blood supply
      a. Arterial supply
         I. Main artery of the organ,
         II. Origin of the artery,
         III. Important relations,
         IV. Peculiarities if any,
         V. Relevant applied anatomy.
      b. Venous drainage
         I. Main veins &
         II. Draining veins.
   F. Nerve supply
      a. Sympathetic
         I. Origin of the fiber
         II. Function
         III. Action on
            i. Smooth muscle
            ii. Blood vessels
            iii. Sphincter
      b. Parasympathetic
         I. Origin of the fibers
         II. Function
         III. Action on
            i. Smooth muscle

              ii.   Glands

              iii.   Sphincter

        IV.   Movement

    c.   Somatic

        I.   Origin of the fibers

        II.   Action at various site

  G.   Lymphatic

    a.   Lymph nodes draining the organ and situation

    b.   Afferent lymphatic

    C.   Efferent lymphatic

2. **Histology**

  A.   Staining character

  B.   Type of the cell

  C.   Position of nuclei

  D.   Identifying features

3. **Development**

  A.   Chronological age

  B.   Germ layer

  C.   Site

  D.   Source

  E.   Anomalies

4. **Applied anatomy**

  A.   Obstruction : Congenital or acquired

    a.   Cause

    b.   Effect

  B.   Vulnerable blood supply

  C.   Important relations of the structure helping to diagnose the disease.

  D.   Operative procedures

    a.   Removal or resection

    b.   Anastomosis

    c.   Exposures

  E.   Diagnostics methods of examination

LAQ on solid organ

1. **Gross anatomy (e.g. Liver, spleen, pancreas, kidney, suprarenal gland, thyroid gland, lung, ovary and tonsil):** It includes everything about a particular organ excluding *Histology, Development and Applied anatomy*

It includes

  A.   Introduction : Brief information about the organ.

    a.   Location and orientation

    b.   Shape

    c.   Dimension :

        I.   Length,

        II.   Breadth and

        III.   Weight of the organ.

B. External features :
   a. Subdivision
   b. Ends or poles
   c. Borders
   d. Surfaces
   e. Lobes
   f. Capsule / coverings
   g. Hilum / structures in the hilum and the position of the hilum
   h. Side determination (for paired organ)
   i. Fissure
   j. Bare area
C. Relations
   a. Peritoneal
   b. Visceral
   c. Neurovascular
   d. Fascial
D. Blood supply
   a. Arterial supply
      I. Main artery of the organ
      II. Origin of the artery
      III. Important relations
      IV. Peculiarities if any
      V. Relevant applied anatomy
   b. Venous drainage
      I. Main veins
      II. Draining veins
E. Nerve supply
   a. Sympathetic
      I. Origin of the fiber,
      II. Functions of the nerve &
      III. Action on.
         i. Smooth muscle,
         ii. Blood vessels &
         iii. Sphincter.
   b. Parasympathetic
      I. Origin of the fibers,
      II. Function &
      III. Action on
         i. Smooth muscle,
         ii. Glands,
         iii. Sphincter.
   c. Somatic
      I. Origin of the fibers
      II. Action at various site

F. Lymphatic
    a. Lymph nodes draining the organ and situation,
    b. Afferent lymphatic &
    c. Efferent lymphatic.
G. Duct system

2. **Histology**
A. Staining character,
B. Type of the cell,
C. Position of nuclei &
D. Identifying features.

3. **Development**
A. Chronological age,
B. Germinal layer,
C. Site,
D. Source &
E. Anomalies.

4. **Applied anatomy**
A. Relations of the structure helping to diagnose the disease.
B. Diagnostic methods of examination
C. Operative procedure

LAQ on tubular structure

1. **Gross anatomy of tubular, long structure (e.g. Oesophagus, Ureter, vas deferens fallopian tube, thoracic duct):** It includes everything about a particular organ excluding *Histology, Development and Applied anatomy*
It includes
A. Introduction : Brief information about the organ.
    a. General introduction
    b. Measurement :
        I. Length,
        II. Diameter &
    c. Constrictions,
B. Internal features (interior)
C. Course
D. Relations
    a. Peritoneal,
    b. Visceral.
E. Blood supply
    a. Arterial supply
        I. Main artery of the organ,
        II. Origin of the artery,
        III. Important relations,

   IV. Peculiarities if any &
   V. Relevant applied anatomy.
  b. Venous drainage
   I. Main veins &
   II. Draining veins.
 F. Nerve supply
  a. Sympathetic
   I. Origin of the fiber,
   II. Function(s) &
   III. Action on.
    i. Smooth muscle,
    ii. Blood vessels &
    iii. Sphincter.
  b. Parasympathetic
   I. Origin of the fibers,
   II. Function(s),
   III. Actions on
    i. Smooth muscle,
    ii. Glands &
    iii. Sphincter.
  c. Somatic
   I. Origin of the fibers &
   II. Action at various site.
 G. Lymphatic
  a. Lymph nodes draining the organ and situation,
  b. Afferent lymphatics &
  c. Efferent lymphatics.

2. Histology
 A. Staining character,
 B. Type of the cell,
 C. Position of nuclei &
 D. Identifying features.

3. Development
 A. Chronological age,
 B. Germinal layer,
 C. Site,
 D. Source &
 E. Anomalies.
  a. Common anomalies
  b. Sex,
  c. Incidence.

4. Applied anatomy
 A. Relations of the structure helping to diagnose the disease.
 B. Investigation carried out diagnose the disease.

SN on muscle
1. **Introduction :**
   A. Position
   B. Compartment
2. **Peculiarity(ies)**·
   A. Subcutaneous
   B. Intra capsular
   C. Synovial attachment
   D. Comminuting to joint space
   E. Divides the artery
   F. Peripheral heart
   G. Contents (venous sinus)
3. **Morphology**
   A. Shape
   B. Direction of fibers
   C. Type of fibers
4. **Origin**
   A. Site
        a. Bone
        b. Ligament of fascia
   B. Mode
        a. Fleshy
        b. Tendinus or aponeurosis
        c. Insertion
5. **Insertion**
   A. Site
   B. Mode
6. **Relations**
   A. Superficial surface
   B. Deep surface
   C. Upper border
   D. Lower border
   E. Bursae
   F. Sesamoid bone
7. **Nerve supply**
   A. Segments, root value
   B. Source
   C. Point of entry
8. **Actions**
   A. As a prime mover
   B. As a synergist
   C. As an antagonist
   D. As a fixator muscle
9. **Applied anatomy**

LAQ on diaphragm

1. **Gross anatomy :**
   A. Introduction :
   B. Origin :
   C. Insertion :
   D. Relations
      a. Superior surface
      b. Inferior surface
   E. Action :
   F. Blood supply
      a. Arterial supply
      B. Venous drainage
   G. Nerve supply :
      a. Sensory
      b. Motor
2. **Openings in the diaphragm**
   A. Major openings
   B. Minor openings
3. **Development :**
4. **Applied anatomy :**

Histology connective tissue (Bone, cartilage and muscle)
1. **Types of the fibers**
2. **Arrangement of cells**
3. **Staining character**
4. **Proportion of the cell and fibers**
5. **Special features**

Histology G I T: (oesophagus, stomach, duodenum jejunum, ilium, appendix, colon)
1. **Layers**
2. **Contents of each layer**
3. **Lining epithelium**
4. **About glands**
   A. Classification
   B. Staining character
   C. Situation of the gland
5. **About muscles**
   A. Types of muscles
   B. Layout of the muscle
   C. Arrangement of the muscle
6. **Special features of the organ**
7. **Staining characters**

Histology lymphatic organ (palatine tonsil, thymus, lymph node, spleen, appendix)
1. About capsule
2. Division of the gland : cortex medulla
3. Types of cell
4. Lining epithelium
5. Arrangement of cell
6. Specific cells of the organ
7. Particular features of the organ
8. Staining characters

Histology blood vessels
1. Coats
2. Contents of each coat
3. Lining of the blood vessels
4. Proportion of the smooth muscle
5. Presence of vasa vasorum

Histology organs which are divided into cortex and medulla (kidney, suprarenal gland,)
1. Capsule
   A. Extension
   B. Types of the fiber
2. Cortex
   A. Layers
   B. Types of the cell
3. Medulla
   A. Description about the cell
      a. Shape of the cell
      b. Staining character of the cell
      c. Shape and position of the nucleus
      d. Any special features

Histology tube, duct (Ureter, vas deferens)
1. Layers
2. Contents of each layer
3. Proportion of each layer
4. Relation of the lumen and wall of the duct
5. Lining epithelium
6. Type of the lumen

CONTENTS

Foreword viii

Acknowledgements ix

Special thanks xi

Syllabus xii

Prototype description of question xiii

Section One
INFEX

SN-1	Sciatic notch	3
SN-2	Ischial tuberosity	3
SN-3	Organs related to hipbone	4
SAQ-1	Linea aspera	4
SAQ-2	Adductor tubercle	5
SN-4	Iliac crest	5
SN-5	Structure attached to spines of hipbone	6
LAQ-1	Great saphenous vein	6
SN-6	Superficial inguinal lymph nodes	8
SN-7	Fascia lata	9
SN-8	Iliotibial tract	10
SAQ-3	Saphenous opening	10
LAQ-2	Femoral triangle	11
SN-9	Femoral sheath	13
SN-10	Femoral canal	14
LAQ-3	Femoral artery	15
LAQ-4	Femoral nerve	17
LAQ-5	Adductor canal	18
LAQ-6	Obturator nerve	20
SN-11	Gluteus maximus	22
LAQ-7	Structure under cover of gluteus maximus	23
SAQ-4	Trochanteric anastomosis	25

SAQ-5	Cruciate anastomosis	26
SN-12	Gluteus medius	26
SN-13	Hamstring muscles	27
LAQ-8	Popliteal fossa	28
LAQ-9	Popliteal artery	30
LAQ-10	Sciatic nerve	31
SN-14	Soleus	33
SN-15	Dorsalis pedis artery	34
SN-16	Popliteus	35
SN-17	Plantar aponeurosis	36
SN-18	Layers of sole	37
LAQ-11	Hip joint	38
SN-19	Classify knee joint (genual)	40
SN-20	Capsule of knee joint	41
SAQ-6	Enumerate intra-articular structure of knee joint	41
SN-21	Cruciate ligament	42
SN-22	Meniscus	42
SAQ-7	Meniscofemoral ligament	44
SAQ-8	Oblique popliteal ligament	44
SAQ-9	Transverse ligament	44
SAQ-10	Synovial membrane	45
SAQ-11	Coronary ligament	45
SAQ-12	Arcuate ligament	45
SAQ-13	Ligamentum patellae	45
SN-23	Collateral ligament	45
SN-24	Relation of knee joint	46
SAQ-14	Movements of knee joint and muscles bringing the movement	47
SN-25	Bursae around knee joint	48
SN-26	Locking and unlocking of knee joint	49
LAQ-12	Ankle joint	49
SN-27	Deltoid ligament	52
SAQ-15	Lateral ligament of ankle joint	52
LAQ-13	Inversion	53
LAQ-14	Eversion	54

SN-28 Compare pronation, supination with inversion, eversion 55

LAQ-15 Medial longitudinal arch 55

SAQ-16 Spring ligament 57

LAQ-16 Lateral longitudinal arch 58

SN-29 Lateral plantar nerve 59

Section Two
ABDOMEN

SN-1 Spina bifida 63

SAQ-1 Sacral hiatus 63

SAQ-2 Transpyloric plane 63

SAQ-3 Caput medusae 64

SN-2 Inguinal ligament 64

SN-3 Rectus abdominis 65

LAQ-1 Rectus sheath 66

LAQ-2 Inguinal canal 68

SAQ-4 Superficial inguinal ring 71

SAQ-5 Deep inguinal ring 72

SAQ-6 Coverings of spermatic cord 72

SN-4 Spermatic cord 72

SN-5 Hesselbach's triangle 73

SN-6 Inguinal hernia 74

LAQ-3 Testis 75

SN-7 Blood supply of testis 76

SN-8 Histology of testis 77

SAQ-7 Development of testis 78

LAQ-4 Testis 80

SAQ-8 Epididymis 81

SN-9 Foramen of Winslow 81

SN-10 Lesser sac 83

LAQ-5 Stomach 84

SN-11 Stomach bed 90

LAQ-6 Second part of duodenum 91

SN-12	Duodenal cap	
SN-13	Ligament of Treitz	95
SN-14	Meckel's diverticulum	96
LAQ-7	Caecum	96
LAQ-8	Appendix	99
LAQ-9	Coeliac trunk	103
LAQ-10	Portal vein	105
LAQ-11	Extrahepatic biliary apparatus	109
LAQ-12	Spleen	113
LAQ-13	Liver	116
SAQ-9	The bare area	120
LAQ-14	Head of pancreas	121
LAQ-15	Kidney	124
LAQ-16	Ureter	130
LAQ-17	Suprarenal gland	137
LAQ-18	Diaphragm	140
LAQ-19	Abdominal aorta	143
LAQ-20	Inferior vena cava	145
SN-15	Cisterna chyli	148
SN-16	Perineal body	148
SN-17	External anal sphincter	149
LAQ-21	Ischiorectal fossa	150
SN-18	Pudendal canal	152
SN-19	Perineal membrane	153
SN-20	Urogenital diaphragm	155
LAQ-22	Superficial perineal pouch	156
LAQ-23	Deep perineal pouch	158
LAQ-24	Urinary bladder	159
LAQ-25	Male urethra	164
LAQ-26	Ovary	168
SAQ-10	Ovarian fossa	171
LAQ-27	Uterine tube	172
LAQ-28	Uterus	174
LAQ-29	Prostate	178

LAQ-30 Rectum 182

LAQ-31 Anal canal 186

SN-21 Internal iliac artery 189

Section Three
GENERAL HISTOLOGY

SAQ-1 Simple saphenous epithelium 193

SN-1 Columnar epithelium 193

SN-2 Pseudostratified epithelium 194

SN-3 Stratified squamous epithelium 194

SN-4 Transitional epithelium 195

SAQ-2 Loose areolar tissue 196

SN-5 Hyaline cartilage 197

SN-6 Articular cartilage 198

SN-7 Fibrocartilage 198

SN-8 Elastic cartilage 199

SN-9 Compact bone 199

SAQ-3 Sarcomere 201

SN-10 Cardiac muscle 201

SN-11 Elastic artery 202

SN-12 Muscular artery 203

Section Four
GENERAL EMBRYOLOGY

SN-1 Mitosis 207

SN-2 Meiosis 209

SN-3 Spermatogenesis 211

SAQ-1 Spermiogenesis 213

SAQ-2 Sperms 213

SN-4 Capacitation of sperms 214

SN-5 Oogenesis 214

SN-6 Graafian follicle 215

SN-7 Fertilization 216

SN-8	Implantation	218
SN-9	Blastocyst	219
SN-10	Decidua	220
SN-11	Amnion	221
SN-12	Yolk sac	223
SN-13	Primitive streak	224
SN-14	Notochord	226
SN-15	Connecting stalk	227
SN-16	Somites	228
SN-17	Umbilical cord	228
SN-18	Intraembryonic mesoderm	229
SN-19	Allantois	230
SN-20	Trophoblast	231
SN-21	Placenta	232
SN-22	Types of placenta depending upon shape	235
SN-23	Types of placenta depending upon attachment	235
SAQ-3	Placenta praevia	236
SN-24	Chorion	237
SN-25	The maternal foetal barrier	238
SN-26	Coelomic wall epithelium	239
SAQ-4	Surface ectoderm epithelium	239
SAQ-5	Septum transversum	240
SN-27	Neural crest	240

Section Five
GENERAL ANATOMY

SN-1	Long bone	243
SAQ-1	Short bone	243
SN-2	Pneumatic bone	244
SN-3	Sesamoid bone	244
SAQ-2	Growing end	245
SAQ-3	Primary centre	246
SAQ-4	Secondary centre	246

SN-4	Metaphysis	246
SN-5	Diaphysis	247
SN-6	Epiphysis	247
SN-7	Blood supply of the long bone	248
SN-8	Suture	250
SN-9	Syndesmoses	251
SN-10	Primary cartilaginous joint	252
SN-11	Secondary cartilaginous joint	252
SN-12	Pivot joint	253
SN-13	Typical synovial joint	253
SN-14	Prime movers	255
SN-15	Antagonist	256
SN-16	Synergist	256
SN-17	Fixators	257
SN-18	Bursa	257
SN-19	Anastomosis	258
SN-20	End arteries	258

Section Six
GENETICS

SN-1	Gene	261
SN-2	Barr body	262
SN-3	Structure of chromosome	263
SN-4	Classification of chromosomes	264
SN-5	Chromosomal aberrations	264
SN-6	Chromosome banding	266
SN-7	Trisomy 21	266
SN-8	Autosomal dominant inheritance	267
SN-9	Autosomal recessive inheritance	267
SN-10	X-linked recessive traits	268
SN-11	Turner's syndrome (45 X)	270
SN-12	Klinefelter syndrome (47 XXY)	270
SN-13	Cru-de-chat syndrome 45 5p	271

SN-14   Non-disjunction 271

SN-15   Aneuploidy 272

SN-16   Karyotyping 273

Key to memory 275

Appendix 287

INFEX

SECTION ONE: INFEX

SN-1	Sciatic notch	3
SN-2	Ischial tuberosity	3
SN-3	Organs related to hipbone	4
SAQ-1	Linea aspera	4
SAQ-2	Adductor tubercle	5
SN-4	Iliac crest	5
SN-5	Structure attached to spines of hipbone	6
LAQ-1	Great saphenous vein	6
SN-6	Superficial inguinal lymph nodes	8
SN-7	Fascia lata	9
SN-8	Iliotibial tract	10
SAQ-3	Saphenous opening	10
LAQ-2	Femoral triangle	11
SN-9	Femoral sheath	13
SN-10	Femoral canal	14
LAQ-3	Femoral artery	15
LAQ-4	Femoral nerve	17
LAQ-5	Adductor canal	18
LAQ-6	Obturator nerve	20
SN-11	Gluteus maximus	22
LAQ-7	Structures under cover of gluteus maximus	23
SAQ-4	Trochanteric anastomosis	25
SAQ-5	Cruciate anastomosis	26
SN-12	Gluteus medius	26
SN-13	Hamstring muscles	27
LAQ-8	Popliteal fossa	28
LAQ-9	Popliteal artery	30
LAQ-10	Sciatic nerve	31
SN-14	Soleus	33
SN-15	Dorsalis pedis artery	34
SN-16	Popliteus	35
SN-17	Plantar aponeurosis	36
SN-18	Layers of sole	37
LAQ-11	Hip Joint	38
SN-19	Classify knee joint (genual)	40
SN-20	Capsule of knee joint	41
SAQ-6	Enumerate intra articular structures of knee joint	41
SN-21	Cruciate ligament	42
SN-22	Meniscus	42
SAQ-7	Menisco femoral ligament	44
SAQ-8	Oblique popliteal ligament	44
SAQ-9	Transverse ligament	44
SAQ-10	Synovial membrane	45
SAQ-11	Coronary ligament	45
SAQ-12	Arcuate ligament	45
SAQ-13	Ligamentum patellae	45
SN-23	Collateral ligament	45
SN-24	Relations of knee joint	46
SAQ-14	Movements of knee joint and muscles bringing the movement	47
SN-25	Bursae around knee joint	48
SN-26	Locking and unlocking of knee joint	49
LAQ-12	Ankle joint	49
SN-27	Deltoid ligament	52
SAQ-15	Lateral ligament of ankle joint	52
LAQ-13	Inversion	53
LAQ-14	Eversion	54
SN-28	Compare pronation, supination with inversion, eversion	55
LAQ-15	Medial longitudinal arch	55
SAQ-16	Spring ligament	57
LAQ-16	Lateral longitudinal arch	58
SN-29	Lateral plantar nerve	59

SN-1   Sciatic notch

Posterior border of ilium presents two notches divided by ischial spine. The notch above the ischial spine is called greater sciatic notch and below is called lesser sciatic notch. The greater sciatic notch is divided by the piriformis. Following are the structures passing through greater sciatic notch.

1. **Structures above piriformis**
   A. Superior gluteal vessels and
   B. Superior gluteal nerve.

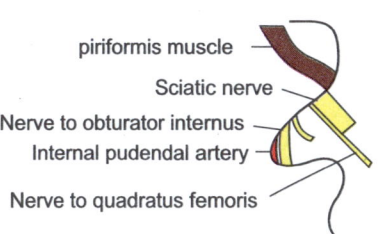

2. **Structures below piriformis (from medial to lateral)**
   They are divided into three groups:
   A. Structures which reenter into lesser sciatic notch
      a. Internal pudendal vessels and
      b. Pudendal nerve.
   B. Structures going to gluteal region
      a. Sciatic nerve,
      b. Nerve to obturator internus and
      c. Inferior gluteal vessels and nerve.
   C. Structure going to thigh region: Posterior femoral cutaneous nerve.

Fig. 1.1 Structures passing through the greater sciatic notch

SN-2   Ischial tuberosity

It is a tuberosity present on lower area of the dorsal surface of ischium.
Ischial tuberosity is rough and divided by a transverse ridge into upper quadrilateral & lower

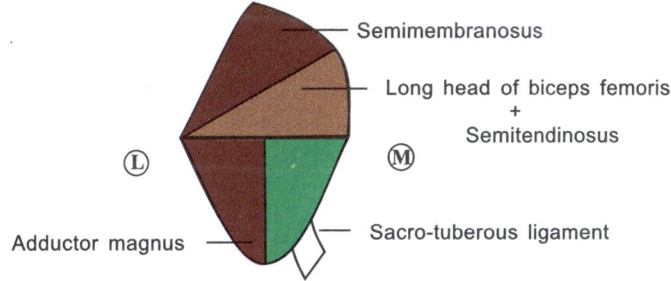

Fig. 1.2 Muscles attached to the ischial tuberosity

Table 1.1 Showing muscles and ligament attached to ischial tuberosity

Part	Attachments
A. Upper	
a. Upper lateral	Semimembranosus.
b. Lower medial	Semitendinosus and long head of biceps femoris.
B. Lower	
a. Lateral	Ischial fibers of adductor magnus.
c. Medial	Medial margin gives attachment to sacrotuberous ligament covered with fibrofatty tissue & transmits the body weight in sitting position.

SN-3   Organs related to hipbone

Pelvis and related organs

Table 1.2 Showing organs related to the bones of pelvis

Bone	Organs	
	Male	**Female**
Pelvic part of pubic bone	Urinary bladder Prostate gland	Urinary bladder
Anterior margin of greater sciatic notch	Ureter	Ovary and ureter
Transtubercular plane	Appendix and caecum on right side of pelvis.	
Pubic tubercle	Spermatic cord	Round ligament of uterus

SAQ-1   Linea aspera

(*linea* line, *aspera* thick & irregular)

It is irregular thick and line present on the posterior border of femur. It forms the apex of adductor canal. It gives attachment to intermuscular septum, which divides into extensor, adductor and flexor compartments of the thigh. Following are the structures attached to linea aspera (from lateral to medial). **I** love **B**, **Mr** **B** love **me**

1. Vastus **i**ntermedius.
2. Vastus **l**ateralis.
3. Short head of **b**iceps femoris.
4. Adductor **m**agnus.
5. Adductor **b**revis.
6. Adductor **l**ongus.
7. Vastus **m**edialis.

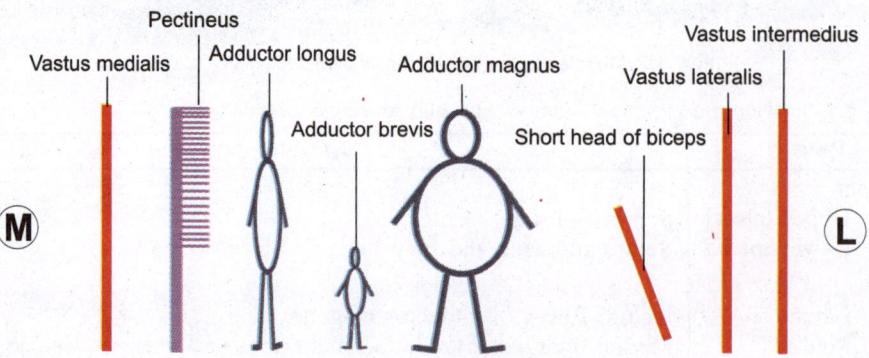

Fig. 1.3 Muscles attached to linea aspera.

SAQ-2 — Adductor tubercle

1. **Introduction:** It is first bony prominent felt on the medial side of thigh.

2. **Attachment:** It gives attachment to
   A. Ischial fibers of adductor magnus muscle and
   B. Tibial collateral ligament.

3. **Applied anatomy:**
   A. The epiphyseal line of lower end passes through the tubercle.
   B. It forms a bony landmark for surface anatomy.

SN-4 — Iliac crest

1. **Introduction:** It is a 'S' shaped curvature present on the upper border of ilium. It is divided into:
   A. Ventral segment which is subdivided into:
      a. Anterior 2/3rd: It gives attachment (from lateral to medial) to
         I. External oblique,
         II. Internal oblique and
         III. Transversus abdominis.
      b. Posterior one-third: It gives attachment to (from lateral to medial) to
         I. Latissimus dorsi and
         II. Quadratus lumborum.
   B. Dorsal segment is divided into
      a. Outer sloping area gives attachment to gluteus maximus.
      b. Inner sloping area gives attachment to erector spinae.

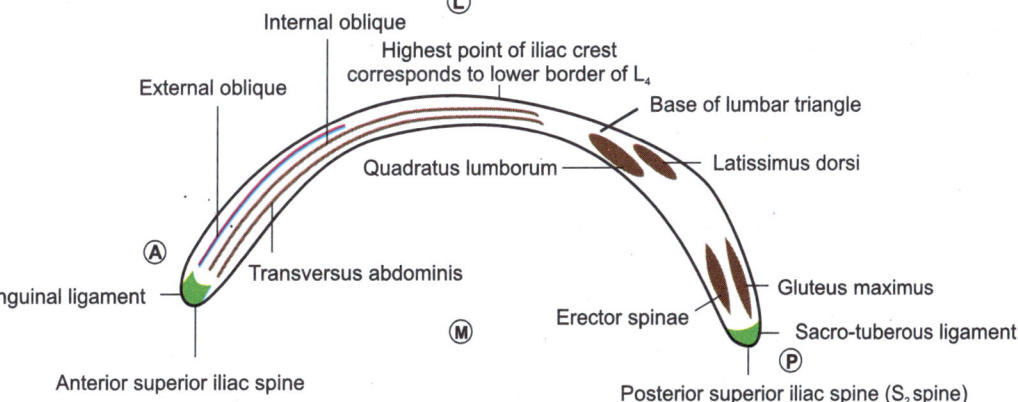

Fig. 1.4 Structure attached to Iliac crest.

2. **Applied anatomy:**
   A. Iliac crest is used for bone grafting.
   B. Bone marrow examination.

SN-5 — Structures attached to spines of hipbone

Table 1.3 Showing structures attached to spines of hipbone

Spines	Attachments	
	Muscles	**Ligament**
1. Anterior superior iliac spine	Sartorius in lower part	Lateral end of inguinal ligament in upper part
2. Anterior inferior iliac spine	Straight head of rectus femoris in upper part	Ilio femoral ligament in lower part
3. Posterior superior iliac spine	Erector spinae	Posterior sacroiliac ligament and sacrotuberous ligament
4. Posterior inferior iliac spine	piriformis	Sacrotuberous ligament
5. Ischial spine	Posterior fibers of levator ani	Sacrospinous, coccygeal ligament

LAQ-1 — Describe great saphenous vein under 1. Introduction, 2. Formation, 3. Course & relations, 4. Peculiarities, 5. Perforating veins, 6. Termination, 7. Tributaries, 8. Communicating veins and 9. Applied anatomy.

1. **Introduction:** The great saphenous (*Saphes* easily seen) vein is the longest vein of the body. It drains the lower extremity except the medial side of leg between tendo calcaneus and tibia.

2. **Formation:** It is formed by the medial end of dorsal venous arch and medial marginal vein.

3. **Course and relations:** It begins at   🗝 **M** for **m**
    A. **M**edial end of the dorsal venous arch.
    B. It is supplemented by **m**edial marginal vein.
    C. It runs in front of **m**edial malleous and crosses obliquely on **m**edial surface of lower third of tibia.
    D. It ascends behind the **m**edial border of tibia to reach knee.
    E. It runs along the **m**edial side of thigh to drain in saphenous opening present in cribriform fascia.

4. **Peculiarities:** It contains 10 to 15 valves, which prevents back flow of venous blood. One of the valve is always present at sapheno femoral junction.

5. **Perforating veins:** They connect saphenous vein to deep vein. They are 3 in number.
    A. Above the ankle,
    B. Below the knee and
    C. In the adductor canal.
    The perforating veins are provided with valves, which permit the flow of blood only from superficial to deep.

6. **Termination:** It terminates into upper part of femoral vein by piercing fascia lata.

7. **Tributaries:**

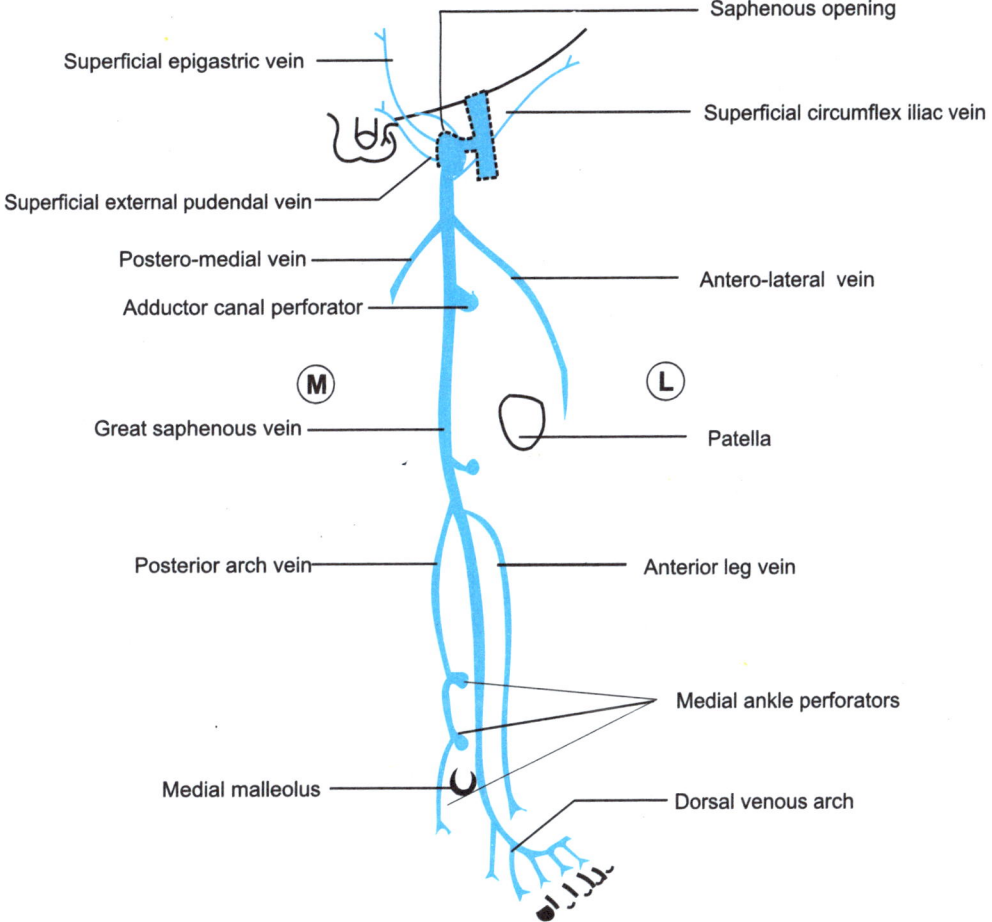

Fig. 1.5 Course and tributaries of great saphenous vein.

A. At the beginning: Medial marginal vein
B. Just below knee:
    a. Anterior vein of leg
    b. Posterior arch vein of calf
C. In the thigh:
    a. Accessory saphenous vein.
    b. Anterior cutaneous vein of thigh.
D. Before piercing cribriform fascia:
    a. Superficial epigastric vein.
    b. Superficial circumflex iliac vein.
    c. Superficial external pudendal vein.
E. Before termination: Deep external pudendal.

8. **Communicating veins:** Small saphenous vein.

9. **Applied anatomy:**
   A. Varicosity (torturous, dilated, enlarged and visible vein) of the veins is more common in people who are standing for long time (e.g. traffic police). The valve become incompetent & the flow of the blood is reversed. The defective veins become 'high pressure leaks'. The blood is stagnated in the depending veins and there is gradual degeneration of their valves. It produces varicose veins and varicose ulcers.
   B. Great saphenous vein is used for arterial grafting in coronary artery bypass surgery.

| SN-6 | **Superficial inguinal lymph nodes** |

1. **Introduction:** The lymph vessels accompany the great saphenous vein from the foot, leg and thigh, drains all the structures superficial to deep fascia of lower limb.

2. **Arrangement:** They are arranged in the form of T.

3. **Location:** Along the great saphenous vein and inguinal ligament.

4. **Afferent & efferent lymphatics:**

Table 1.4 Showing afferent & efferent lymphatics of superficial inguinal lymph nodes

Lymph node	Site	Afferent	Efferent
A. Lower vertical	Along great saphenous vein	It receives lymphatic from all the structures superficial to deep fascia of lower limb except buttock and popliteal nodes.	Drains into deep inguinal lymph node, which lie along upper part of femoral vessels.
B. Upper lateral group	Lateral part of inguinal ligament	Buttock, flank and back	

C. Upper medial group	Medial end of ligament along the superficial epigastric vessel	a. Anterior abdominal wall below the umbilicus.
		b. Perineum including external genitalia except glans.
		  I. The part of the anal canal below the pectinate line.
		  II. The vagina below the hymen.
		  III. The penile part of the male urethra.
		c. The superolateral angle of the uterus.	

5. **Applied anatomy:**
   A. The upper group of the superficial inguinal nodes are enlarged due to spread of infection or malignant growth from
      a. Superolateral part of uterus,

b.   Penile part of urethra,

C.   The vagina below the hymen &

d.   Part of the anal canal below the pectinate line.

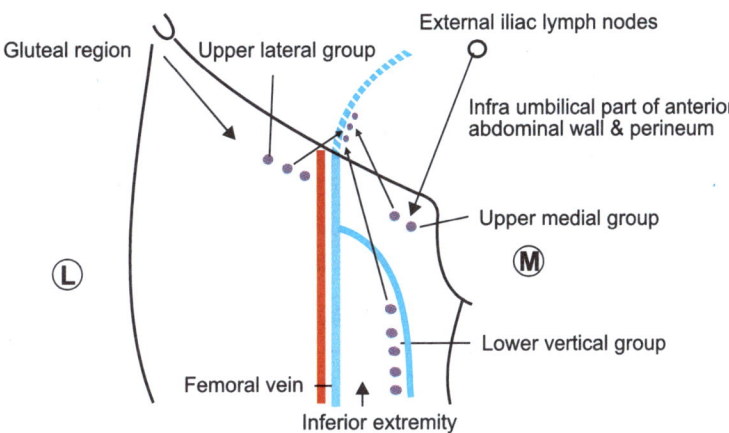

Fig. 1.6 Superficial inguinal lymph nodes

B.   In syphilitic lesion of the prepuce involves medial upper group of the superficial nodes.

SN-7	**Fascia lata**

1.   **Introduction:** It is a tough, fibrous, deep fascia which envelops the thigh like the stockings.

2.   **Modifications:**

A.   Iliotibial tract.

B.   Saphenous opening.

3.   **Attachments:**

A.   Proximally: It is attached to pubic tubercle, under surface of inguinal ligament, outerlip of entire iliac crest, splitting to enclose the tensor fascia lata and gluteus maximus, dorsal surface of sacrum, coccyx, sacrotuberous ligament and ischial tuberosity.

B.   Anteromedially: It is attached to ischiopubic ramus, anterior margin of pubic symphysis, pubic crest, pubic tubercle, anterior surface of pectineus muscle and pectin pubis.

C.   Distally: It is attached to the patella and the inferior margin of the tibial condyles and the head of the fibula.

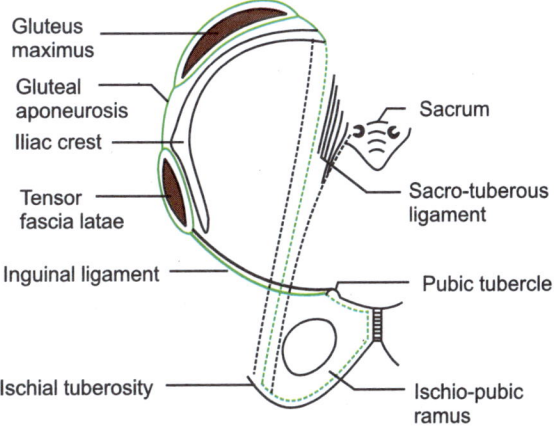

Fig. 1.7 Extent and attachments of fascia lata

4. **Encloses:** It encloses
   A. Gluteus maximum and
   B. Tensor fascia lata.

5. **Functions:**
   A. It protects the deeper structures and
   B. It keeps deeper structures in position.

SN-8   Iliotibial tract

It is a modified thick fascia of thigh (fascia lata) measuring about 2 inch

1. **Situation:** Lateral aspect of thigh.

2. **Extent:**
   A. Superiorly
       a. Superficial lamina is attached to tubercle of iliac crest.
       b. Deep lamina is attached to capsule of hip joint.
   B. Inferiorly: it is attached to smooth area on the anterior surface of lateral condyle of the tibia.

2. **It gives insertion to:**
   A. Greater part of gluteus maximum and
   B. Tensor fascia lata.

3. **Nerve supply:** Superior gluteal nerve (L_4, L_5).

4. **Functions:**
   A. It stabilizes the knee both in extension & partial flexion & therefore used constantly during walking & running.
   B. It is the main support of knee against gravity.

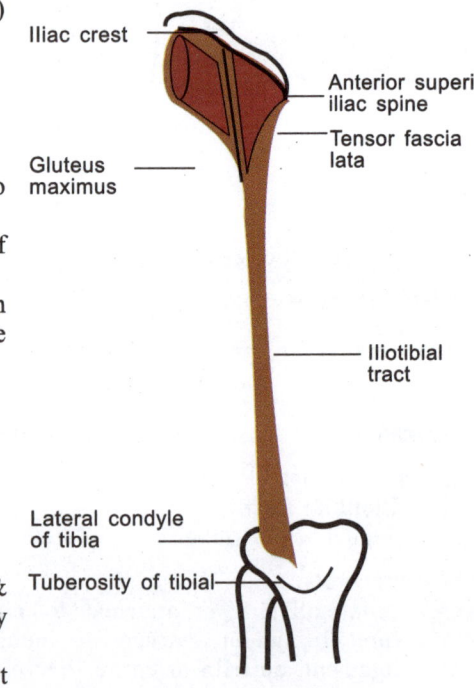

Iliac crest

Anterior superior iliac spine

Tensor fascia lata

Gluteus maximus

Iliotibial tract

Lateral condyle of tibia

Tuberosity of tibial

Fig. 1.8 Iliotibial tract

SAQ-3   Saphenous opening

Saphenous easily seen

1. **Introduction:** It is an oval opening present in the fascia lata.

2. **Location:** It is situated 4 cm below & 4 cm lateral to pubic tubercle. The vertical height is 4cm. Saphenous opening has 2 margins: Lateral & medial margin
   A. The lateral margin is superficial and well defined. It is half moon shaped and is present in front of femoral sheath. It is also called falciform margin.
   B. Medial margin is deep and ill defined.

3. **Opening:** It is closed by areolar membrane called cribriform fascia. This fascia is pierced by number of structures & give sieve like appearance hence it is called cribriform fascia. The structure passing through saphenous opening are
   A. Vein: Great saphenous vein.
   B. Artery:
      a. Superficial external pudendal artery,
      b. Superficial epigastric artery and
      c. Superficial circumflex iliac artery.
      (**Note:** Corresponding veins do not pass through the saphenous opening. Superficial circumflex iliac artery usually emerges lateral to the saphenous opening.)
   C. Lymph vessels: They connect superficial & deep inguinal lymph nodes.
   D. Nerve:
      a. Medial femoral cutaneous nerve.
      b. Few branches of medial femoral cutaneous nerve.

LAQ-2 **Describe femoral triangle (Scarpa's triangle) under**
1. **Boundaries,** 2. **Roof,** 3. **Floor,**
4. **Contents,** 5. **Relations &** 6. **Applied Anatomy.**

1. **Boundaries:**
   A. Laterally: Medial border of sartorius.
   B. Medially: Medial border of adductor longus.
   C. Base: Inguinal ligament.
   D. Apex: Meeting point of medial and lateral borders.

2. **Roof:**
   A. Skin.
   B. Superficial fascia containing
      a. Lymph nodes: Superficial inguinal lymph nodes and lymphatics.
      b. Nerves
         I. Femoral branch of genito femoral nerve and
         II. Femoral branch of ilio inguinal nerve.
   C. Vessels: superficial branches of femoral vessels
      a. Superficial circumflex iliac,
      b. Superficial external pudendal and
      c. Superficial epigastric.
   D. Deep fascia: Saphenous opening with cribriform fascia.

3. **Floor:** (From medial to lateral) Adductor longus, pectineus, psoas major & iliacus covered by fascia.

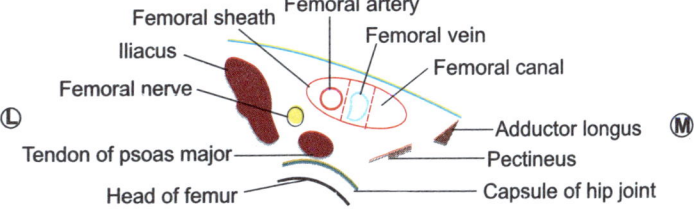

Fig. 1.9 Floor of the femoral triangle

4. **Contents:**
    A. Femoral artery with it branches
        a. Superficial
            I.   Superficial epigastric.
            II. Superficial circumflex iliac.
            III. Superficial external pudendal.
        b. Deep
            I.   Profunda femoris,
            II. Deep external pudendal &
            III. Muscular branches.
    B. Femoral vein & its tributaries.
    C. Femoral sheath containing upper 4 cm of femoral vessels.
    D. Nerves:
        a. Femoral nerve outside the femoral sheath.
        b. Nerve to pectineus passing posterior to femoral vessels & supplying pectineus.
        c. Femoral branch of genito femoral nerve.
        d. Lateral cutaneous nerve of thigh.
    E. Deep inguinal lymph nodes (Gland of Cloquet or Rosen Muller).

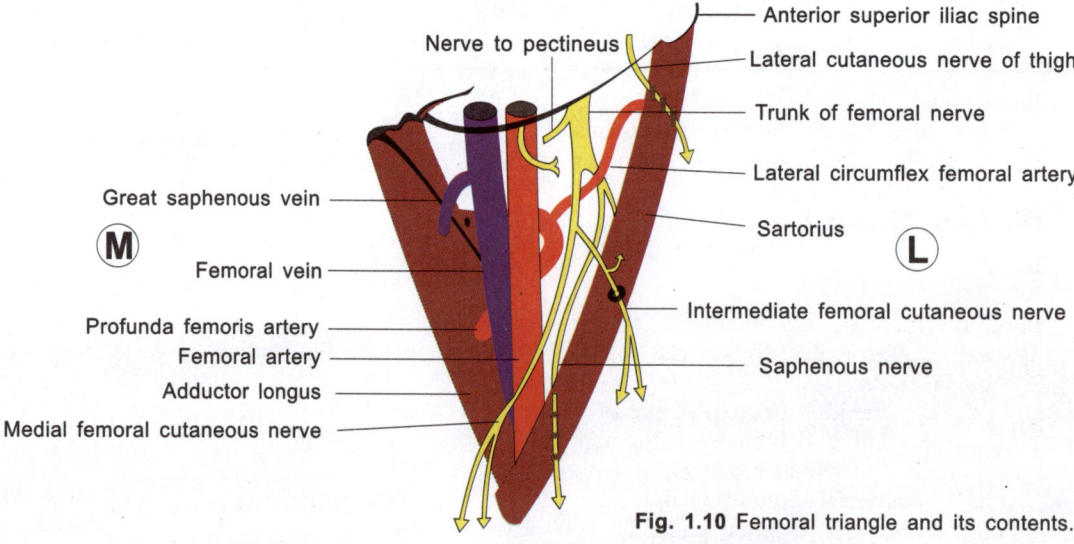

Fig. 1.10 Femoral triangle and its contents.

5. **Relations of vessels**
    A. At base: (from medial to lateral)
         **VAN**
        a. Femoral **V**ein,
        b. Femoral **A**rtery and
        c. Femoral **N**erve.
    B. At apex: (from anterior to posterior)
        a. Femoral artery,
        b. Femoral vein,
        c. Profunda femoris vein and
        d. Profunda femoris artery.

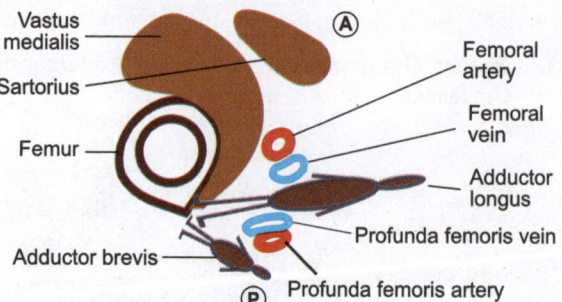

Fig. 1.11 Relations of the structures at the apex of the femoral triangle

6. **Applied:**
  A. Enlargement of lymph nodes in femoral triangle indicate infection of
    a. Skin below umbilicus .
    b. Skin of gluteal region.
    c. Cancer of fundus of uterus.
    d. Skin of leg, sole and external genitalia.
  B. Pulsation's of femoral artery can be felt at the midinguinal point against head of femur and tendon of psoas major.
  C. Intravenous injection can be given by feeling the pulsations of femoral artery and going medially to it.
  D. Stab wounds at the apex of femoral triangle nay be fatal injury as it cuts all vessels of lower limb.

SN-9   Femoral sheath

1. **Introduction:** It is the fascia covering femoral vessels in thigh region.

2. **Gross:**
  A. Length: 4 cm.
  B. Shape conical (Funnel).
    a. Lateral wall is vertical
    b. Medial wall is oblique directed downwards & laterally.

3. **Formation:**
  A. Anterior wall: Fascia transversalis.
  B. Posterior wall: Fascia iliacus.

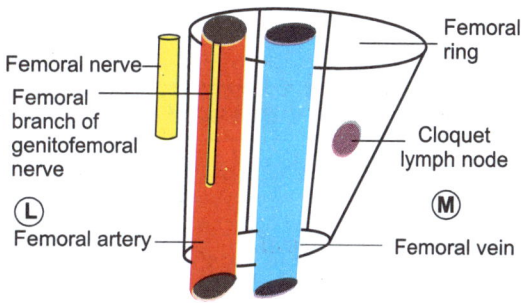

Fig. 1.12 Femoral sheath and its contents

4. **Communication:**
  A. Superiorly opens into abdomen.
  B. Inferiorly merges with tunica adventitia of femoral vessels.

5. **Division:** It is divided into 3 compartments by two vertical septa.
  A. Medial compartment: It is also called femoral canal.
    a. Fatty connective tissue.
    b. Cloquet lymph nodes which drains.
      I. Male: Glans penis.
      II. Female: Clitoris.
    c. Cloquet lymph vessels.
  B. Intermediate or venous compartment which contains femoral vein.
  C. Lateral or arterial compartment which contains
    a. Femoral artery and
    b. Femoral branch of genitofemoral nerve.

6. **Functions:** It allows free gliding in and out behind inguinal ligament during movements of the hip joint.

7. **Age changes:** It is rudimentary in new born and is prolonged after one year.

8. **Structures piercing femoral sheath:**
   A. Laterally it is pierce by femoral branch of genitofemoral nerve.
   B. In front it is pierce by
      a. Superficial epigastric artery.
      b. Superficial circumflex artery.
      c. Superficial external pudendal artery.
   C. Medially it is pierce by great saphenous vein.

9. **Applied anatomy:**
   A. Femoral canal is a potential weak point through which abdominal contents are passing Femoral hernia is common in females because of following reasons
      a. Pelvis is wider and
      b. Vessels are smaller.
   B. In cases of strangulated femoral hernia, the surgical reduction is possible only by c cutting lacunar ligament because all other boundaries of femoral ring contains important structures and cannot be sacrificed.
      While cutting the lacunar ligament one should remember the possibility of an abnormal obturator artery which is present in 30% cases.

SN-10   Femoral canal

1. **Introduction:** It is a potential weakness present in medial compartment of femoral sheath.

2. **Gross:**
   A. Shape: Conical.
   B. Base is wider and is called as femoral ring.
      a. Shape: Oval.
      b. Diameter: ½"
      c. Boundaries:
         I. Anteriorly: Inguinal ligament.
         II. Posteriorly: Pectineus & fascia covering it.
         III. Medially: Lacunar ligament.

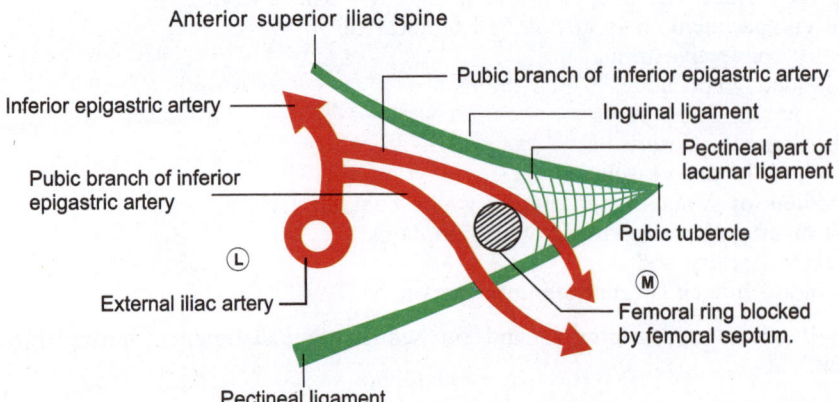

Fig. 1.13 Two different positions of the pubic branch of the inferior epigastric artery. (abnormal artery) in relation to the femoral ring.

    IV. Laterally: Septum separating femoral vein.
- d. Relations: Inferior epigastric vessels are closely related to the junction of anterior & lateral wall of ring.
- e. Closure of ring is by condensation of extraperitoneal connective tissue called femoral septum.

  C. Apex is narrow.

  D. Dimension: ½" x ½"

3. Function: Provides space for distension of femoral vein.

4. Applied anatomy:
- A. Femoral hernia
  - a. Introduction: It is the protrusion of abdominal contents through the femoral canal.
  - b. It is more common in female because of wider pelvis and narrower vessels.
  - c. Precepitating causes
    - I. Increased intra-abdominal pressure.
    - II. Chromic cough.
    - III. Constipation.
    - IV. Multiparity.
    - V. Tumors in the abdomen.
    - VI. Old age.
- B. Hernioraphy: Repair of the femoral canal during repair of strangulated hernia, position of accessory obturator artery should be kept in mind.

LAQ-3 — Describe femoral artery under
1. Origin,   2. Extent,   3. Course,   4. Relations,   5. Branches,   6. Terminations &   7. Applied Anatomy.

1. Origin: Femoral artery is continuation of an external iliac artery below inguinal ligament.

2. Extent: It extends from midinguinal point to adductor canal.

3. Course: It passes downward and medially first in the femoral triangle & then in adductor canal. At the apex of the adductor canal it continues as popliteal artery.

4. Relations:
- A. With other vessels
  - a. At the base of femoral triangle from medial to lateral
    - I. Femoral <u>v</u>ein,
    - II. Femoral <u>a</u>rtery and   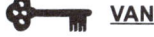 <u>VAN</u>
    - III. Femoral <u>n</u>erve.
  - b. At the apex of femoral triangle from anterior to posterior
    - I. Femoral artery,
    - II. Femoral vein,
    - III. Profunda femoris vein and
    - IV. Profunda femoris artery.
- B. Anterior: Skin, superficial fascia and deep fascia (fascia lata).
- C. Posterior: From above downwards
  - a. Psoas major,
  - b. Pectineus and
  - c. Adductor longus.

5. **Branches:**
   A. Superficial:
       a. Superficial epigastric artery,
       b. Superficial circumflex iliac artery and
       c. Superficial external pudendal artery.
   B. Deep:
       a. Profunda femoris gives following branches:
           I. Lateral circumflex femoral gives following branches:
               i.   Ascending branch takes part in spinous anastomosis.
               ii. Transverse branch takes part in cruciate anastomosis.
               iii. Descending branch takes part in anastomosis around knee joint.
           II. Medial circumflex femoral artery gives following branches:
               i.   Ascending branch takes part in the trochanteric anastomosis. It is chief artery of head and neck of femur
               ii. Transverse branch takes part in cruciate anastomosis.
           III. Perforating branches are 4 in number. They perforate adductor magnus.
       b. Deep external pudendal supplies the scrotum or labium.
       c. Muscular.
       d. Descending genicular artery.

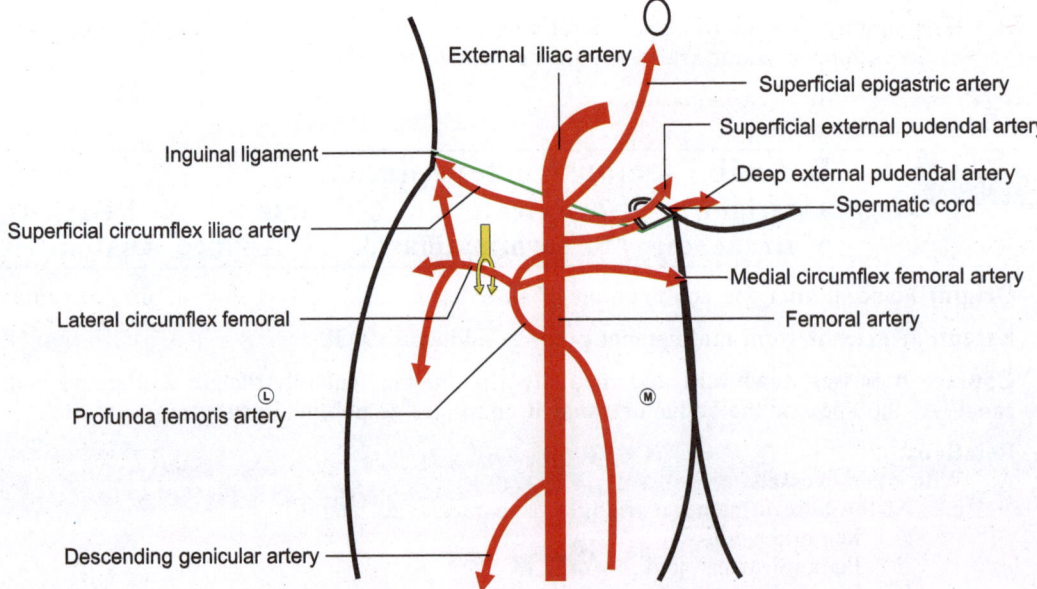

Fig. 1.14 Femoral artery and its branches.

6. **Termination:** It continues as popliteal artery through an opening present in the adductor magnus.

7. **Applied anatomy:**
   A. Femoral vein can be located by feeling the pulsations of femoral artery and going medial to it.
   B. Femoral artery is used for angiography of lower limb.

LAQ-4 **Describe femoral nerve under**
1. **Root value,**   2. **Branches,**
3. **Course and relation and 4. Applied Anatomy.**

1. **Root value:** It is formed by dorsal division of ventral rami of L_2, L_3 & L_4 spinal nerve

2. **Branches:**
   A. From the trunk
      a. Branch to iliacus.
      b. Branch to pectineus.
      c. Vascular branches to femoral artery.

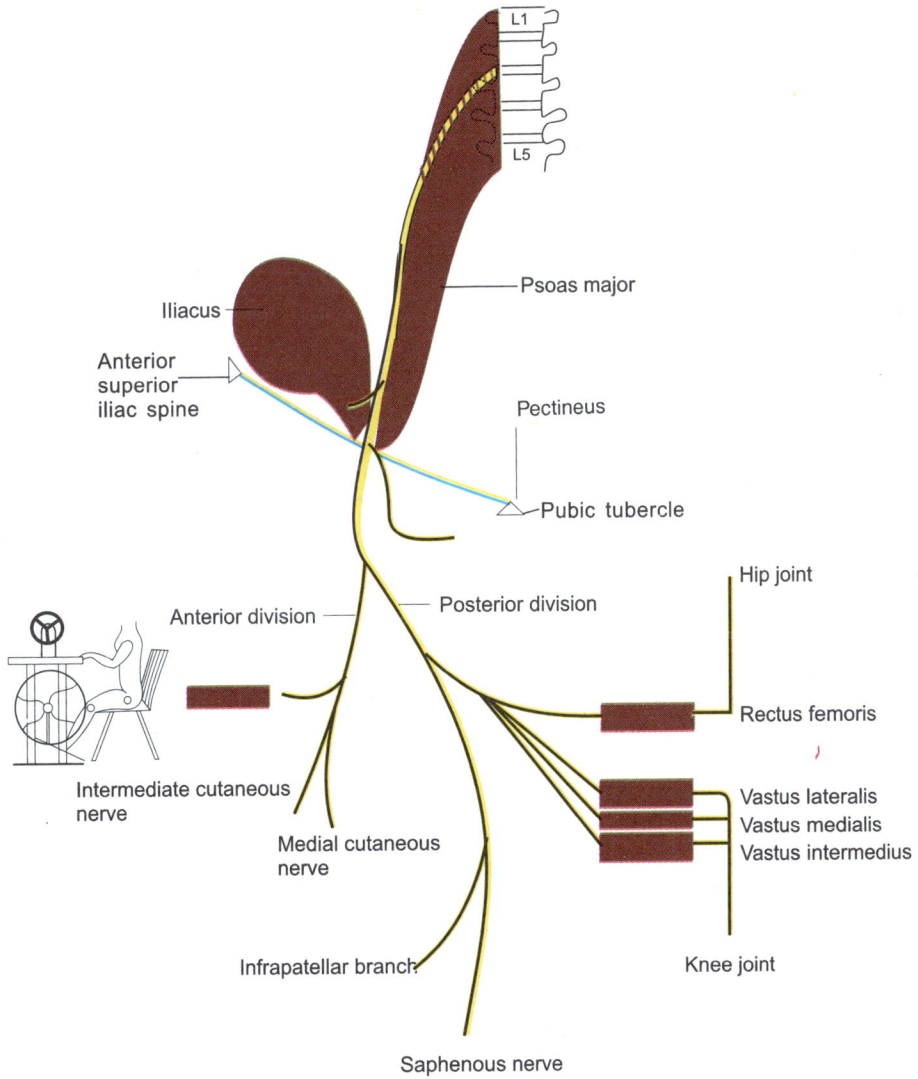

Fig. 1.15 Femoral nerve and its branches.

B.   From the divisions
   a.   Anterior division: ☘━━ SHORT CUT (S = <u>s</u>artorius, CUT = <u>cut</u>aneous)
      I.   Muscular: <u>S</u>artorius.
      II. <u>Cut</u>aneous:
        i.   Medial cutaneous nerve of thigh supplies skin of medial side of thigh.
        ii. Intermediate cutaneous nerve of thigh.
          -   Supplies front of thigh.
          -   Patellar plexus.
   b.   Posterior division:

      ☘━━ Quadri saph - J (Quadri = <u>quadri</u>ceps femoris, saph = <u>saph</u>enous, J = <u>j</u>oint)
      I.   Muscular:
        <u>**i.**</u>   Rectus femoris,
        <u>**ii.**</u>   Vastus lateralis,
        <u>**iii.**</u> Vastus medialis and
        <u>**iv.**</u>   Vastus intermedius.
      II. Cutaneous: <u>**Saph**</u>enous nerve forms subsartorial plexus and supplies skin on the medial side of leg.
      III. Articular:
        i.   Knee <u>j</u>oint and
        ii. Hip <u>j</u>oint.

3.   Course and relations:
   A.   In the pelvis: The nerve is formed in the substance of psoas major and runs on its lateral border and lies between psoas major & iliacus.
   B.   In the thigh: It enters thigh by passing deep to inguinal ligament
      a.   It lies on lateral side of femoral artery and outside the femoral sheath.
      b.   The nerve divides 4 cm below inguinal ligament.
   The nerve splits into anterior and posterior division by lateral circumflex femoral artery.

Relations
   A.   Anterior: Skin, superficial fascia and deep fascia.
   B.   Posterior & medial: Psoas major.
   C.   Posterior & lateral: Iliacus.

4.   Applied anatomy:
   A.   Disease of hip joint may be referred to knee joint & on the medial side of thigh.
   B.   Injury to femoral nerve causes paralysis of quadriceps femoris and affects extension of knee joint.

LAQ-5	**Describe adductor canal OR Subsartorial canal OR Hunter's canal under**
	1. Gross anatomy and 2. Applied anatomy.

1.   Gross anatomy: It is musculo aponeurotic passage or tunnel present in the middle third of thigh.
   A.   Length 6 inches or 15 cms
      a.   Extent: It extends from apex of femoral triangle to fifth osseo-aponeurotic opening of adductor magnus.

    b.   Lo1cation: It is situated on the middle third of medial side of thigh.

    c.   Shape: It is triangular in cross section.

B. Boundaries: Anterolateral wall is formed by vastus medialis.

C. Roof or medial wall is

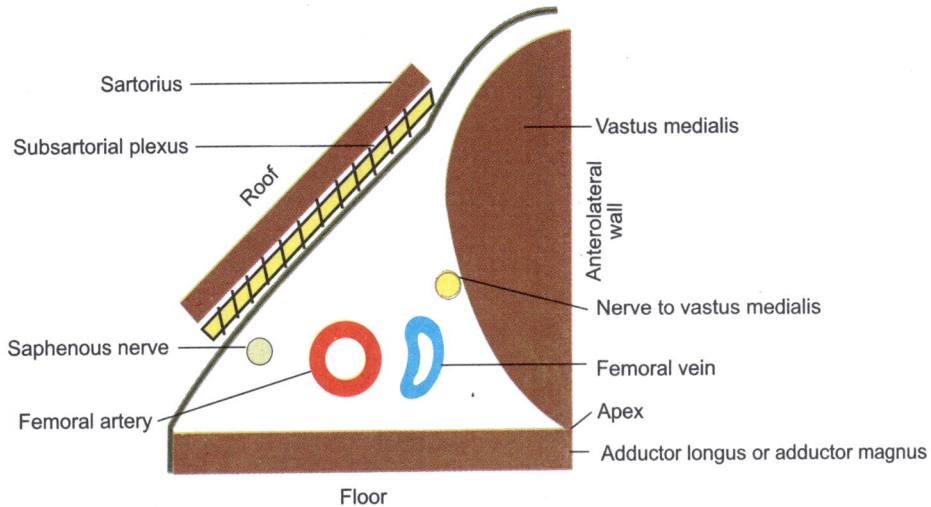

Fig. 1.16 Relations in subartorial canal

    a.   By strong fascia which extends across vastus medialis to adductor longus in the upper part and vastus medialis to adductor magnus in the lower part.

    b.   By sartorius muscle.

    c.   Subsartorial plexus which is formed by 🔑 **PAS**

        I.   **P**osterior branch of medial femoral cutaneous nerve.

        II.   **A**nterior division of obturator nerve.

        III.   **S**aphenous nerve.

           This plexus supplies

           i.   Fascia lata and

           ii.   Skin on medial side of knee.

D. Floor: In the upper part it is formed by adductor longus muscle and in the lower part it is formed by adductor magnus muscle.

E. Apex is formed by meeting point of vastus medialis & adductor muscle on linea aspera of femur.

F. Function: It provides the passage for femoral vessels.

G. Contents:

    a.   Femoral artery lies anterior to the femoral vein in upper part and medial to the vein in the lower part.

    b.   Femoral vein.

    c.   Descending genicular artery, branch of femoral artery.

    d.   Anterior & posterior divisions of obturator nerve.

    e.   Nerve to vastus medialis lies lateral to the femoral artery.

    f.   Saphenous nerve crosses the femoral artery anteriorly from lateral to medial side.

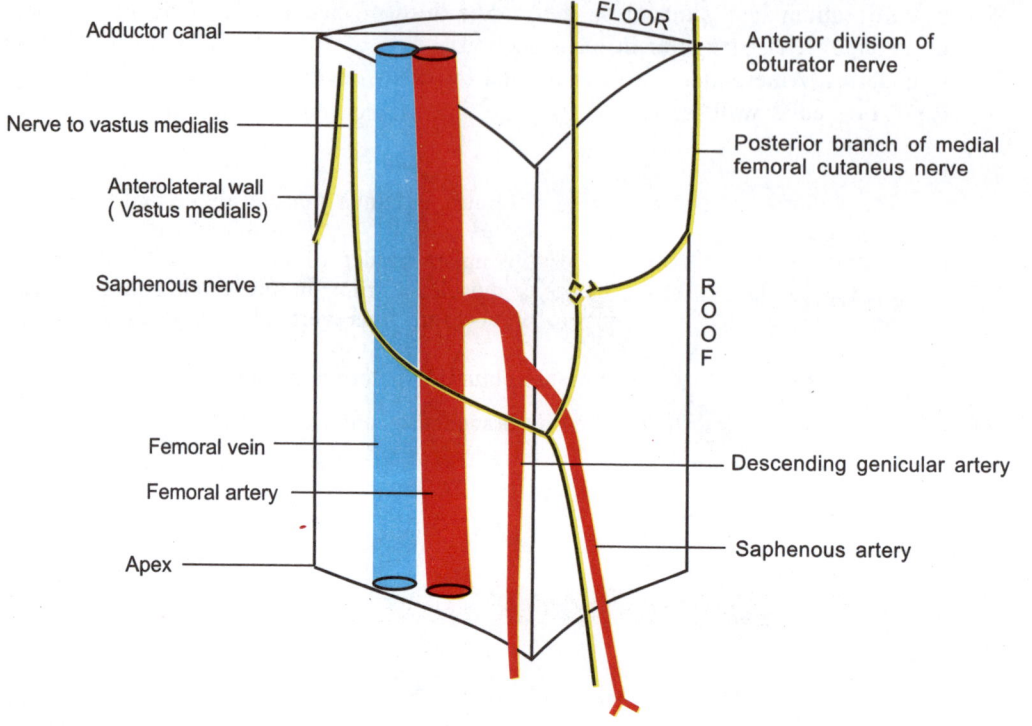

Fig. 1.17 Adductor canal and its content.

2. **Applied anatomy:**
    A. A tourniquet is applied against the linea aspera to arrest bleeding of popliteal vessels in rupture of aneurysm of popliteal artery & during surgery below the amputation of knee.
    B. In amputation of the lower limb, below the knee joint, blood vessels are compressed by tourniquet.
    C. Canal is the site of ligation of femoral artery for the treatment of aneurysm of popliteal artery.

LAQ-6 **Describe obturator nerve under**
1. **Introduction,**   2. **Root value,**   3. **Course**
4. **Branches,**   5. **Relations &**   6. **Applied anatomy.**

1. **Introduction:** It is a nerve of the adductor compartment of the thigh, supplies the adductor muscle and the skin over the medial side of thigh.

2. **Root value:** It arises from ventral division of ventral rami of L_2, L_3 & L_4. It extends from pelvis to knee joint.

3. **Course:**
    A. In the pelvis:
        a. It arises within the substance of psoas major muscle.
        b. It passes on the medial border of psoas major.

    c.   It lies behind the common iliac vessels.

    d.   It runs lateral to internal iliac vessels.

    e.   It passes along the lateral wall of pelvis.

    e.   It passes through obturator foramen and divides into anterior & posterior divisions in the obturator notch.

B.   In the thigh

    a.   The anterior divisions lies on obturator externus muscle above and adductor brevis muscle below.

    b.   The posterior division pierces the upper border of obturator externus and gives a branch to the obturator externus muscle. It runs in the thigh and lies behind the posterior surface of adductor brevis and runs vertically downwards on adductor magnus.

    c.   The posterior division perforates obturator externus muscle.

4.   **Branches:** The branches are described as branches of anterior and posterior division

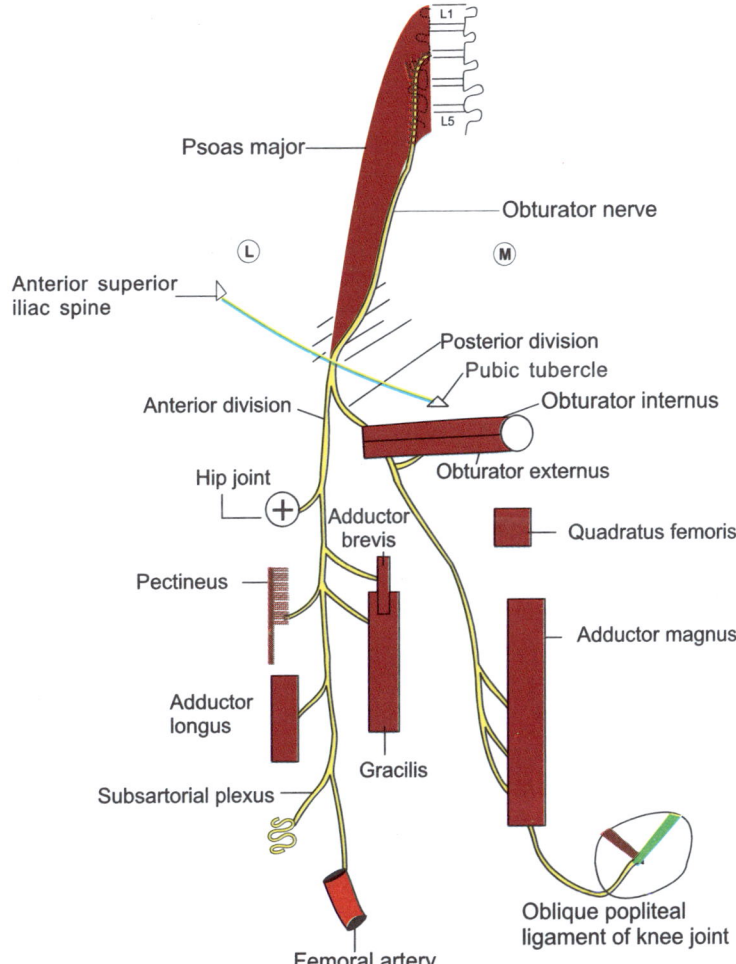

Fig. 1.18 Obturator nerve with its distribution (Diagramatic)

Table 1.5 Showing branches and distribution of obturator nerve

Particulars	Anterior	Posterior
A. Muscular	Pectineus, Gracilis, Adductor longus and Adductor brevis.	Adductor brevis, Adductor magnus and Obturator externus.
C. Vascular	Femoral artery	Popliteal artery
D. Articular	Hip joint	Knee joint
E. Miscellaneous	Subsartorial plexus supplying a. Fascia lata and b. Skin of the medial side of thigh.	Capsule of knee joint

5. **Relations:** The anterior and posterior relation of the obturator nerve are as follows

Table 1.6 Showing relations of obturator nerve

Division	Anterior	Posterior
Anterior	Adductor longus and pectineus.	Adductor brevis.
Posterior	Adductor longus and adductor brevis.	Adductor magnus.

6. **Applied anatomy:**
   A. The obturator nerve supplies both hip & knee joint. So disease of one joint gives referred pain to other joint.
   B. Injury to obturator nerve is uncommon. A penetrating wound may injure obturator nerve and results in the weakness of adduction of the hip joint.

SN-11   Gluteus maximus

1. **Introduction:** It is a large, quadrilateral muscle present in the gluteal region.

Table 1.7 Showing origin, insertion and nerve supply of gluteus maximus

2. Origin ⚷ SCST	3. Insertion	4. Nerve supply
A. Aponeurotic: Aponeurosis of erector spinae	A. The superficial major part is inserted into iliotibial tract.	Inferior gluteal nerve (L_5, S_1, S_2)
B. Bony: a. Posterior gluteal line. b. Area posterior to the posterior gluteal line. c. Outer sloping area of the dorsal segment of the iliac crest. d. Dorsal surface of lower part of sacrum. e. Side of coccyx.	B. The deep, lower part is inserted into gluteal tuberosity.	
C. Ligamentous: Sacrotuberous ligament		
D. Fascial: Fascia covering the gluteus medius.		

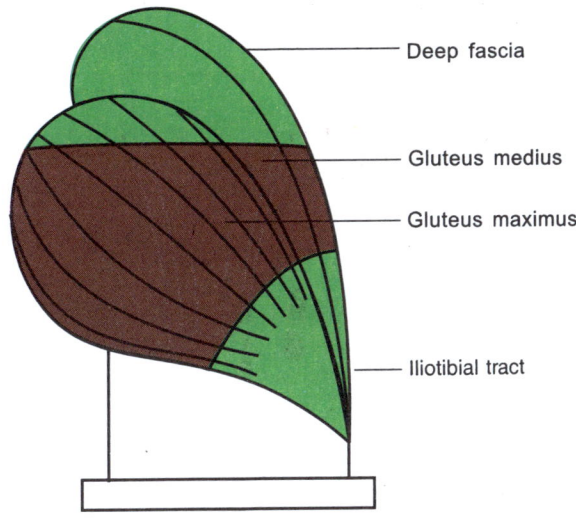

Fig. 1.19 Guteus maximus

5. **Actions:**
    A. It is the powerful extensor of the hip joint.
    B. It is the powerful lateral rotator of the thigh.
    C. It acts in rising from sitting position and in climbing the staircase.
    D. It supports the extended knee.
    E. It is abductor of the thigh.

LAQ-7	**Describe the structures under cover of gluteus maximus**
	1. Muscles, 2. Vessels, 3. Nerves, 4. Bones, 5. Joints, 6. Ligaments, 7. Bursae.

1. **Muscles:** (key ½, 1,2,3,4)
    A. **Key** muscle is piriformis.
    B. **½** muscle is reflected head of rectus femoris.
    C. The muscle which is **single**, quadratus femoris.
    D. The muscles which are in group of **two**:
        a. Gamelli
            I.   Superior and
            II. Inferior.
        b. Obturator
            I.   Internus &
            II. Externus.
    E. The muscles which are in group of **three**:
        a. Gluteus minimus.
        b. Gluteus medius.
    F. The muscle which are in group of **four**:
        a. Semimembranous.
        b. Semitendinosus.

  c. Ischial fibers of adductor magnus.
  d. Biceps femoris.

2. **Vessels** can be remembered by pneumonic 'SIATICA' 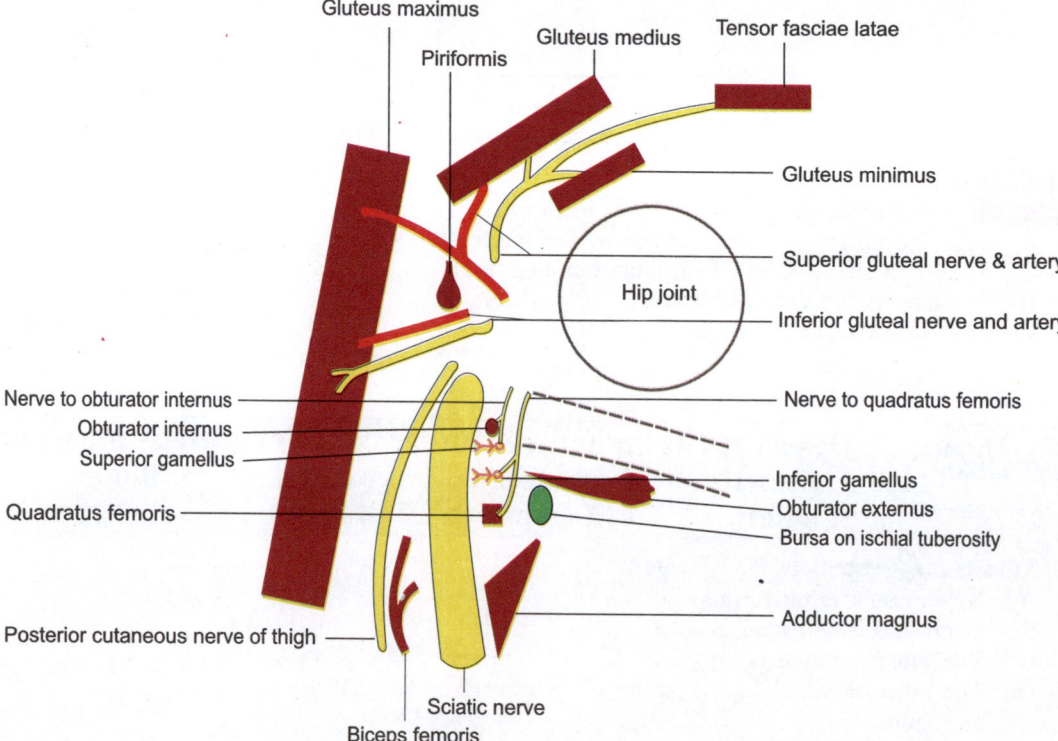 **SIATICA**
 A. **S**uperior gluteal artery.
 B. **I**nferior gluteal artery.
 C. **A**scending branch of medial and lateral circumflex femoral artery (profunda femoris).
 D. **T**rochanteric anastomosis.
 E. **I**nternal pudendal vessels.
 F. **C**ruciate anastomosis.
 G. **A**scending branch of first perforating artery.

3. **Nerves:** The key nerve in this region is sciatic nerve. The other nerves under cover of gluteus maximus are recollected by remembering the muscles & their nerve supply.

Fig. 1.20 Structures under cover of the gluteus maximus.

 A. Key nerve is sciatic nerve ($L_{4, 5}$, $S_{1, 2, 3}$).
 B. Nerve to quadratus femoris ($L_{4, 5}$, S_1).
 C. Nerve to obturator internus (L_5, $S_{1, 2}$).
 D. Superior gluteal nerve ($L_{4, 5}$, S_1).
 E. Inferior gluteal nerve (L_5, $S_{1, 2}$).
 F. Pudendal nerve ($S_{2, 3, 4}$).
 G. Posterior cutaneous nerve of thigh ($S_{2, 3}$)
 H. Perforating cutaneous nerve ($S_{2, 3}$) branch of posterior cutaneous nerve of thigh.

4. **Bones:**
   A. Part of hip bone:
      a. Ilium and
      b. Ischium.
   B. Sacrum and coccyx.
   C. Upper end and greater trochanter of femur.

5. **Joint:** Hip and sacroiliac.

6. **Ligaments:**
   A. Sacrotuberous,
   B. Sacrospinous and
   C. Ischiofemoral ligament.

7. **Bursae:** Under cover of gluteus maximus
   A. Trochanteric bursa: Bursa present at greater trochanter.
   B. Bursa over ischial tuberosity.
   C. Bursa between gluteus maximus & vastus lateralis.

SAQ-4   Trochanteric anastomosis

1. **Site:** Trochanteric fossa

2. **Arteries** taking part
   A. Descending branch of superior gluteal artery.
   B. Ascending branch of medial circumflex femoral artery.
   C. Ascending branch of lateral circumflex femoral artery.
   D. Inferior gluteal artery.
   E. Internal pudendal artery.

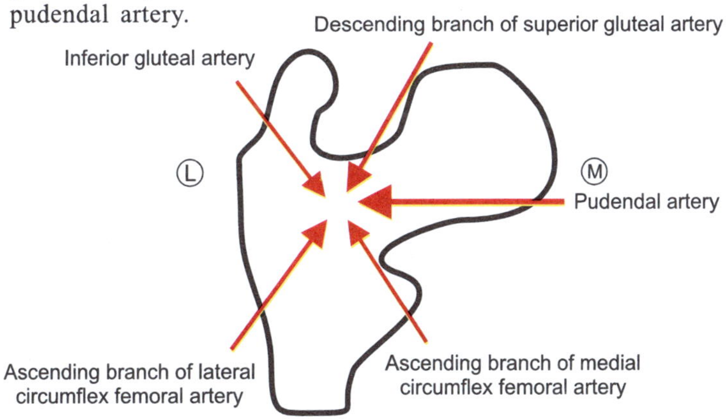

Fig. 1.21 Arteries forming trochanteric anastomosis

3. **Applied anatomy:**
   A. It provides chief source of blood supply to the head of femur.
   B. Since trochanteric anastomosis is between branches of internal iliac and femoral artery, so that in case of blockage of one of the artery, the collateral circulation is developed to maintain the blood supply to this region.

SAQ-5 Cruciate anastomosis

1. **Site:** Root of the greater trochanter between quadratus femoris and adductor magnus.

2. **Arteries** taking part
   A. Transverse branch of medial circumflex femoral artery.
   B. Transverse branch of lateral circumflex femoral artery.
   C. Descending branch of inferior gluteal artery.
   D. Ascending branch of first perforating artery.

3. **Applied anatomy:** This establishes the collateral circulation between internal iliac artery and profunda femoris artery in case of ligature of the femoral artery proximal to the origin of profunda femoris artery.

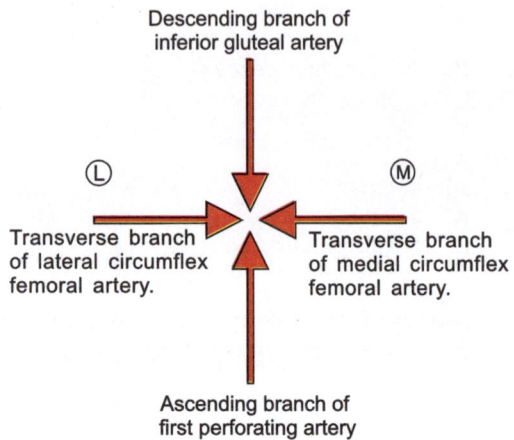

Fig. 1.22 Arteries forming cruciate anastomosis.

SN-12 Gluteus medius

1. **Introduction:** It is a fan-shaped muscle & covers the lateral surface of the bony pelvis.

2. **Origin:** gluteal surface of ilium between anterior & posterior gluteal lines.

3. **Insertion:** into the lateral surface of greater trochanter of femur along and oblique line that slopes downward and forward. Its tendon of insertion gives a strong expansion that crosses the capsule of hip joint.

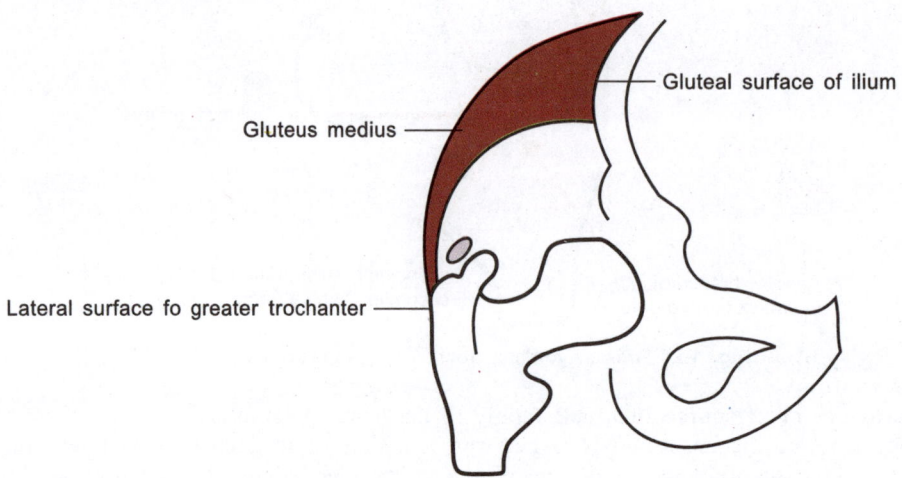

Fig. 1.23 Origin and insertion of gluteus medius

4. **Nerve supply:** superior gluteal nerve (L_5, S_1).

5. **Structures:** Deep to the gluteus medius.
   A. Superior gluteal nerve,
   B. Deep branch of the superior gluteal artery,
   C. Gluteus minimus &
   D. Trochanteric bursa of the gluteus medius.

6. **Actions:**
   A. It is an abductor of the hip joint.
   B. It prevents the sagging of the pelvis on the unsupported side.
   C. It is a lateral rotator of hip joint.

7. **Applied anatomy:** The stability of the hip joint when a person stands on one leg depends on three factors
   A. The gluteus medius & minimus must be functioning normally.
   B. The head of the femur must be located normally within the acetabulum.
   C. The neck of the femur must be intact and must have a normal angle with the shaft of the femur.
   If any one of these factors is defective, then the pelvis will sink downward on the opposite, unsupported side, the patient is then said to exhibit a positive Trendelenberg's sign.

SN-13   Hamstring muscles

Ham Posterior aspect of thigh, *string* Thread like.
1. **Introduction:** These are thread like muscles present on the posterior aspect of thigh and includes
   A. Semimembranosus: The upper part of the muscle is membrane like and measures about 15 cm in length. It arises from smooth facet present on the lateral part of ischial tuberosity.
   B. Semitendinosus: The lower part of the muscle is tendon like. It arises from medial facet of ischial tuberosity.
   C. Biceps femoris: It has two heads
      a. Ischial head and
      b. Femoral head.
   D. Ischial fibers of adductor magnus.

2. **Characters:**
   A. All the muscle arise from ischial tuberosity.
   B. They get inserted into one of bone of leg (either tibia or fibula).
   C. They are supplied by the tibial division of sciatic nerve (L_5 $_{S1}$).
   D. They are extensors of the hip joint and flexor of the knee joint.

Note: The semimembranosus and the semitendinosus are true hamstrings. The biceps femoris and the adductor magnus are modified hamstring muscles. The biceps arises from the iliac crest and the part extending from ilium and sacrum to ischial tuberosity is converted into sacrotuberous ligament. The adductor magnus is inserted into tibial tuberosity. The part of the adductor magnus extending from adductor tubercle to tibial tuberosity is converted into tibial collateral ligament. Hence biceps femoris and adductor magnus are called modified hamstring muscles.

LAQ-8   Describe popliteal fossa under
1. **Boundaries,**   2. **Content,**
3. **Relations and**   4. **Applied anatomy.**

1. **Boundaries:**
   A. Introduction: It is a diamond shaped fossa present on posterior aspect of knee joint. It is homologous with cubital fossa, present in front of the elbow joint. It is bounded by
      a. Superomedially: Semimembranosus and semitendinosus.
      b. Superolaterally: Tendon of biceps femoris.
      c. Inferolaterally: Lateral head of gastrocnemius
      d. Inferomedially: Medial head of gastrocnemius

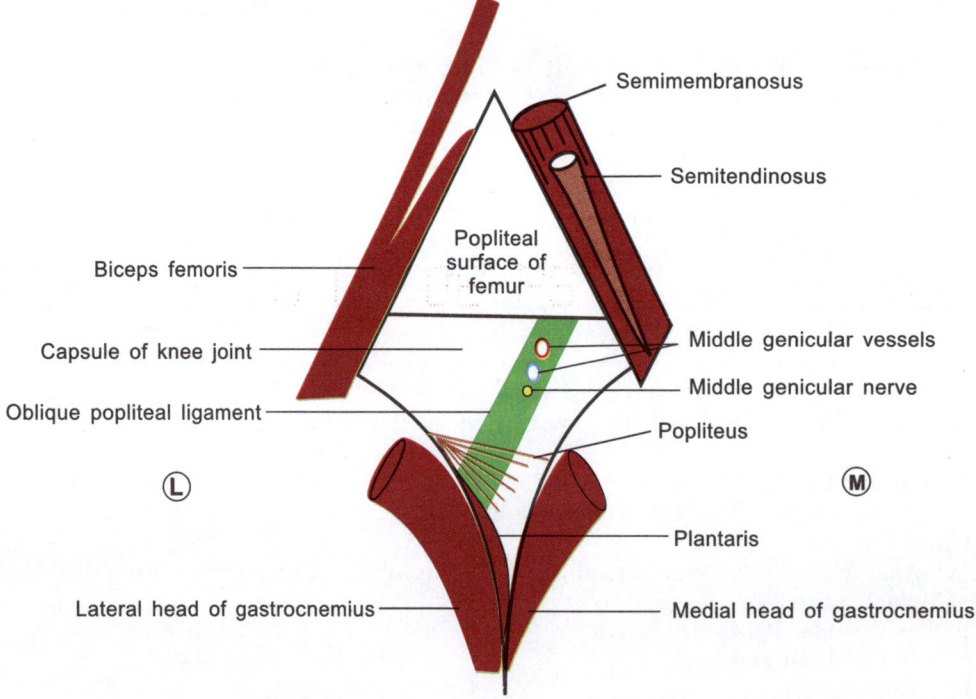

Fig. 1.24 Boundaries and floor of the popliteal fossa.

   B. Roof is formed by following structures from superficial to deep
      a. Skin.
      b. Superficial fascia.
      c. Strong popliteal fascia (continuity between fascia lata & fascia cruris) which is pierced by
         I. Sural nerve (cutaneous branch of tibial nerve).
         II. Posterior femoral cutaneous nerve of thigh.
         III. Short saphenous vein.
   C. Floor (anterior wall) is from by following structures above downward.
      a. Popliteal surface of femur.
      b. Capsule of knee joint.
      c. Oblique popliteal ligament.

      d.   Fascia covering popliteus muscle.
      e.   Floor is pierced by
          I.   Middle genicular vessels.
          II.   Middle genicular nerve.
          III. Genicular branch of posterior division of obturator nerve.

2.   Contents:
    A.   The most important structure are branches of sciatic nerve namely
       a.   Tibial nerve and
       b.   Common peroneal nerve.
    B.   The other contents are
       a.   Posterior division of obturator nerve,
       b.   Posterior cutaneous nerve of thigh,
       c.   Popliteal artery,
       d.   Popliteal vein,
       e.   Popliteal lymph nodes,
       f.   Pad of fat and
       g.   Small saphenous vein.

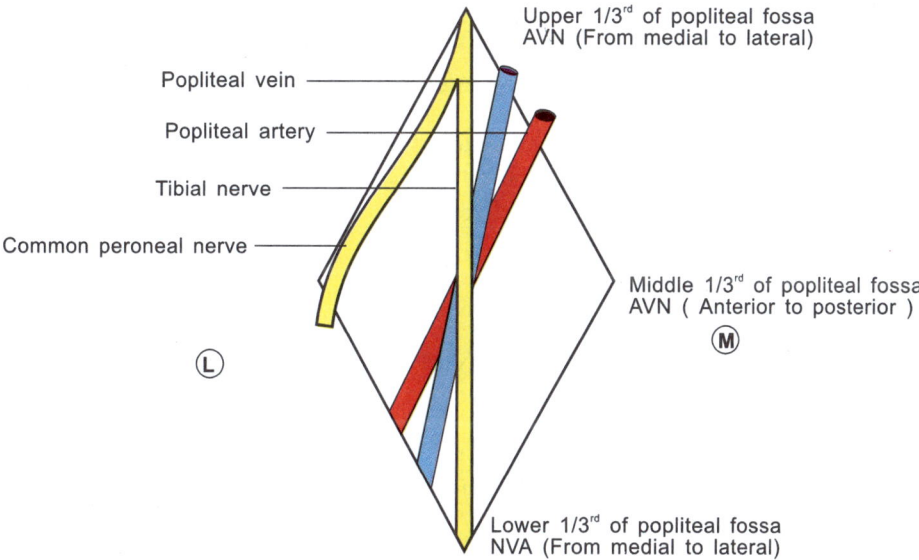

Fig. 1.25 Relations of the structures in the popliteal fossa.

3.   Relations: The relations of the contents with each other are described at three different levels in following table:

Table 1.8 Showing relations of structures in the popliteal fossa

In upper part	In middle part	In lower part
Relations from medial to lateral 🔑 AVN	Relations from anterior to posterior 🔑 AVN	Relations from medial to lateral 🔑 NVA
A. Popliteal **a**rtery	A. Popliteal **a**rtery	A. Tibial **n**erve
B. Popliteal **v**ein	B. Popliteal **v**ein	B. Popliteal **v**ein
C. Tibial **n**erve	C. Tibial **n**erve	C. Popliteal **a**rtery

4. **Applied anatomy:** The division of tibial nerve in popliteal fossa is associated with motor paralysis of muscles supplied by it
   A. Foot is dorsi flexed at ankle joint and held in eversion.
   B. There is a sensory loss on entire sole of foot.

LAQ-9 **Describe popliteal artery under**
1. **Course and relations,** 2. **Branches &**
3. **Applied anatomy.**

1. **Course:** The popliteal artery is a continuation of the femoral artery at the fifth osseoaponeurotic opening in adductor magnus. It runs downwards and laterally and passes in between two condyles and reaches the lower border of popliteus where it terminates into anterior and posterior tibial arteries.

   Relations: The relations of the contents with each other are described at three different levels in following table

   Table 1.9 Showing relations of popliteal artery with other structures

In upper part	In middle part	In lower part
Relations from medial to lateral	Relations from anterior to posterior	Relations from medial to lateral
A. Popliteal <u>a</u>rtery	A. Popliteal <u>a</u>rtery	A. Tibial <u>n</u>erve
B. Popliteal <u>v</u>ein	B. Popliteal <u>v</u>ein	B. Popliteal <u>v</u>ein
C. Tibial <u>n</u>erve	C. Tibial <u>n</u>erve	C. Popliteal <u>a</u>rtery

2. **Branches:**

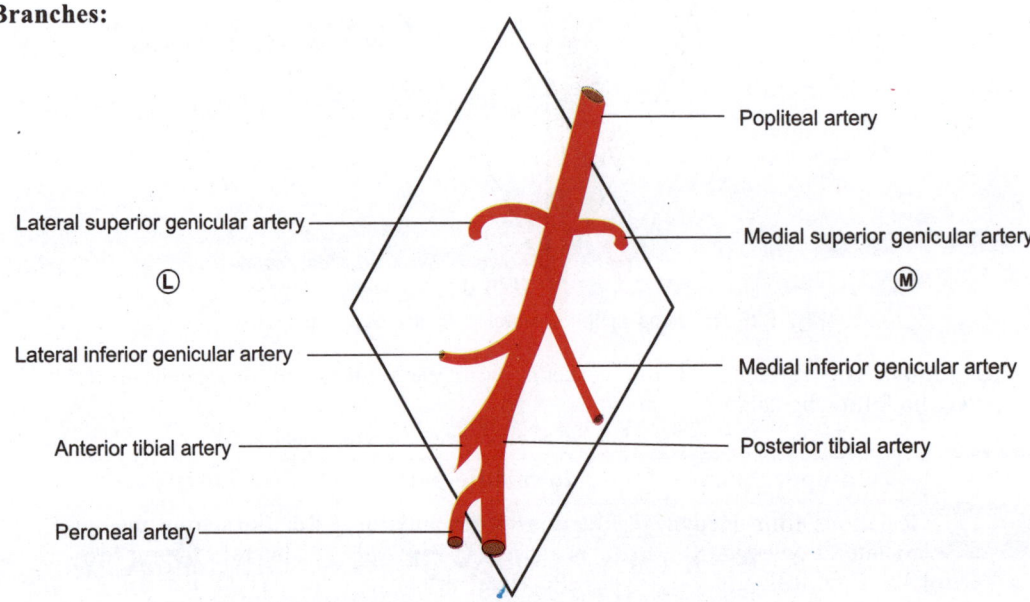

Fig. 1.26 Branches of the popliteal artery

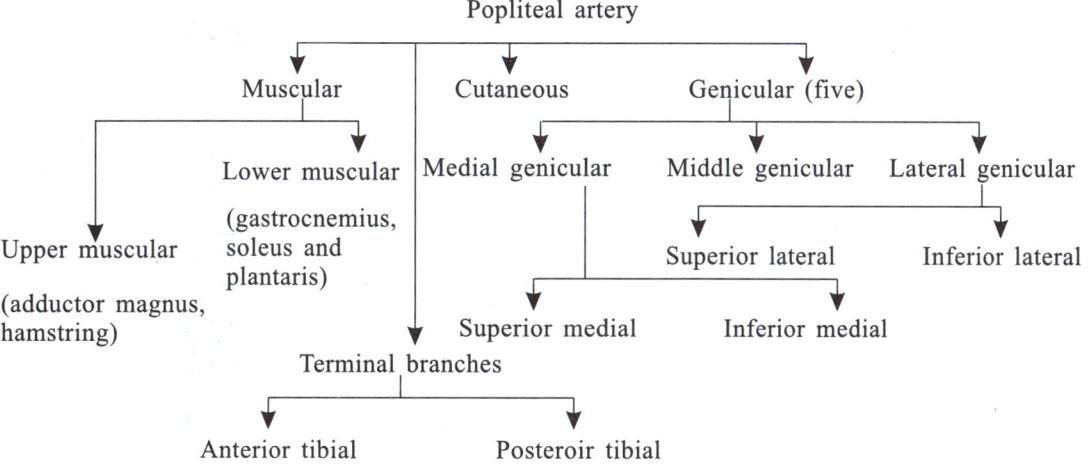

Popliteal artery
- Muscular
  - Upper muscular (adductor magnus, hamstring)
  - Lower muscular (gastrocnemius, soleus and plantaris)
- Cutaneous
- Genicular (five)
  - Medial genicular
    - Superior medial
    - Inferior medial
  - Middle genicular
  - Lateral genicular
    - Superior lateral
    - Inferior lateral
- Terminal branches
  - Anterior tibial
  - Posteroir tibial

3. **Applied anatomy:**
A. The blood pressure in the lower limb is recorded by the auscultation of popliteal artery.
B. In atherosclerosis of popliteal artery the graft can be tried from the lower part of popliteal artery as it is patent.
C. The popliteal artery is more prone to aneurysm than any other arteries of the body.

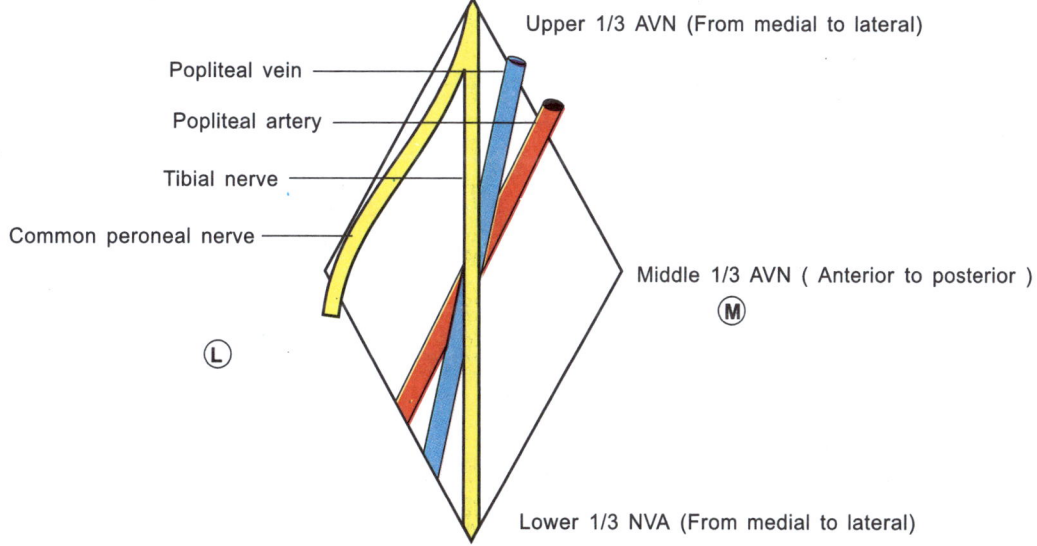

Popliteal vein
Popliteal artery
Tibial nerve
Common peroneal nerve

Upper 1/3 AVN (From medial to lateral)

Middle 1/3 AVN (Anterior to posterior)
Ⓜ

Ⓛ

Lower 1/3 NVA (From medial to lateral)

Fig. 1.27 Relations of popliteal artery with other structures in the popliteal fossa.

LAQ-10 Describe the sciatic nerve under
1. **Root value,** 2. **Course and relations,**
3. **Distribution &** 4. **Applied anatomy.**

1. **Root value:** It arise from ventral and dorsal divisions of ventral rami of $L_{4, 5}$, $S_{1, 2, 3}$.

2. **Course & relations:**
   A. Course: It is thickest nerve in the body. The course and relation of the sciatic nerve is as follows
      a. In pelvis: It lies in front of piriformis
      b. It enters gluteal region through greater sciatic foramen (below piriformis) and passes between ischial tuberosity & greater trochanter.
         It emerges from lower border of gluteus maximus and passes downward deep to the long head biceps.
   B. Relations
      a. Superficial: Gluteus maximus.
      b. Deep:
         I. Body of ischium.
         II. Ascending branch of medial circumflex femoral artery.
         III. Tendon of obturator internus with the gamelli.
         IV. Nerve to quadratus femoris.
         V. Capsule of the hip joint is present deep to all these muscles.
      c. Medial:
         I. Inferior gluteal nerve & vessels.
         II. The posterior cutaneous nerve of thigh.
         At the junction of upper 2/3 & lower 1/3 the sciatic nerve divides into tibial and common peroneal nerve.

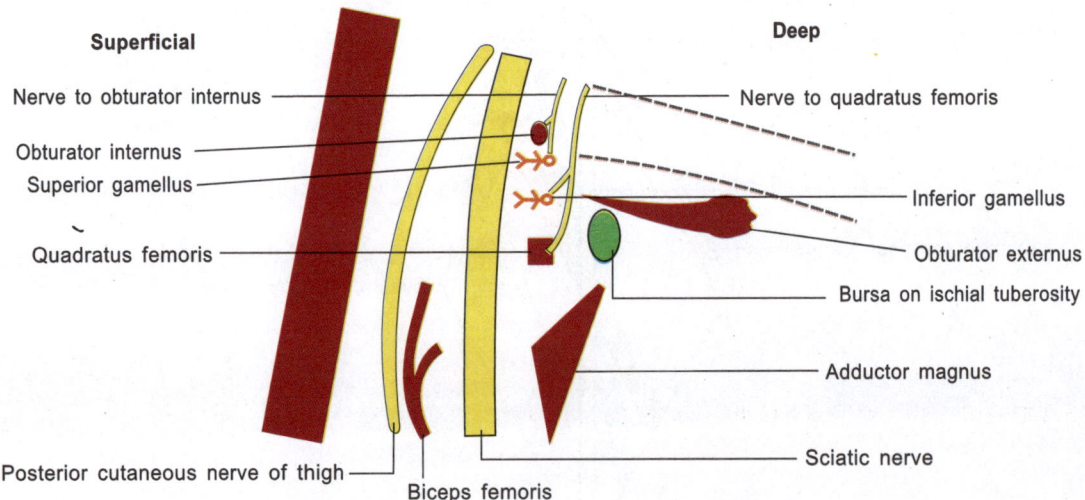

Fig. 1.28 Course and relations of sciatic nerve.

3. **Distribution:**
   A. The tibial part of sciatic nerve supplies hamstring muscles and the muscles of posterior compartment of leg.
   B. Tibial nerve divides between heel and medial malleolus into medial and lateral plantar nerve. The medial plantar nerve supplies all the muscles present on the medial side of foot except adductor hallucis and the lateral plantar nerve supplies all the muscles present on the lateral side of foot and adductor hallucis.

4. **Applied anatomy**
   A. Sciatica: it is due to compression and irritation of nerve roots of sciatic nerve. The patient gets shooting pain along the cutaneous distribution of the sciatic nerve. The pain begins in the gluteal region and radiates along the back of thigh, lateral side of the leg and to the dorsum of foot.
   B. The deep intramuscular injection in the lower medial quadrant of gluteal region causes injury to the sciatic nerve.
   C. The sciatic nerve is injured by penetrating wounds and dislocation of hip joint.

SN-14   Soleus

1. **Introduction:** It is sole like, & multipennate superficial muscle of posterior compartment of leg situated deep to the gastrocnemius.

2. **Peculiarities:**
   A. The soleus contains a rich plexus of small veins. The contraction of the soleus squeezes the vessels and facilitates venous return from the lower extremity. Hence it is often called peripheral heart.
   B. It is an important postural muscle. It contains about 80% type I (red or slow) oxidative fibers. As the body weight acts along a line that passes a few centimeters anterior to the ankle joint, the tonic contractions of type I fibers of the plantar flexor is important to balance the effect of gravity during standing erect.

3. **Origin:** It arises from
   A. The back of head and upper $1/4^{th}$ of posterior surface of fibula,
   B. Soleal line and middle $1/3^{rd}$ of medial border of shaft of tibia,
   C. Deep transverse fascia of leg and
   D. Soleal arch which stretches between tibia and fibula.

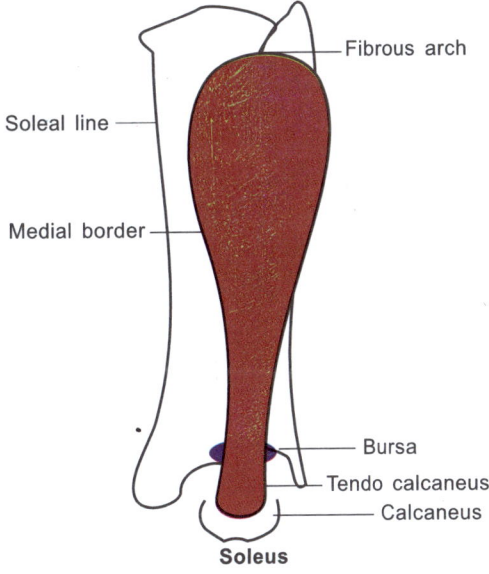

Fig. 1.29 Origin and insertion of soleus muscle

4. **Insertion:** The tendon of soleus fuses with tendon of gastrocnemius to form tendocalcaneus which is inserted into middle $1/3^{rd}$ of posterior surface of calcaneus. The tendocalcaneus is thickest and strongest tendon in the body.

5. **Nerve supply:** Tibial nerve (S_1, S_2)

6. **Action:**
   A. Plantar flexion of ankle joint. When the knees flexed, the soleus is the main muscle for plantar flexion at ankle because the action of gastrocnemius becomes ineffective.
   B. In standing position it steadies the leg.
   C. In walking, it acts as a bottom or first gear and so it overcomes the inertia of body weight.

7. **Relations:** It is pierced by the tibial nerve.
   A. Superficial: Gastrocnemius and plantaris.
   B. Deep:
      a. Flexor digitorum longus,
      b. Flexot hallucus longus,
      c. Tibialis posterior and
      d. Posterior tibial vessels and tibial nerve.
   C. Structures passing deep to soleal arch are popliteal vessels.

| SN-15 | **Dorsalis pedis artery** |

1. **Introduction:** It is the chief artery of dorsum of foot.

2. **Origin:** It is a continuation of anterior tibial artery.

3. **Course and relation:** It begins in front of the ankle joint between two malleoli. It passes along the medial side of the dorsum of the foot to reach the proximal end of first intermetatarsal space. Here it pierces first dorsal interosseous muscle.

4. **Termination:** It forms plantar arterial arch in the sole.

5. **Branches:**
   A. Lateral tarsal artery,
   B. Medial tarsal branches,
   C. Arcuate artery and
   D. First dorsal metatarsal artery.

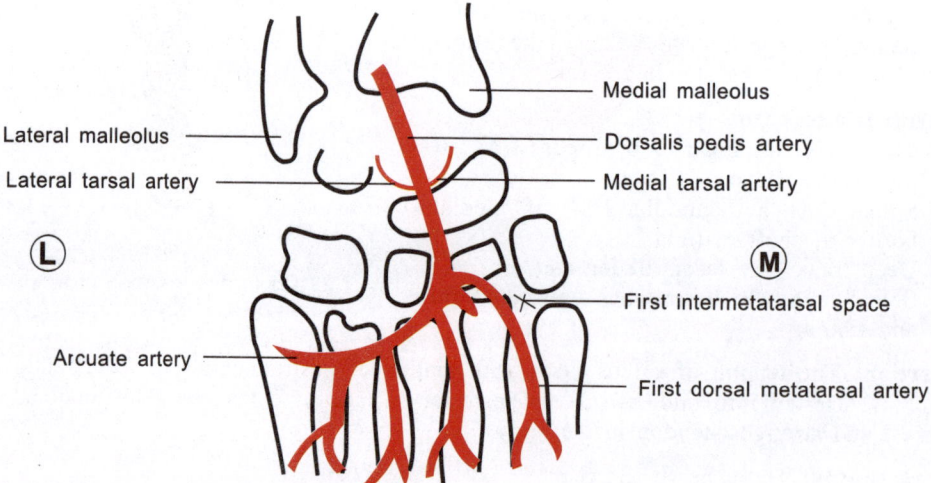

Fig. 1.30 Course and branches of dorsalis pedis artery.

6. **Applied anatomy:** Pulsations of dorsalis pedis artery are felt between tendons of extensor hallucis longus and extensor digitorum longus.

SN-16   **Popliteus**

Pop ham posterior aspect of knee.

1. **Introduction:** It is a flat, triangular muscle present in the floor of lower part of popliteal fossa.

2. **Peculiarities:**
   A. It has tendinous origin and fleshy insertion.
   B. The origin is intracapsular.

3. **Origin:** It arises from
   A. The anterior part of the popliteal groove present on the lateral surface of the lateral condyle of femur.
   B. Arcuate ligament
   C. The outer margin of lateral meniscus of the knee joint.

4. **Insertion:**
   A. Posterior surface of tibia into medial 2/3rd of the triangular area above the solial line.
   B. Fascia covering it.

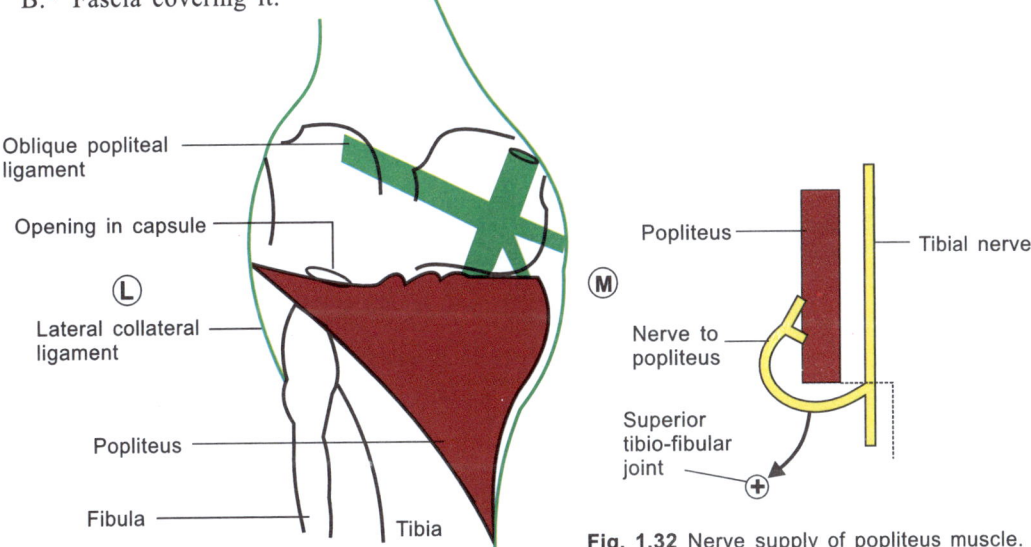

Fig. 1.32 Nerve supply of popliteus muscle.

Fig. 1.31 Origin and insertion of popliteus muscle.

5. **Nerve supply:** It is supplied by a branch of tibial nerve.

6. **Action:**
   A. It unlocks the knee in initial phase of flexion, i.e.
      a. Medial rotation of tibia on the femur when foot is off the ground, or
      b. Lateral rotation of femur on fixed tibia when foot is on the ground.
   B. Flexes the knee joint
   C. It **p**ulls the lateral meniscus **p**osteriorly and **p**revents it from being trapped at the beginning of the flexion. **PPPP** - Popliteus, pulls, posteriorly, prevents.

7. **Applied anatomy:** Injury to tibial nerve may result in to inability of unlocking.

SN-17   Plantar aponeurosis

1. **Introduction:** It is a thickened central part of deep fascia.

2. **Formation:** It is formed by longitudinal displayed compact bundles of collagen fibers.

3. **Parts:** It has following parts
   A. Lateral part: It covers the abductor digiti minimi and extends from lateral tubercle of calcaneum to the base of proximal phalanx of fifth toe.
   B. Medial part: It covers abductor hallucis and distally attached to the base of proximal phalanx of great toe. Both lateral and medial parts are thinner.
   C. Central part: It is the thickest part and most prominent part and in reality it is the plantar aponeurosis.

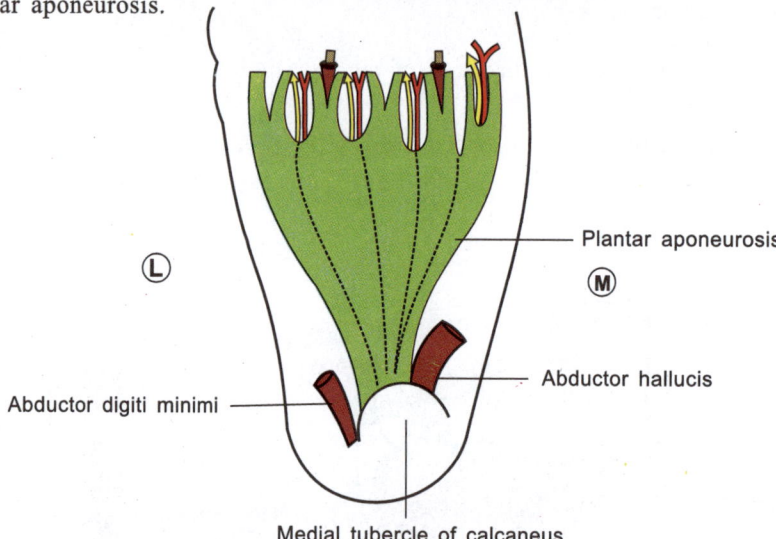

Fig. 1.33 Plantar aponeurosis

4. **Shape: It is triangular in shape having the base and apex.**
   A. The apex is the proximal part and is attached to medial tubercle of calcaneum.
   B. The base is distal part and divides opposite the head of metatarsal bones into five slips or processes which are connected by transverse fibers. In between the gaps of five processes digital vessels and nerves and lumbricals pass.

5. **Each slip or process divides into**
   A. Superficial part: It is attached to transverse sulcus of the skin at the toes of foot.
   B. Deep part: It again splits into two parts and transmits the flexor tendons. Finally they are attached to
      a. Transverse metatarsal ligament.
      b. Fibrous sheaths of flexor tendons.
      c. Lateral and medial borders of proximal & middle phalanx.

6. **Morphology:** It is continuation of the plantaris muscle and homologous to palmar aponeurosis.

7. **Functions:** 🔑 **MAPP**
   A. It **m**aintains the longitudinal arch.

B. It **a**cts as tie beam.

C. It **p**rovides origin to superficial plantar muscles.

D. It **p**rotects plantar vessels and nerves.

SN-18   Layers of sole

1. **First layer**
   A. Abductor hallucis,
   B. Abductor digiti minimi and
   C. Flexor digitorum brevis.

2. **Second layer**
   A. Tendons of
      a. Flexor digitorum longus.
      b. Flexor hallucis longus.
   B. Flexor accessorius.
   C. Lumbricals.

3. **Third layer**
   A. Flexor hallucis brevis,
   B. Adductor hallucis and
   C. Flexor digiti minimi brevis.

4. **Fourth layer**   TIP
   A. **T**ibialis posterior.
   B. **I**nterossei: Three plantar & four dorsal.
   C. Tendon of **p**eroneus longus.

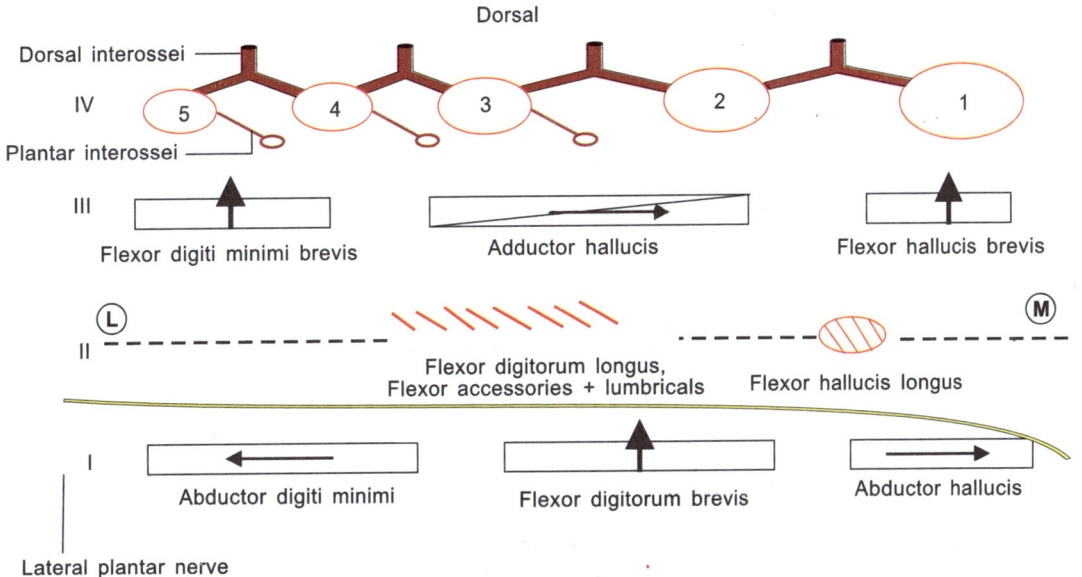

Fig. 1.34 Layers of the sole showing the structures.

LAQ-11 Describe hip joint under
1. Classification, 2. Ligaments, 3. Relations,
4. Blood supply, 5. Nerve supply,
6. Movements and muscles bringing movements &
7. Applied anatomy.

1. **Classification:**
   A. Structural: Simple, ball and socket, multi axial type of synovial joint.
   B. Functional: Diarthrosis.

2. **Ligaments:**
   A. Capsule
      a. Attachment
         I. Superiorly: It is attached superiorly 5 to 6 mm above the acetabular margin of hip bone.
         II. Inferiorly:
            i. Anteriorly: On the intertrochanteric line.
            ii. Posteriorly: One cm medial to intertrochantric crest.
      b. Variation in thickness
         I. Anterosuperiorly: It is thick and attached firmly. It is subjected to maximum tension in standing.
         II. Posteroinferiorly: It is thin and loosely attached to bone.
      c. Types of fibers: There are two types of fibers
         I. The outer fibers are longitudinal and are best developed anterosuperiorly to form retinacula. The blood vessel supplying head & neck travel along these retinacula.
         II. The inner fibers are circular and are called zona orbicularis.
   B. Synovial membrane: It lines
      a. The inner surface of fibrous capsule, intracapsular portion of neck of femur.
      b. Both surface of acetabular labrum.
      c. Transverse ligament.
      d. Fat in the acetabular fossa.
   C. Acetabular labrum (*labrum* edge, brim). It is fibrocartilagenous.
      Functions: 🔑 **DMP**
      a. **D**eepens the acetabular cavity
      b. **M**aintains the bony contacts
      c. **P**rotects the edges.
   D. Iliofemoral ligament (ligament of Bigelow)
      a. It is Y shaped, strongest ligament in the body extends from the anterior inferior iliac spine to the intertrochanteric line.
      b. It prevents backwards falling
   E. Pubofemoral ligament it is triangular and extends from iliopubic eminence, obturator crest & obturator membrane to inferior part of capsule.
   F. Ischio femoral ligament: It should be ideally called as ischio capsular because it is attached to inner layer of capsule. It is weak and extends from posterior inferior surface of acetabular margin to posterior part of neck of femur and is continues with zona orbicularis.
   G. Ligament of head of femur (ligamentum teres or round ligament)
      a. It is flat & triangular ligament.

    b. Its apex is attached to the depression present on the head of femur called fovea centralis & base is attached to:
        I. Transverse acetabular ligament and
        II. Margins of acetabular notch.
    c. It transmits arteries of head of femur (from acetabular branches of the obturator & medial circumflex femoral arteries).
  H. Transverse ligament of the acetabulum
    a. Is a part of acetabulum and
    b. It bridges the notch.

3. Relations:
  A. Anterior:
    a. Pectineus,   ⎫ Floor
    b. Iliopsoas,   ⎬ of femoral triangle
    c. Rectus femoris,
    d. Femoral vein,   ⎫ Contents
    e. Femoral artery,   ⎬ of femoral triangle
    f. Femoral nerve.   ⎭
  B. Posterior:
    a. Tendon of obturator externus,
    b. Tendon of obturator internus, ⎫ Structures under
    c. Gamelli,   ⎬ cover of gluteus
    d. piriformis.   ⎭ maximus
  C. Superior:
    a. Reflected head of rectus femoris and
    b. Gluteus minimus.
  D. Inferior:
    a. Pectineus and
    b. Obturator muscle.

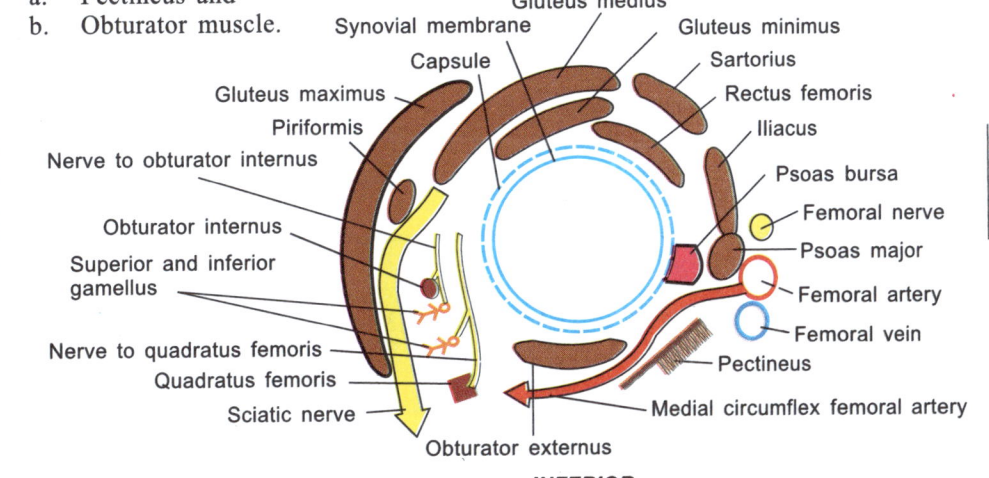

Fig. 1.35 Relations of hip joint

4. Blood supply:
  A. Obturator artery, a branch of posterior division of internal iliac artery.
  B. Medial circumflex femoral, a branch of profunda femoris.
  C. Lateral circumflex femoral, a branch of profunda femoris.

5. **Nerve supply:** (All should reads questions often)
   A. Accessory obturator nerve   B. Sciatic nerve   C. Nerve to rectus femoris
   D. Nerve to quadratus femoris   E. Obturator nerve.

6. **Movements:**

Action	Muscles
A. Flexion:	Psoas major, iliacus.
B. Extension:	a. Gluteus maximus and
	b. Hamstring muscles
	I. Adductor magnus,
	II. Biceps femoris,
	III. Semimembranosus and
	IV. Semitendinosus.
C. Adduction:	a. Adductor magnus,
	b. Adductor longus and
	c. Adductor brevis.
D. Abduction:	a. Gluteus medius and
	b. Gluteus minimus.
E. Medial rotation:	Tensor fascia lata.
F. Lateral rotation:	a. Gluteus maximus,
	b. Obturator internus and externus,
	c. Superior and inferior gamelli,
	d. piriformis and
	e. Quadratus femoris.

7. **Applied anatomy:**
   A. Congenital dislocation is more common in hip than in any other joint.
   B. Dislocation may be posterior which is (more common) & anterior is (less common), central is very (rare).
   C. Fracture of neck of femur occurs between 40 to 60 years.
   D. Disease may produce shortening of limb.
   E. Disease of hip may cause referred pain to knee joint.
   F. The position of the hip joint is weak in flexion and lateral rotation of femur hence posterior dislocation (dash board injuries) is more common.

SN-19   Classify knee joint (genual)

1. **Structurally:**
   A. Compound: More than two bones are involved sharing a common articular capsule.
   B. Complex: Joint is divided into two compartments by a meniscus.
   C. Condylar: Medial and lateral condyles of femur and tibia, are taking part.
   D. Saddle shaped: Between femur & patella, the surface of which is concavoconvex.
   E. Modified hinge joint: The movements permitted are flexion, extension hence hinge joint. But there is a certain amount of axial rotation so it is called modified hinge joint.

2. **Functionally:** Diarthrosis (freely movable)

SN-20   Capsule of knee joint

1. **Attachments:**
   A. To femur: It is attached to the peripheral margin of articular surface of lower end of femur excluding articulating area for patella & including for popliteus tendon.
   B. To tibia: It is attached 1 cm distal to articular margin
      a. Anteriorly it descends along the margin of tibial tuberosity where it is deficient.
      b. Posteriorly it is attached to the intercondylar ridge.
      c. Postero laterally it leaves a gap for popliteal tendon.

2. **Capsule is strengthened**
   A. Medially by tibial collateral ligament.
   B. Laterally by iliotibial tract.
   C. Anteriomedially by medial patellar retinaculum.
   D. Anterio laterally by lateral patellar retinaculum.
   E. Posteriorly by oblique popliteal ligament.

3. **Capsule blends:**
   A. Anteriorly and above with medial and lateral patellar retinaculum.
   B. Anteriorly and below with ligamentum patellae.
   C. Medially with tibial collateral ligament.

Fig. 1.36 Capsular attachment of knee joint.

SAQ-6   Enumerate intra articular structures of knee joint

1. **The most important structure is cruciate ligament,**

2. **The other structures are**

   🔑 The intra-articular structures start with the letters of the days of the week

   A. **M**enisci (**Mon**),
   B. **T**endon of popliteus (**Tue**),
   C. **M**enisco femoral ligament (**Wed**),
   D. **T**ransverse ligament (**Thu**),
   E. Haversian pad of **f**at (**Fri**),
   F. **S**ynovial membrane (**Sat**) and
   G. **C**oronary ligament (**Cun**).

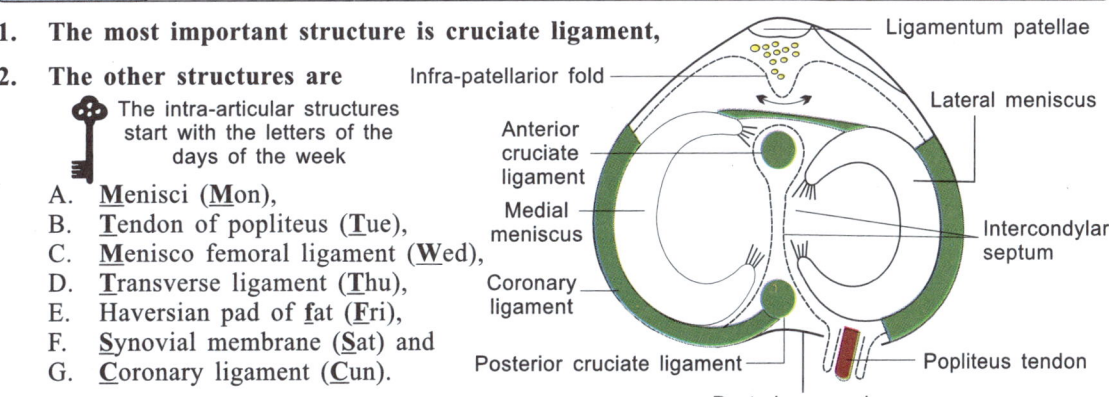

Fig. 1.37 Relations of intra-articular structures of knee joint.

SN-21 Cruciate ligament

1. **Introduction:** It connects the femur & tibia in the form of cross. Hence it is called cruciate ligaments. The nomenclature is based on the attachments to the tibia.

2. **Functions:**
   A. It is key stabilizer of knee joint.
   B. It checks anterior and posterior movements of the femur on tibia.

3. **Attachment:** 🗝 **LAMP**
   A. **A**nterior cruciate ligament extends from anterior part of upper surface of tibia to the **l**ateral condyle of femur.
   B. **P**osterior cruciate ligament extend from posterior part of upper surface of tibia to the **m**edial condyle of femur.

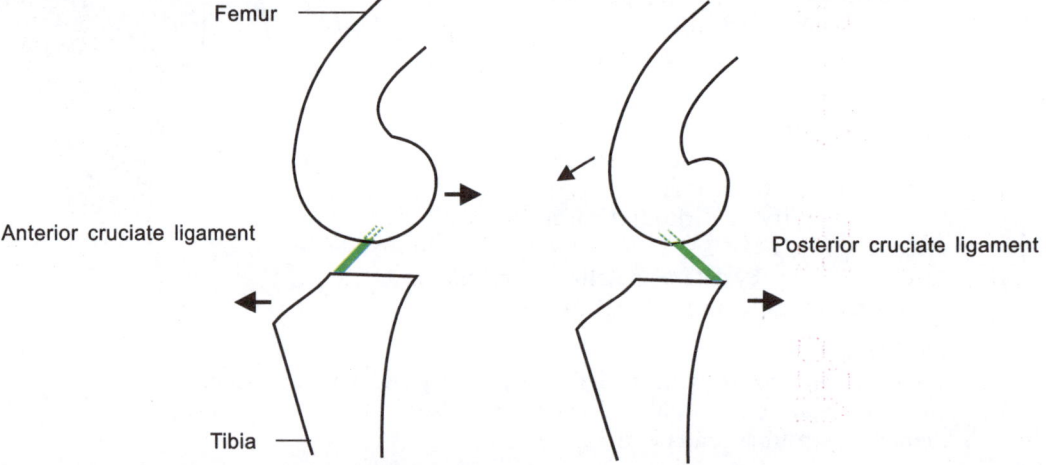

Fig. 1.38 Attachments of cruciate ligament

4. **Morphology:** Anterior and posterior cruciate ligaments can be compared as follows:
   The posterior cruciate ligament is stronger, shorter and less oblique. In weight bearing, flexed knee, posterior cruciate ligament is the only stabilizing factor.

5. **Functions:**
   A. Anterior cruciate ligament prevents the anterior displacement of tibial condyle on femur. It prevents sliding of the femur backwards on tibia.
   B. Posterior cruciate ligament prevents the posterior displacement of tibial condyle on femur. It prevents femur from sliding forward.
   Both cruciate ligaments prevent side to side displacement of tibia and femur.

SN-22 Meniscus

Menisco crescent, half moon

1. **Introduction:** It is a semilunar, fibrocartilagenous ring, triangular in cross section, covers the articular surfaces of the condyles of tibia.

2. **Functions: The chief role of meniscus is to**
   A. Rotate the femur and to
   B. Spread the synovial fluid uniformly.
   Note: They are never subjected to weight bearing.
   The functions of meniscus can be summarized by using "meniscus" word as mnemonics.
   Maintains the bony contact and potential joint space.
   Escorts the articular surfaces.
   Nourishes the articular surface.
   Increases the concavity of tibial condyle for better adaptation with femoral condyle.
   Serves as a cushion and overcomes the thrust.
   Deepens the joint **c**avity.
   Spreads the synovial fluid **u**niformly.
   Saves from the shock during weight transmission and locomotion between two long bones of the body.

3. **Number:** There are two menisci. Medial and lateral.

4. **Attachment:**
   A. Each meniscus has anterior and posterior horns. Both the horn of both the menisci are attached to the anterior and posterior intercondylar area respectively.
   B. The medial margin of the medial meniscus and lateral margin of lateral meniscus is attached to the capsule of the knee joint.
   C. The medial margin of the medial meniscus is also attached to the tibial collateral ligament.
   D. The posterior horn of lateral meniscus provided attachment to
      a. The menisco femoral ligament and
      b. Fibers of the popliteus.

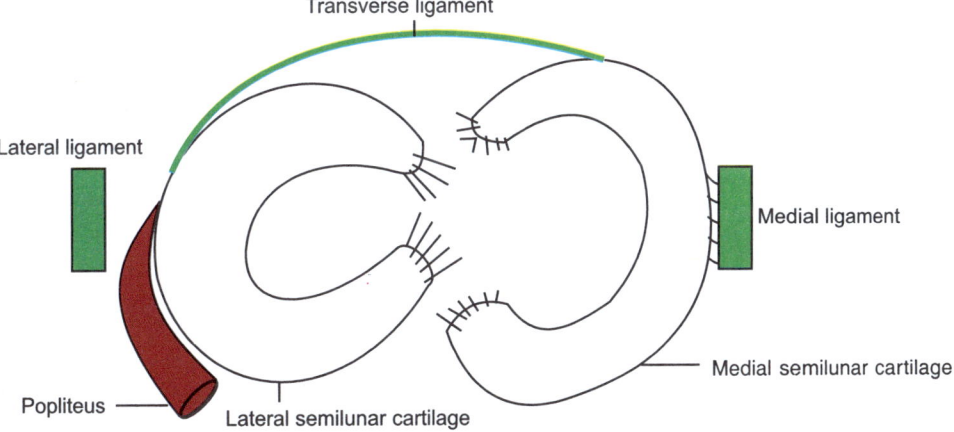

Fig. 1.39 Attachment of the meniscus.

5. **Movements:**
   A. The flexion and extension movements occur in the upper compartment.
   B. The rotation movement occurs in the lower compartment.

6. **Applied anatomy:** *The medial meniscus is more prone for injury as it is more firmly attached to the capsule and tibial collateral ligament.*

SAQ-7   Menisco femoral ligament

1. **Introduction:** They connect the lateral meniscus to medial condyle of femur.

2. **Attachment:**
   A. They arise from posterior horn of lateral meniscus and get attached to medial condyle of the femur.
   B. They are named as anterior and posterior menisco femoral ligament. The anterior menisco femoral ligament passes anterior to the posterior cruciate ligament and posterior menisco femoral ligament passes posterior to the posterior cruciate ligament.

3. **Function:** They regulate the forward movement of the lateral meniscus during extension of the knee.

SAQ-8   Oblique popliteal ligament

The oblique popliteal ligament is an expansion of semimembranosus muscle and extends from posterior surface of medial condyles of tibia to lateral part of intercondylar line of femur. This forms the floor of popliteal fossa. It is pierced by
1. Middle genicular vessels and nerves.

2. Genicular branch of posterior division of obturator nerve.

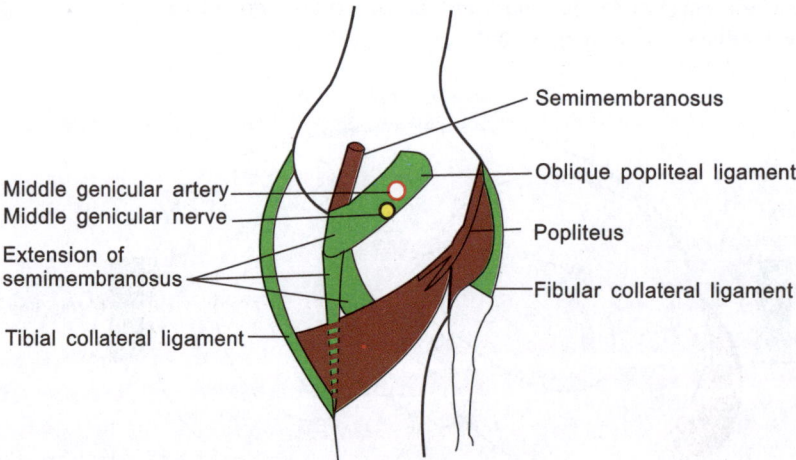

Fig. 1.40 Oblique popliteal ligament

SAQ-9   Transverse ligament

It connects anterior horn of medial meniscus to anterior margin of lateral meniscus. It is present in 40% of individuals.

SAQ-10   Synovial membrane

It lines the inner surface of capsule and extends on patella. It is a mere capillary film. The amount of synovial fluid 0.5 ml.

SAQ-11   Coronary ligament

It is a part of fibrous capsule and provides attachment to peripheral margin of medial and lateral meniscus.

SAQ-12   Arcuate ligament

Introduction: It is Y shaped fibrous band.
1. The stem of the arcuate ligament is fixed to styloid process of fibula.

2. The anterior band is attached to lateral condyle of femur.

3. The posterior band is attached to lateral condyle of tibia.

SAQ-13   Ligamentum patellae

Introduction: Ligamentum patellae derived from tendon of quadriceps femoris and extends from the apex of patella to the tibial tuberosity.

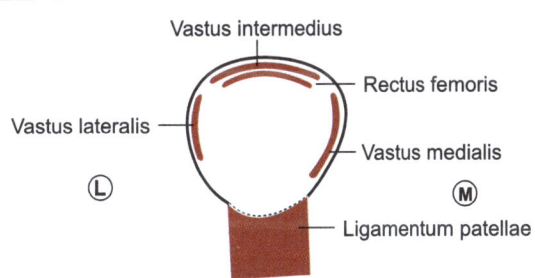

Fig. 1.41 Ligamentum patellae

SN-23   Collateral ligament

The collateral ligaments are present on the medial and lateral side of knee joint. These can be described as follows:

Table 1.10 Showing details of collateral ligament

Particulars	Medial collateral ligament	Lateral collateral ligament
1. Origin	Arises from medial femoral epicondyle	Arises from lateral femoral epicondyle
2. Insertion	Inserted into shaft of tibia	Inserted into styloid process of the head of fibula

	Particulars	Medial collateral ligament	Lateral collateral ligament
3.	Shape	It is broad and fan shaped	It is strong, narrow and cord like
4.	Palpable	It is not palpable	It is palpable
5.	Functions	It prevents excessive abduction	It prevents excessive adduction
6.	Phylogenetically	It represents ischial fibers of adductor magnus	It represents peroneus longus
7.	Attachment to capsule	It is fused to joint capsule	It is relatively free
8.	Attachment to meniscus	It is attached to meniscus	It is not attached to meniscus

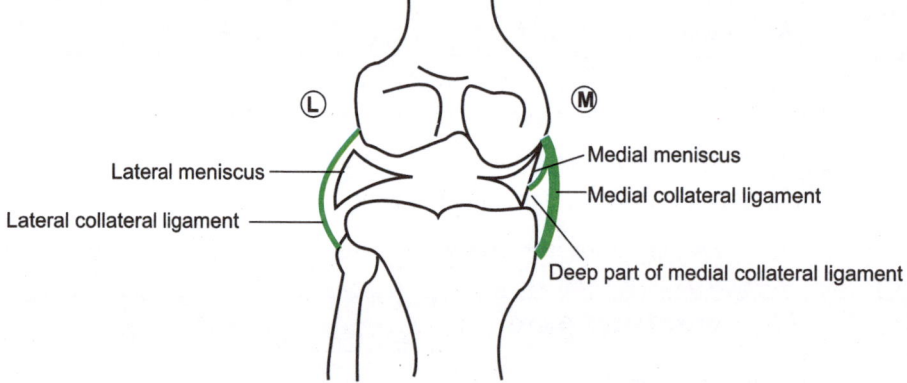

Fig. 1.42 Collateral ligaments and their attachments.

SN-24   Relations of knee joint

1. **Anterior:** Quadriceps femoris

2. **Posterior:**
   A. Popliteal vessels,
   B. Tibial nerve and
   C. Lateral and medial head of gastrocnemius.

3. **Medially:**
   A. Medial patellar retinaculum,
   B. Sartorius, gracilis,
   C. Semimembranosus and
   D. Semitendinosus.

4. **Laterally:**
   A. Common peroneal nerve,
   B. Lateral patellar retinaculum and
   C. Tendon of biceps femoris.

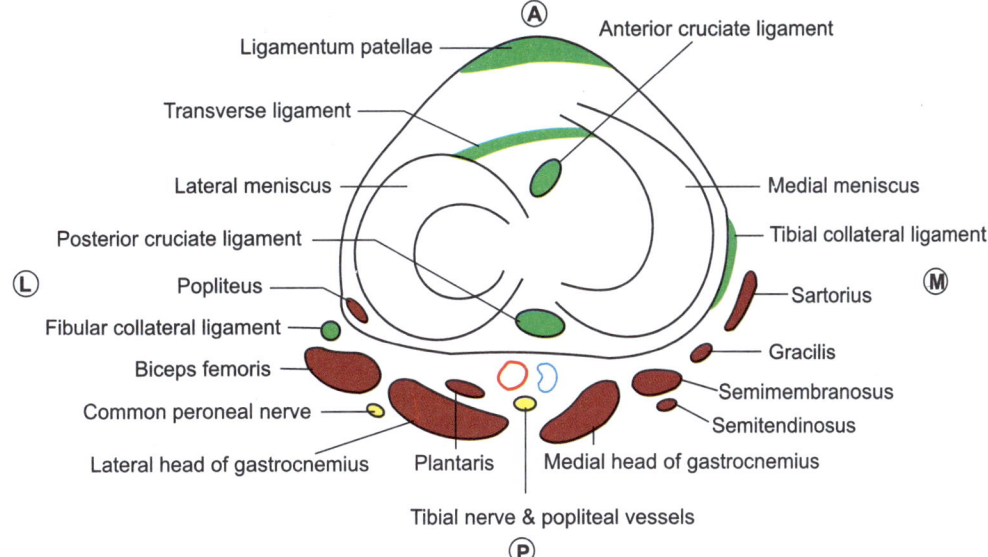

Fig. 1.43 Relations of knee joint.

SAQ-14 **Movements of knee joint and muscles bringing the movement**

Table 1.11 Showing movements of knee joint and muscles bringing movement.

Movements	Muscles	Accessory muscles

1. **Flexion**	A. Hamstring muscles
	   a. Semimembranosus
	   b. Semitendinosus
	   c. Biceps femoris
	B. Sartorius
	C. Gracilis
		Gastrocnemius, plantaris

2. **Extension**	Quadriceps femoris, tensor fascia lata	Articularis genu

3. **Locking**
  A. Medial rotation of the femur on fixed tibia OR
  B. Lateral rotation of tibia on fixed femur.
	Quadriceps femoris,	--------

4. **Unlocking**
  A. Lateral rotation of femur on fixed tibia OR
  B. Medial rotation of tibia on fixed femur.
	Popliteus	--------

The stability of knee joint is maintained by following structure
A.   The crutiate ligaments are indispensable for anteroposterior stability in flexion.
B.   Vastus medialis is indispensable to the stability of patella.
C.   Spines of tibia prevent side way gliding.
D.   Ilio tibial tract, gluteus maximus and tensor fascia lata stabilizes slightly flexed knee joint.
E.   Bones do not play any role.

SN-25 Bursae around knee joint

1.   **Anterior bursae**
    A.   Suprapatellar
    B.   Infrapatellar　🗝 **SICK**
        a.   *Subcutaneous: Clergymans knee*
        b.   *Deep*
    C.   *Prepatellar subcutaneous: Housemaid's knee* 🗝 **PPH**

2.   **Lateral bursae** between
    A.   Lateral condyle of tibia and tendon of popliteus,
    B.   Popliteus and fibular collateral ligament,
    C.   Fibular collateral ligament and biceps femoris and
    D.   Deep to lateral head of gastrocnemius.

3.   **Medial**
    A.   Deep to medial head of gastrocnemius.
    B.   Ansarine bursa: Complicated bursa separates sartorius, semitendinosus, and gracilis from one another and from tibia and tibial collateral ligament.
    C.   Deep to tibial collateral ligament
    D.   Deep to semimembranosus
    E.   Between semimembranosus and semitendinosus.

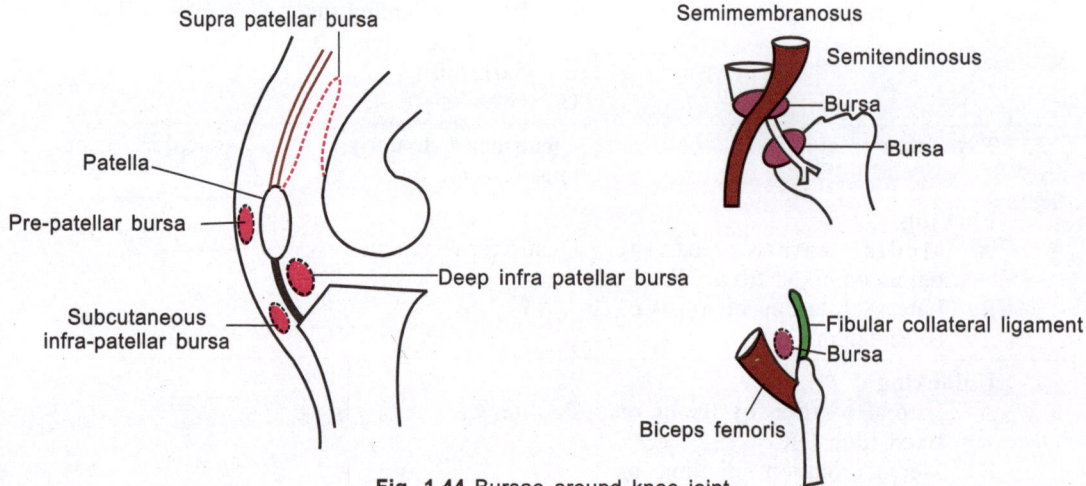

Fig. 1.44 Bursae around knee joint.

SN-26   Locking and unlocking of knee joint

1. **Necessity:** The function of locking and unlocking of knee joint is to keep the knee in full extension without muscular effort. It occurs due to
   A. Medial rotation of femur on fixed tibia during terminal stage of extension.
   B. Lateral rotation of femur on fixed tibia during early stage of flexion

2. **Necessity of the movement of locking and unlocking:**
   A. The surface area of articular surfaces of tibia and femur are not proportionate.
   B. The articular surfaces of tibia and femur are incongruent.
   C. During the terminal part of extension of knee joint, the small articular surface of the tibia is used up by the femur. To accommodate the unused articular surface of femur on tibia, the femur or tibia is required to rotate to have the stable movement.

3. **Difference between locking and unlocking:**
   Table **1.12** Showing difference between locking and unlocking of knee joint.

Particulars		Locking	Unlocking
A.	Position of bone a. When tibia is fixed b. When femur is fixed	**MRF** Medial rotation of femur. Lateral rotation of tibia.	Lateral rotation of femur. Medial rotation of tibia.
B.	Muscles bringing	Quadriceps femoris.	Popliteus.
C.	Ligaments bringing	Oblique popliteal, Medial collateral, Lateral collateral.	
D.	Position of the joint	In terminal part of extension of knee joint.	In Initial flexion from extreme extension of knee joint.

LAQ-12   Describe ankle joint (talo crural) under
1. Bones taking part,   2. Classification,   3. Ligaments,
4. Movements and muscles producing movements,
5. Relations,   6. Arterial supply,
7. Nerve supply &   8. Applied Anatomy.

1. **Bones taking part:**
   A. Lower end of fibula with lateral malleolus.
   B. Medial malleolus of tibia.
   C. Superior surface of talus.

2. **Classification:**
   A. Structural:
      a. Compound (articulating bones are tibia, fibula and talus).
      b. Uniaxial, modified hinge (since the axis of movement is basically transverse with a slight downward inclination on the lateral side) variety of synovial joint.
   B. Functional: Diarthrosis (freely mobile).

3. **Ligaments**
    A. Fibrous capsule covers the joint completely
        a. Attachment
            I. It is attached superiorly to the peripheral margins of the articular surfaces of lower end of tibia and fibula.
            II. It is attached inferiorly to
                i.   The peripheral margin of articular surface of the superior surface of talus.
                ii. The peripheral margin of comma shaped facet present on the medial surface.
                iii. The peripheral margin of the triangular facet present on the lateral surface of talus.
        b. Variations in thickness:
            I. Thin in front, thin behind.
            II. Thick laterally, thick medially.
        c. Fate: It blends with collateral ligament.
    B. Synovial membrane lines the inner surface of the fibrous capsule but stops at the periphery of the articular cartilage. A small synovial recess extends upwards in the inferior tibio fibular joint.
    C. Deltoid ligament: It is a strong triangular ligament present on the medial side of the ankle joint. It is superficial and deep part.
    D. Lateral ligament: It is a ligament present on the lateral side of ankle joint connects talus and calcaneum and fibula.

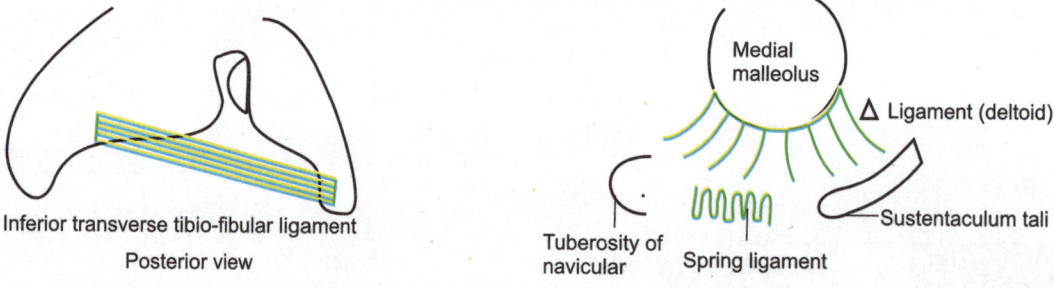

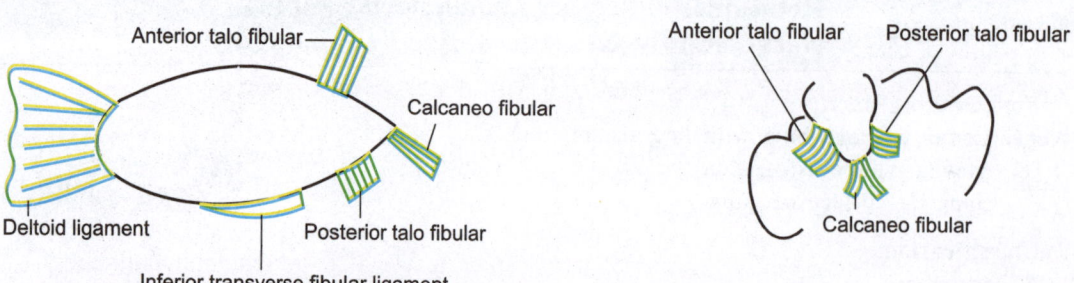

Fig. 1.45 Ligaments of the ankle joint.

4. **Movements and muscles producing movements:**
   A. Dorsi flexion: (The range of movement is 10° and extends upto 20°) All muscles present in the anterior or extensor compartment of the leg bring dorsi flexion of the ankle joint i.e.
      a. Tibialis anterior,
      b. Extensor hallucis longus and
      c. Extensor digitorum longus.
   B. Plantar flexion: (The range of movement is 20° and increased upto 40°) All the muscles of flexor compartment of the leg are plantar flexors of ankle joint.
      The gastrocnemius with soleus act as prime mover. *The peroneus longus and brevis come into play in extreme plantar flexion.* The muscles bringing plantar flexion are
      a. Peroneus tertius,
      b. Tibialis posterior,
      c. Flexor digitorum longus,
      d. Flexor hallucis longus,
      e. Tendocalcaneus.
   C. In symmetrical standing the line of gravity passes slightly in front of the ankle joint therefore there is a natural tendency for forward dislocation which is prevented by:
      a. Broader anterior part of trochlear surface of talus and
      b. Tonic contraction of triceps surae.

5. **Relations:**
   A. Anterior: (From medial to lateral)   Tall Himalayas are never dry places
      a. Tendon of tibialis anterior,
      b. Extensor hallucis longus,
      c. Anterior tibial vessels,
      d. Deep peroneal nerve,
      e. Extensor digitorum longus &
      f. Peroneus tertius.
   B. Posterior: Behind tibial malleolus   Talented Doctors are never hungry
      (From anterior to posterior)
      a. Tendon of tibialis posterior,
      b. Flexor digitorum longus,
      c. Posterior tibial artery,
      d. Tibial nerve &
      e. Tendon of flexor hallucis longus.
   C. Behind the fibular malleolus: Tendon of peroneus brevis and peroneus longus. The peroneus brevis is situated deep and peroneus longus is situated superficially.

6. **Arterial supply:** Malleolar branches of anterior tibial and peroneal arteries.

7. **Nerve supply:** Branches from deep peroneal and tibial nerves.

8. **Applied anatomy:**
   A. Ankle sprain: It is due to over inversion of foot, which is one of the common manifestation. The anterior talo fibular and calcaneo fibular ligaments are some time torn and in severe cases the anterior part of the capsule of the ankle joint is ruptured.
   B. Pott's fracture: The forceful eversion of the foot causes avulsion of the deltoid ligament, fracture of the tibia and fibula. This is described in three degrees
      a. In first degree there is a avulsion (tearing) of deltoid ligament.
      b. In second degree there is a avulsion (tearing) of deltoid ligament and fracture of medial malleolus of tibia.

c. In third degree there is a avulsion fracture of the deltoid ligament, fracture of medial malleolus of tibia and oblique fracture of the lower part of the fibula.

C. The ankle sprains usually occur when the foot is plantar flexed.

D. *The sprains of the ankle joint are almost always abduction sprains of the subtalar joints.*

SN-27   Deltoid ligament

Introduction: It is a strong triangular ligament present on the medial side of the ankle joint. It is superficial and deep part.

1. **Superficial part:** It is triangular. The base of the triangle is attached to tarsal bones i.e. Navicular, calcaneum and talus. The apex is attached to the tip of medial malleolus. It extends from tip of medial malleolus to

   A. Tuberosity of navicular bone and to the medial margin of spring ligament. These fibers are present anteriorly, hence they are called anterior fibers of deltoid ligament or tibio navicular ligament.

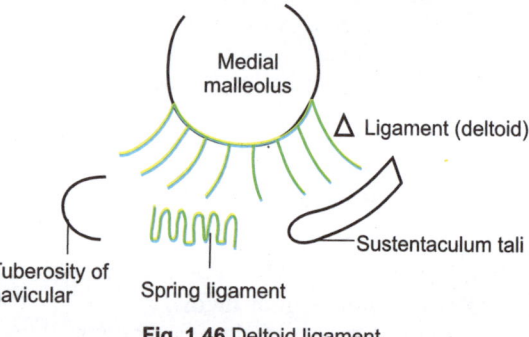

Fig. 1.46 Deltoid ligament

   B. Sustantaculum tali are middle fibers. They are called tibiocalcanean ligament.

   C. The medial tubercle of talus. These are the posterior fibers and are also called superficial tibiotalar ligament.

2. **Deep part** blends with fibrous capsule. It is connects tibial malleolus to anterior part of medial surface of talus below comma shaped facet. This is also called deep tibiotalar ligament.

SAQ-15   Lateral ligament of ankle joint

Table 1.13 Showing details of lateral ligaments of knee joint

	Particulars	Direction	Attachment
A.	Anterior talofibular ligament (Weak)	Forward and medially	It extends from the anterior margin of the tibial malleolus to the lateral surface of neck of talus.
B.	Posterior talofibular ligament	Backward and medially	It extends from the posterior margin of fibular malleolus to the posterior tubercle of talus.
C.	Calcaneofibular	Downwards and backwards	It extends from notch on the lower border of the lateral malleolus to the tubercle on the lateral surface of calcaneum.

LAQ-13   **Describe inversion under**
1. Introduction,   2. Bones taking part,
3. Joints and classification of joints,
4. Axis,   5. Combination of action,
6. Range of movement, 7. Muscles bringing movement,
8. Functions &   9. Applied anatomy.

1. **Introduction:** It is a movement in which the medial border of foot is elevated so that the sole or plantar surface of the foot faces medially. Inversion and eversion are best demonstrated when the foot is off the   ground. When the foot is on the ground typical inversion and eversion are not observed. The malleoli lock the talus and suspended foot inverts and everts around it.

2. **Bones taking part:** Talus, calcaneus and navicular.

3. **Joints and classification of joints:**
   A.   Talocalcaneonavicular: Ball and socket variety of synovial joint.
   B.   Subtalar: Plane synovial joint.

4. **Axis:** An oblique axis which runs forwards, upwards and medially passes from the back of lateral tubercle of calcaneus, through sinus tarsi to emerge at the supero-medial aspect of neck of talus.
   This axis corresponds to abduction, adduction, plantar flexion and dorsi flexion and medial and lateral rotation of calcaneus occurs on the axis.

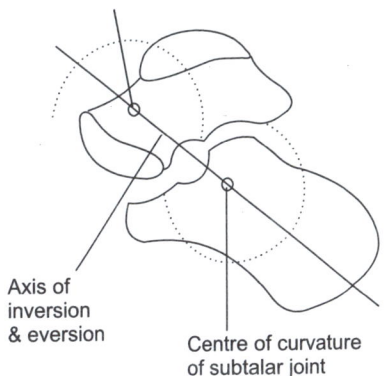

5. **Combination of movements:** Adduction, plantar flexion, rotation and gliding movements.

6. **Range of movements:** It is more free as compared to the eversion.

7. **Muscles bringing movements:**
   A.   Tibialis anterior,
   B.   Tibialis posterior and
   C.   Flexor hallucis longus.
   Tibialis anterior dorsiflexes and tibialis posterior plantar flexes the foot at the ankle joint and these opposite effects cancel each other when the two muscles combine to produce an uncomplicated inversion of foot. Inversion is the movement of supination and is accompanied by adduction of fore part of foot. The movement begins at midtarsal joint and completes at subtalar joint.

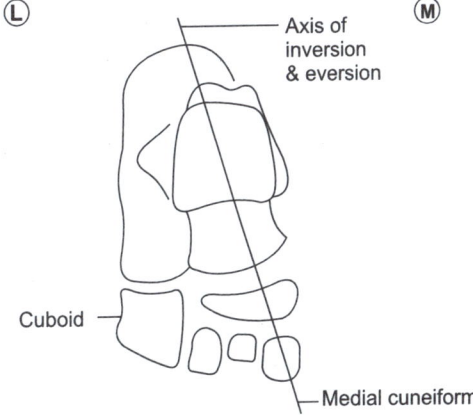

Fig. 1.47 Axis of inversion & eversion.

8. **Functions:**
    A. To walk on slippery & uneven surfaces.
    B. To maintain an efficient shift of weight distribution among the head of metatarsal bones during locomotion.

9. **Applied anatomy:**
    A. Talipes calcaneovarus (*talipes* club foot, *varus* bent inward): *A deformity of the foot in which the heel is turned toward the midline of the body and the anterior part is elevated.*
    B. Talipes calcaneovalgus (*valgus* bent outward): *A deformity of the foot in which the heel is turned outward from the midline of the body and the anterior part of the foot is elevated.*
    C. Talipes equinovalgus: A deformity of the foot in which the heel is elevated and turned outward from the midline of the body.
    D. Talipes equinovarus: A deformity of the foot in which the heel is turned inward from the midline of the leg and the foot is plantar flexed. This is typical club foot.
    E. Inversion sprain is the most common ankle injury, it involves the tearing of lateral collateral ligaments. Usually the anterior talofibular ligament is torn first, then the calcaneofibular ligament and in severe cases, the posterior talofibular ligament.

LAQ-14 **Describe eversion under**
1. **Introduction,** 2. **Bones taking part,**
3. **Axis,** 4. **Combination of action,**
5. **Range of movement,** 6. **Muscles bringing movement,**
7. **Functions &** 8. **Applied anatomy.**

1. **Introduction:** It is a movement in which the lateral border of foot is elevated so that sole or plantar surface of the foot faces laterally when the foot is off the ground. Eversion is a combination of pronation & abduction.

2. **Bones taking part:** Calcaneum, talus and cuboid.

3. **Axis:** An oblique axis which runs forwards, upwards & medially passes from the back of lateral tubercle of calcaneus, through sinus tarsi to emerge at the supero-medial aspect of neck of talus. This axis corresponds to abduction, adduction, plantar flexion and dorsi flexion and medial and lateral rotation of calcaneus occurs on the axis.
    Refer the Fig. 1.47 of inversion.

4. **Combination of movements:** Abduction, dorsi flexion, rotation and gliding.

5. **Range of movements:** It is less free as compared to inversion.

6. **Muscles bringing movements:**
    A. Peroneus longus,
    B. Peroneus brevis and
    C. Peroneus tertius.
    Peroneus longus and brevis whose tendon pass behind lateral malleolus, are plantar flexors and peroneus tertius is dorsiflexor of ankle joint. These opposite effects cancel each other and produce simple eversion movement. Eversion is a movement of pronation and is accompanied by abduction of the fore part of the foot.

7. **Functions:**
   A. To walk on slippery & uneven surfaces.
   B. To maintain an efficient shift of weight distribution among the head of metatarsal bones during locomotion.

8. **Applied anatomy:**
   A. Talipes calcaneovarus: A deformity of the foot in which the heel is turned toward the midline of the body and the anterior part is elevated.
   B. Talipes calcaneovalgus: A deformity of the foot in which the heel is turned outward from the midline of the body and the anterior part of the foot is elevated.
   C. Talipes equinovalgus: A deformity of the foot in which the heel is elevated and turned outward from the midline of the body.
   D. Talipes equinovarus: A deformity of the foot in which the heel is turned inward from the midline of the leg and the foot is plantar flexed. This is typical club foot.
   E. Eversion sprains, which are less common, usually involve tearing of the deltoid ligament.

SN-28   **Compare pronation, supination with inversion and eversion**

Table 1.14 Showing comparison of pronation, supination with inversion and eversion.

Character	Pronation / Supination	Inversion / Eversion
1. Joints	Superior and inferior radioulnar joints.	Subtalar, Talocalcaneonavicular and Transverse tarsal.
2. Axis of movement	A. Vertical axis passes downward and medially. B. It passes through the center of head of the radius & the ulnar attachment of the articular disc.	A. An oblique axis which runs forward & medially. B. It passes from the back of the calcaneum, through the sinus tarsi to emerge at the superomedial aspect of the neck of the talus.
3. Distance between joints	The joints are placed far apart.	The joints are close together.

LAQ-15   **Describe medial longitudinal arch under**
1. Functions,   **2. Formations of the arch,**
3. Factors maintaining arch &   **4. Applied anatomy.**

1. **Functions:** The main functions of the arch are,
   A. It helps to absorb shock, to increase pliability and to bring resilience.
   B. It helps in propulsion of body in walking, running and jumping.

2. **Formation of the arch:**
   A. Ends:
      a.   Anterior end is formed by heads of first, second and third metatarsals.
      b.   Posterior end is formed by medial tubercle of calcaneum (it is short and strong).
   B. Summit is formed by superior articular facet of body of talus.
   C. Pillar:
      a.   Anterior pillar is formed by 3 cuneiform bones, navicular and talus.
      b.   Posterior pillar is formed by medial half of the calcaneum.
   D. Joint: talocalcaneo navicular.
   E. Classification of joints: Ball and socket type of synovial joint.

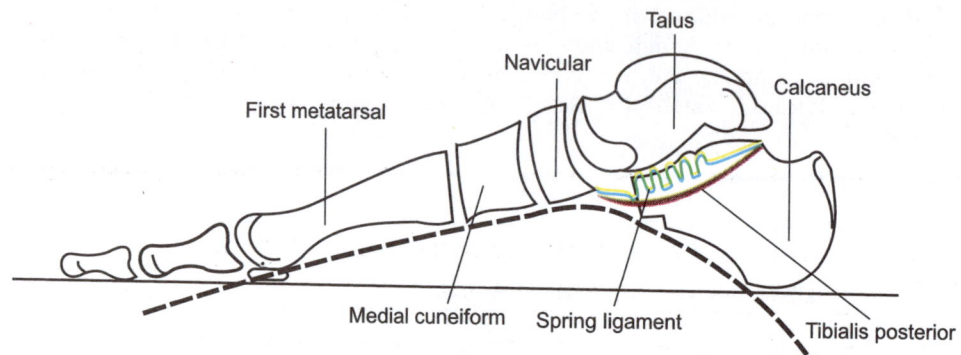

Fig. 1.48 Medial longitudinal arch.

3. **Factors maintaining arch:**
   A. Bones: They are not responsible for maintaining the stability of the arch. The bones are mostly wedge shaped with narrower edge facing plantar surface. The head of talus acts as key stone.
   B. Tie beam (Bow string)
      a.   Plantar aponeurosis: It is a most important ligament stretching like a tie beam. By the contraction it increases the height of the arch.
      b.   Flexor hallucis longus: It also acts as tie beam. It extends from sustantaculum tali to great toe. It gives slip to its weakest sister flexor digitorum longus, which acts on the medial three digits. It is most efficient means of maintaining an arch as it ties the two pillars. This is the bulkiest of the calf muscles, which is multipennate.
      NOTE: For short standing, ligaments support the arch. For prolonged standing, ligaments 'tire', relief is obtained by pressing the pads of the toes to the grounds. During the movements of propulsion and during landing on the feet, the strain is taken by the tendon of flexor hallucis longus.
   C. Inter segmental ties (staples):
      a.   Spring ligament: It extends from sustantaculum. tali of calcaneus to tuberosity of navicular bone. It is next important ligament for maintenance of medial longitudinal arch.
      b.   Flexor hallucis brevis also act as staples.
   D. Slings: They are
      a.   Tendon of tibialis anterior and
      b.   Tendon of peroneus longus.
      They are inserted into the same two bones (medial cuneiform and first metatarsal bone). Tibialis anterior increases and peroneus longus decreases the medial longitudinal arch.

E. Tibialis anterior and posterior have a significant influence on the medial longitudinal arch as they bring out inversion.

4. **Applied anatomy:**
   A. Absence of arches is called as flat foot. It is also called pes planus.
   B. The exaggeration of longitudinal arch of the foot is known as pes cavus.
   C. The deformities of foot:
   - a. Clubfoot (a congenital deformity of the foot, which is twisted out of shapes or position).
   - b. Talipes calcaneus: Person walks on heel (*talipes* club foot).
   - b. Talipes equinus: Person walks on toes.
   - c. Talipes varus: The foot is bent inwards, persons walks on the outer border, the foot is inverted and adducted.
   - d. Talipes valgus: Bent outwards person walks on inner border of foot i.e. Foot everted and abducted.
   - e. Talipes equinovarus: Club foot, inverted, adducted and plantar flexed. It is associated with spina bifida.

SAQ-16   Spring ligament (Plantar calcaneo navicular ligament)

1. **Introduction:** It is a inter segmental tie (staples) and is one of the important ligament in the formation of medial longitudinal arch.

2. **Extent:** It extends from sustantaculum tali of calcaneus to tuberosity of navicular bone.

3. **Function:**
   A. It supports the head of talus.
   B. It provides attachment to deltoid ligament.

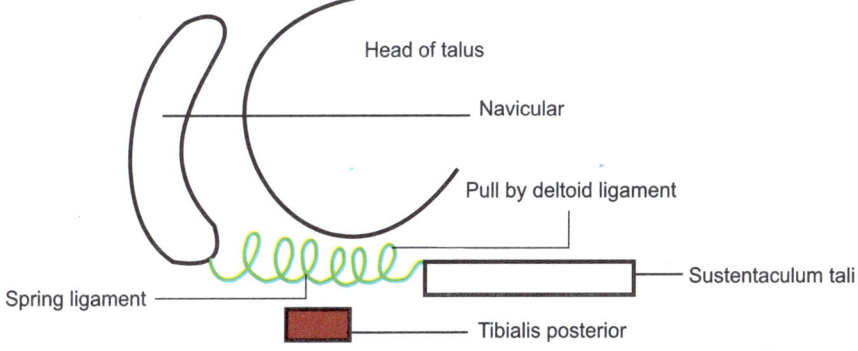

Fig. 1.49 Spring ligament.

4. **Applied anatomy:** If this ligament is stretched, the navicular and calcaneum move away from each other and the head of the talus sinks and arch is flattened. It is supported by tibialis posterior and by the tendons of flexor digitorum brevis, abductor hallucis.

LAQ-16   Describe lateral longitudinal arch under
1. Functions,   2. Formations of the arch,
3. Factors maintaining arch &   4. Applied anatomy.

1. **Functions:** The lateral longitudinal arch is formed by few bones and joints therefore rigidity is more and helps in transmission weight and thrust.

2. **Formations of arch:**
   A. Ends:
      a. Anterior end is formed by cuboid and by the heads of fourth and fifth metatarsal bones.
      b. Posterior end is formed by lateral part of calcaneum, which is short and strong
   B. Summit is formed by articular facet of superior surface of calcaneum.
   C. Pillar
      a. Anterior pillar is formed by fourth, fifth metatarsal and cuboid.
      b. Posterior pillar is formed by lateral half of the calcaneum.
   D. Joint involved is calcaneocuboid.
   E. Classification of joint: saddle type of synovial joint.

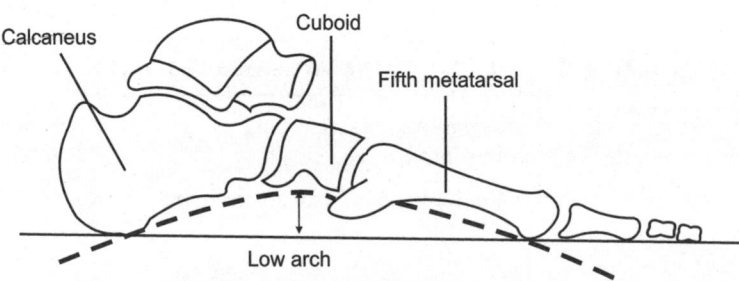

Fig. 1.50 Lateral longitudinal arch.

3. **Factors maintaining arch:**
   A. Bone: Bones do not play any important role in maintenance of the arch. A triangular projection of cuboid called as calcanean angle, occupies the lower part of anterior surface of calcaneum. This bony projection maintains the upward tilt of the long axis of calcaneus.
   B. Tie beam or bow string:
      a. Lateral part of plantar aponeurosis is a main structure acting as tie beam,
      b. The other structures forming the tie beam are
         I. Tendons of flexor digitorum longus of the fourth and fifth toes,
         II. The lateral half of flexor digitorum brevis and
         III. Abductor digiti minimi.
   C. Intersegmental tie or staples:
      a. Short plantar ligament is very thick. It fills the concavities of calcaneus & cuboid.
      b. Long plantar ligament is thin and extends from the heel to both ridges of cuboid. It helps to maintain the concavity of the arch.
   D. Sling: Peroneus longus by contraction increases the height of lateral longitudinal arch. It is the most important single factor in maintaining its integrity.

4. **Applied anatomy:**
   A. Absence of arches is called as flat foot. It is also called pes planus.
   B. The exaggeration of longitudinal arch of the foot is known as pes cavus.

C. The deformities of foot:
   a. Clubfoot: A congenital deformity of the foot, which is twisted out of shapes or position.
   b. Talipes calcaneus: Person walks on heel (talipes club foot).
   c. Talipes equinus: Person walks on toes.
   d. Talipes varus: The foot is bent inwards, persons walks on the outer border, the foot is inverted and adducted.
   e. Talipes valgus: Bent outwards person walks on inner border of foot i.e. foot everted and abducted.
   f. Talipes equinovarus: Club foot, inverted, adducted and plantar flexed. It is associated with spina bifida.

SN-29   Lateral plantar nerve

1. **Introduction:** It is a small terminal branch of tibial nerve which passes between the first and second layer of the sole. It resembles the ulnar nerve in the hand.

2. **Branches:**
   A. From main trunk
      a. Muscular branches to
         I.   Flexor digitorum accessories and
         II. Abductor digiti minimi.
      b. Cutaneous branches to the skin of sole.
          The main trunk divide into superficial and deep branches.
   B. Superficial branche divides into two branches
      a. Lateral branch to
         I.   Flexor digiti minimi brevis,
         II. Third plantar and
         III. Fourth dorsal interossei.
      b. Medial branch: Supplies the skin lining the fourth interdigital cleft.
   C. Deep branches supply nine muscles. This includes
      a. The second, third and fourth lumbricals,
      b. The adductor hallucis and
      c. Five interossei of the first three intermetatarsal spaces.

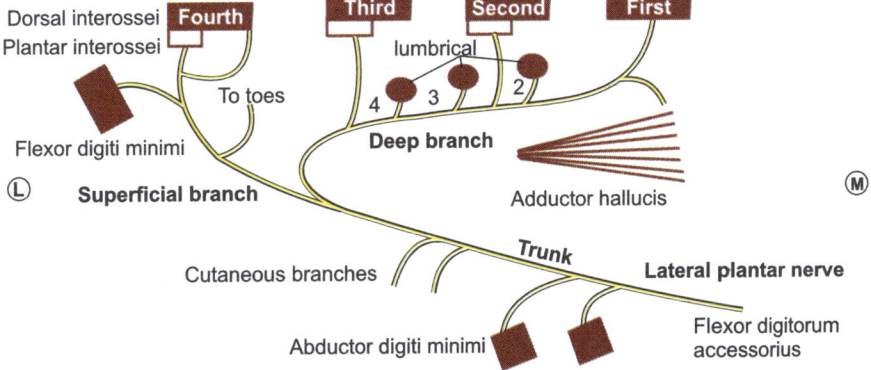

Fig. 1.51 Lateral plantar nerve with its branches.

ABDOMEN

SECTION TWO

SN-1	Spina bifida	63
SAQ-1	Sacral hiatus	63
SAQ-2	Transpyloric plane	63
SAQ-3	Caput medusae	64
SN-2	Inguinal ligament	64
SN-3	Rectus abdominis	65
LAQ-1	Rectus sheath	66
LAQ-2	Inguinal canal	68
SAQ-4	Superficial inguinal ring	71
SAQ-5	Deep inguinal ring	72
SAQ-6	Covering of spermatic cord	72
SN-4	Spermatic cord	72
SN-5	Hesselbach's triangle	73
SN-6	Inguinal hernia	74
LAQ-3	Testis	75
SN-7	Blood supply of testis	76
SN-8	Histology of testis	77
SAQ-7	Development of testis	78
LAQ-4	Testis	80
SAQ-8	Epididymis	81
SN-9	Foramen of Winslow	81
SN-10	Lesser sac	83
LAQ-5	Stomach	84
SN-11	Stomach bed	90
LAQ-6	Second part of duodenum	91
SN-12	Duodenal cap	95
SN-13	Ligaments of Treitz	95
SN-14	Meckel's diverticulum	96
LAQ-7	Caecum	96
LAQ-8	Appendix	99
LAQ-9	Coeliac trunk	103
LAQ-10	Portal vein	105
LAQ-11	Extra hepatic biliary apparatus	109
LAQ-12	Spleen	113
LAQ-13	Liver	116
SAQ-9	The bare are	120
LAQ-14	Head of pancreas	121
LAQ-15	Kidney	124
LAQ-16	Ureter	130
LAQ-17	Suprarenal gland	137
LAQ-18	Diaphragm	140
LAQ-19	Abdominal aorta	143
LAQ-20	Inferior vena cava	145
SN-15	Cisterna chyli	148
SN-16	Perineal body	148
SN-17	External anal sphincter	149
LAQ-21	Ischiorectal fossa	150
SN-18	Pudendal canal	152
SN-19	Perineal membrane	153
SN-20	Urogenital diaphragm	155
LAQ-22	Superficial perineal pouch	156
LAQ-23	Deep perineal pouch	158
LAQ-24	Urinary bladder	159
LAQ-25	Male urethra	164
LAQ-26	Ovary	168
SAQ-10	Ovarian fossa	171
LAQ-27	Uterine tube	172
LAQ-28	Uterus	174
LAQ-29	Prostate	178
LAQ-30	Rectum	182
LAQ-31	Anal canal	186
SN-21	Internal iliac artery	189

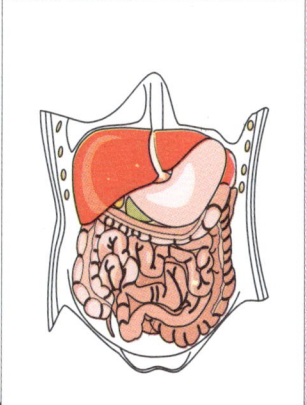

SN-1   Spina bifida

It is a failure of fusion of two neural arches and causes a gap in the midline posteriorly. Meninges and spinal cord may herniate out through the gap. There are different terms used to describe the contents. These are

1. **Meningocoele:** It is a protrusion of only meninges in the form of a cystic swelling. It is filled by cerebrospinal fluid.

2. **Meningomyelocoele:** It is a protrusion of meninges and spinal cord.

3. **Syringomyelocoele:** It is a protrusion of meninges and spinal cord with dilated central canal.

4. **Myelocoele:** It is a protrusion of the substance of the spinal cord through a defect in the vertebral canal.

5. **Spina bifida occulta:** There is a failure of fusion of two neural arches, but there is no protrusion through it so that there is no swelling on the surface. This usually associated with talipes equino varus (or club foot). In this condition the foot is inverted, adducted and plantar flexed.

SAQ-1   Sacral hiatus

It is the opening present at the inferior end of sacral canal formed by failure of laminae of the fifth sacral vertebra. The structures passing through are

1. <u>C</u>occygeal nerves.

2. <u>S</u>acral nerves.

3. <u>F</u>ilum terminale.

SAQ-2   Transpyloric plane

Trans across, *pyloric* pyloric end of the stomach.

1. **Introduction:** It is an horizontal plane passing through the pyloric end of the stomach. It lies midway between suprasternal notch and upper end of pubic symphysis. It roughly corresponds with midpoint between xiphisternal joint and the umbilicus.

2. **Situation:**
   A. Anteriorly at tips of 9th costal cartilages.
   B. Posteriorly lower border of L_1 vertebra.

3. **Structures at the transpyloric plane are**
   A. Pyloric end of the stomach.
   B. Fundus of the gall bladder.
   C. Hila of both kidneys.
   D. Origin of superior mesenteric artery.
   E. Lower end of spinal cord.
   F. Lateral aortic group of lymph node.

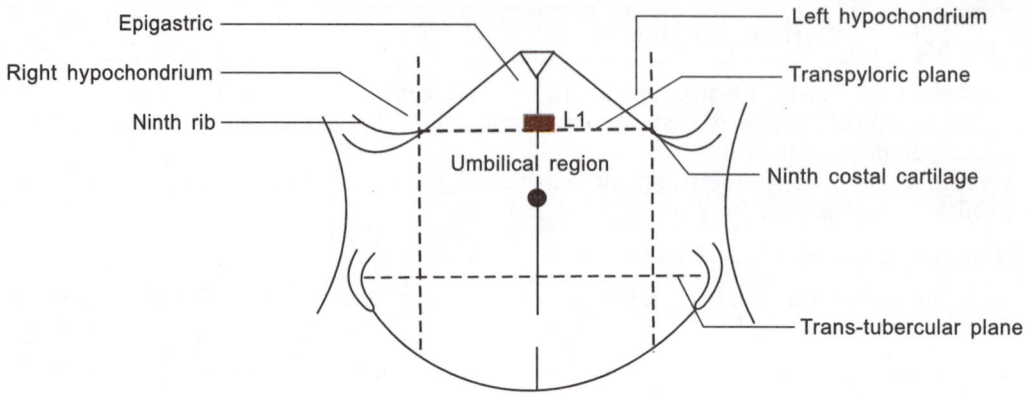

Fig. 2.1 Transpyloric plane

SAQ-3 | Caput medusae

Caput head, *Medusa* Greek myth, female with snaky hair.

The umbilicus is one of the important sites of portocaval anastomosis. The anastomosis takes place between paraumbilical veins in the falciform ligament (tributaries of portal vein) and subcutaneous veins in the anterior abdominal wall (tributaries of epigastric veins which are tributaries of inferior vena cava).

In case of portal hypertension the blood from portal tributaries is directed into the caval tributaries causing their dilatation and tortuosity. This condition is referred to as 'caput medusae' because of its resemblance to the serpents on the head of Medusa, a mythical lady in Greek mythology.

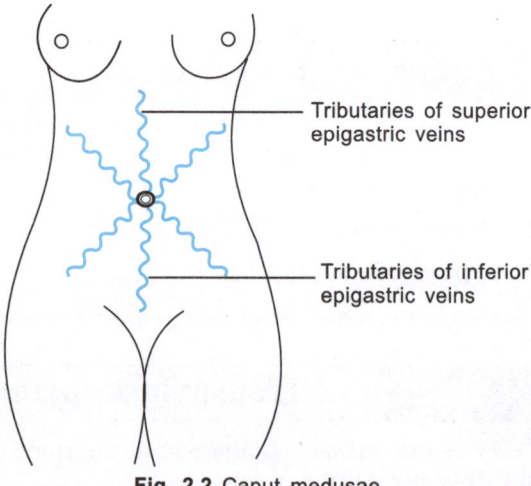

Fig. 2.2 Caput medusae

SN-2 | Inguinal ligament

1. **Synonymous:** Inguinal arch, arcus inguinalis, ligament of Poupart.

2. **Introduction:** It is a thickening of lower border of external oblique aponeurosis. It separates abdomen from thigh.

3. **Extent:** It extends from anterior superior iliac spine to pubic tubercle.

4. **Attachments:**
   A. Upper surface: Gives attachment to
      a. Internal oblique in lateral two third.

b.   Transversus abdominis in lateral one third.
B.   Lower surface: Gives attachment to facia lata.

5.   **Relations:** Medial half of upper groove forms floor of inguinal canal and lodges spermatic cord.

6.   **Extension:**

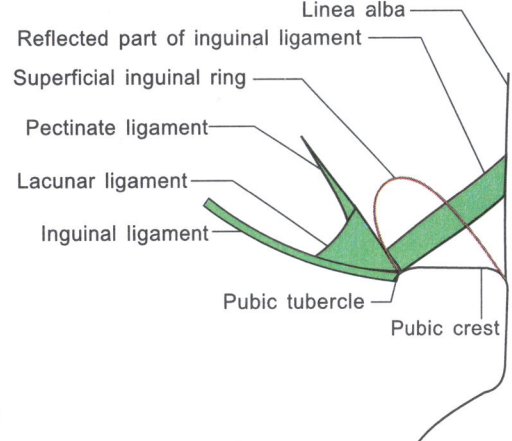

A.   Pectineal part of the inguinal ligament is called lacunar ligament. It is triangular in shape.
   a.   Anteriorly: It is attached to the medial end of the inguinal ligament.
B.   Posteriorly: It is attached to the pecten pubis. It is horizontal in position and supports the spermatic cord.
   c.   Apex is attached to the pubic tubercle.
B.   Pectineal ligament (ligament of Cooper): It is an extension of the inguinal ligament extending from posterior part of base of lacunar ligament. It is attached to the pecten pubis.

Fig. 2.3 Inguinal ligaments and its extensions

C.   The reflected part of inguinal ligament extends from inguinal ligament to linea alba.

| SN-3 | **Rectus abdominis** |

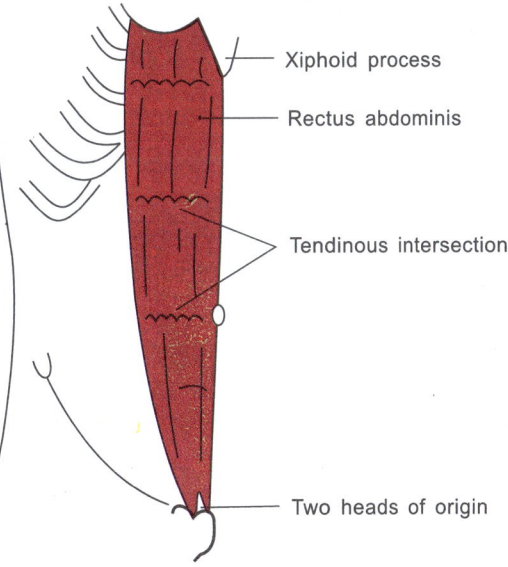

1.   **Origin** : It arises by two tendinous heads as follows:
   A.   Lateral head from the lateral part of the pubic crest.
   B.   Medial head from the anterior pubic ligament.
   C.   The direction of the fibres is vertically and upwards.

2.   **Insertion** : It is inserted along a horizontal line extending from the xiphoid process to the seventh, sixth and fifth costal cartilages.

3.   **Nerve supply** : Intercostal nerves (Lower six or seven thoracic nerves).

4.   **Action** : Flexion of the trunk (lumbar spine).

Fig. 2.4 Rectus abdominis muscle

LAQ-1   Describe rectus sheath under
    1.   Introduction,   2.   Formation,
    3.   Content and   4.   Applied anatomy.

1. **Introduction:** It is an aponeurotic sheath enclosing rectus abdominis muscle and pyramidalis muscle.

2. **Formation:**
   - A. Number: It is one on each side.
   - B. Features:

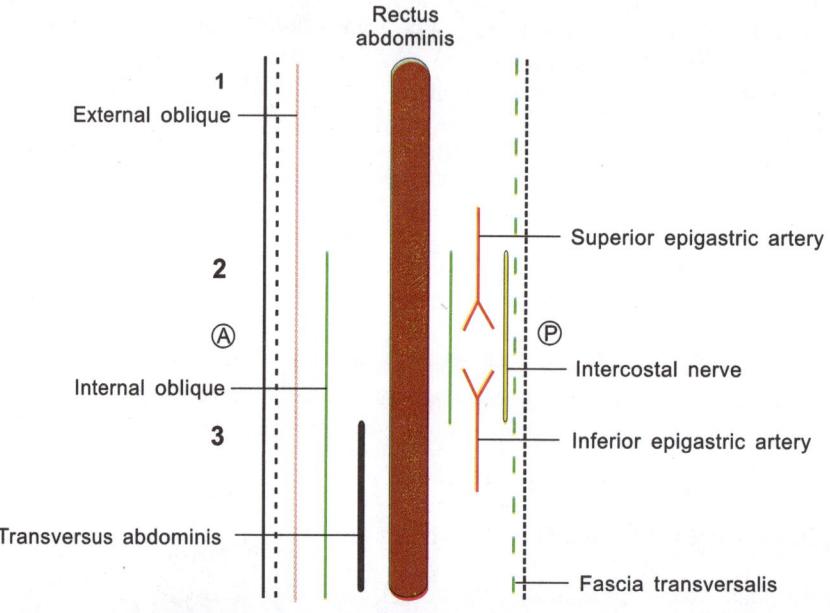

Fig. 2.5 Schemetic diagram through sagittal section of rectus sheath

Table 2.1 Showing formation of rectus sheath.

Particulars	Anterior wall	Posterior wall
a. Wall	Is complete	Is deficient a. Above costal margin b. Below arcuate line
b. Composition	Variable	Uniform
c. Extent	From the costal cartilage to the pubic symphysis	From the lower margins of the ribs to the horizontal line passing through the anterior superior iliac spine (arcuate line).
d. Muscles forming I. Above the costal margin.	Aponeurosis of external oblique	No structures

Particulars	Anterior wall	Posterior wall
II. Below the costal margin to the anterior superior iliac spine.	i. Aponeurosis of external oblique. ii. Anterior lamina of internal oblique.	i. Posterior lamina of internal oblique. ii. Aponeurosis of transversus abdominis.
III. Below the level of anterior superior iliac spine (arcuate line).	i. External oblique ii. Internal oblique & iii. Transversus abdominis.	Fascia transversalis

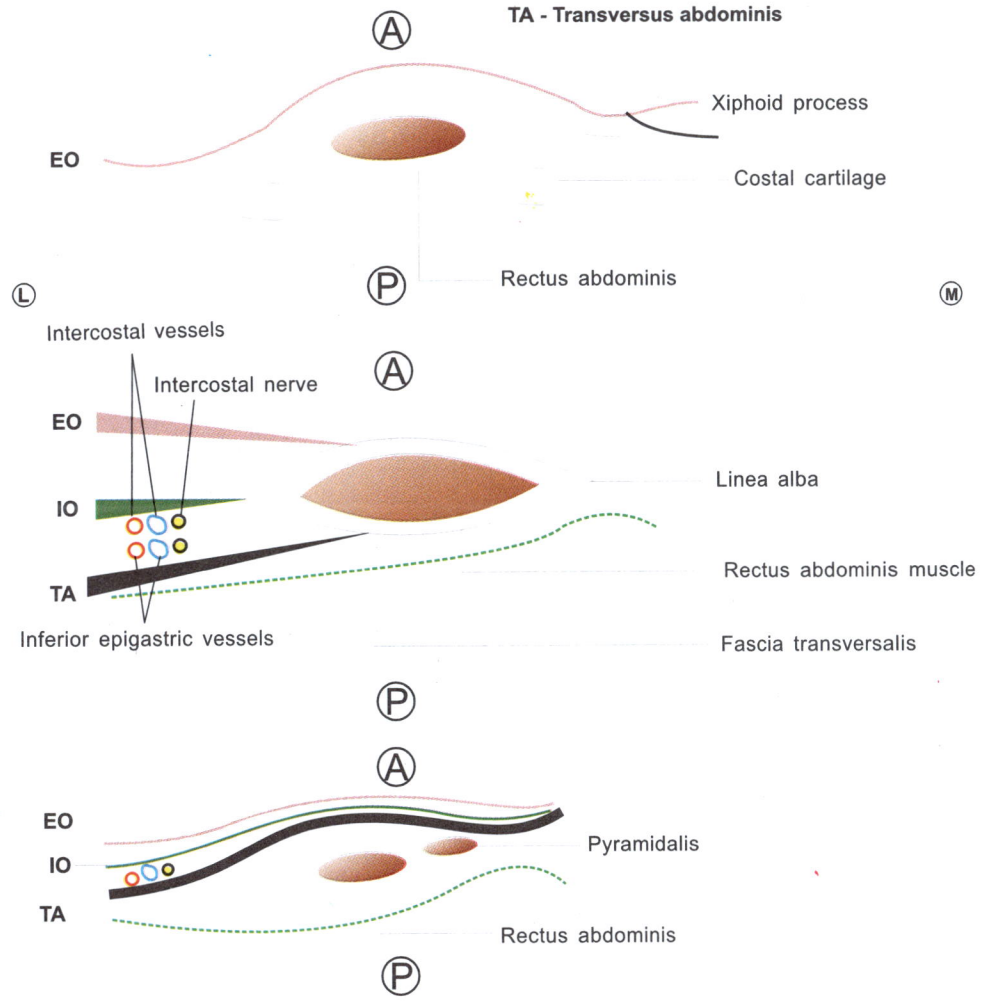

Fig. 2.6 Transverse sections through the rectus sheath at different level
(1) Above the costal margin.
(2) Between costal margin and anterior superior iliac spine.
(3) Below anterior superior iliac spine.

3. **Contents:**
   A. Muscles:
      a. Rectus abdominis.
      b. Pyramidalis.
   B. Arteries:
      a. Superior epigastric artery, branch of internal thoracic artery.
      b. Inferior epigastric artery, branch of external iliac artery.
   C. Veins:
      a. Superior epigastric vein drains into internal thoracic vein-subclavian vein-superior vena cava.
      b. Inferior epigastric vein drains into external iliac vein-common iliac vein-inferior vena cava.
   D. Nerves: Lower five inter costal nerves and sub costal nerve.

4. **Applied anatomy:**
   A. Divarication of recti: In multiparous women and chronic weak children the upper part of linea alba becomes stretched and gap is produced between 2 recti.
   B. Supraumbilical median incisions:
      a. Advantages: It is bloodless area hence there is less bleeding during operation.
      b. Disadvantages:
         I. It leaves a post operative big scar.
         II. There is a delay in healing of the wound.
   C. Infraumbilical median incisions:
      a. Advantages: It prevents ventral hernia.
      b. Disadvantages
         I. There is delay in healing of the wounds because of the less blood supply.
         II. Big scar is formed.
   D. Paramedian incisions
      Advantages: There is an early healing of wound because of rich blood supply.
   E. Incisional hernia.

LAQ-2 — Describe inguinal canal under
1. Gross anatomy,   2. Development &   3. Applied anatomy.

1. **Gross anatomy:**
   A. Introduction:
      a. General introduction: It is an oblique passage or canal present in the lower part of anterior abdominal wall for the
         I. Spermatic cord in male or
         II. Round ligament of uterus in female.
      b. Situation: It is situated just ½″ above the midpoint of inguinal ligament.
      c. Extent: It extends from the deep ring to the superficial inguinal ring.
      d. Length: 1.5 inch (4 cm)
      e. The direction of the inguinal canal is oblique, downwards, forwards and medially (same as the direction of fibers of external oblique muscle).
      f. Sex pre-dilection: The canal is larger in male than female. This is because of larger dimensions of testis in male.

B. Boundaries:
   a. Roof is formed by lower arched fibers of internal oblique & transversus abdominis.
   b. Floor:
      I. Laterally: Grooved surface of inguinal ligament.
      II. Medially:
         i. Grooved surface of inguinal ligament.
         ii. Pectineal part of inguinal ligament.
         iii. Lacunar ligament.
   c. Anterior wall:
      I. Laterally:
         i. Skin.
         ii. Superficial fascia.
         iii. External oblique aponeurosis.
         iv. Internal oblique.

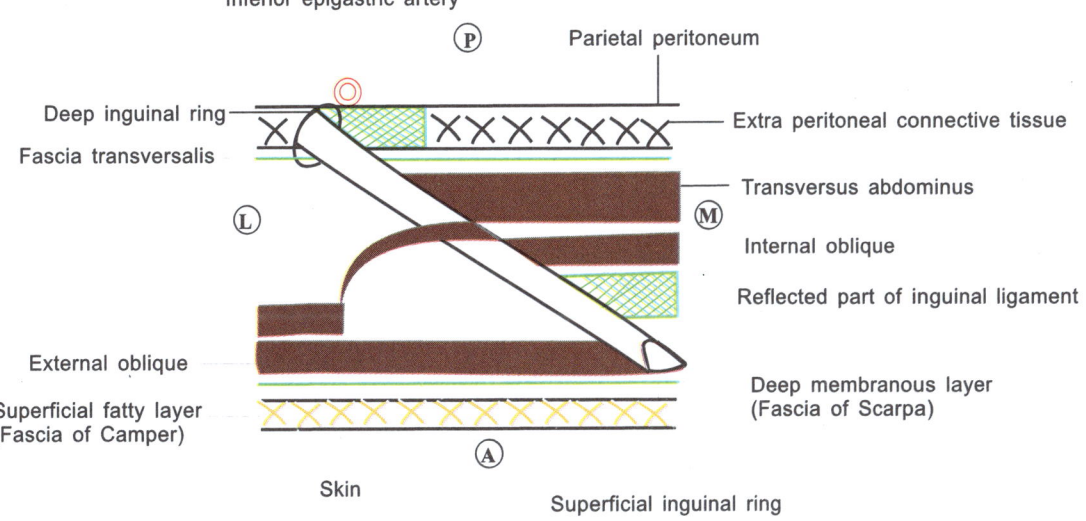

Fig. 2.7 Inguinal canal and its wall, roof and floor

   II. Medially:
      i. Skin.
      ii. Superficial fascia.
      iii. External oblique aponeurosis.
   d. Posterior wall:
      I. Laterally:
         i. Interfoveolar ligament: A thickening in the fascia transversalis present on the medial side of deep inguinal ring. It is connected above to the transversalis muscle and below to the inguinal ligament.
         ii. Fascia transversalis.
         iii. Extraperitoneal connective tissue.
         iv. Parietal peritoneum.

II. Medially:
    i.   Reflected part of inguinal ligament.
    ii. Fascia transversalis.
    iii. Conjoint tendon formed by internal oblique & transversus abdominis.
    iv. Fascia transversalis.
    v. Extraperitoneal connective tissue.
    vi. Parietal peritoneum.

C. Contents:
    a. Spermatic cord in male and round ligament of uterus in females, enters through the deep inguinal ring and passes out through the superficial inguinal ring of inguinal canal.
    b. Ilioinguinal nerve: It is derived from first lumbar nerve. In the anterior abdominal wall it lies in the neurovascular plane between the internal oblique and transversus abdominis muscles, it passes infront of the cord to the superficial inguinal ring. It supplies the skin of the root of the penis and anterior $1/3^{rd}$ of the scrotum. It also supplies small area of thigh below the medial end of the inguinal ligament.

D. Defensive mechanism of inguinal canal: It is the mechanism by which the abdominal contents normally are prevented from entering the inguinal canal. These are as follows:
    a. Flap valve mechanism: The increased intra-abdominal pressure approximates anterior and posterior wall, and obliterates the inguinal canal.
    b. Slit valve mechanism: The contraction of external oblique approximates two crura of the superficial inguinal ring.
    c. Shutter mechanism: The contraction of the internal oblique closes the inguinal canal as a shutter.
    d. Ball valve mechanism: The cremaster contracts and draws upwards the constituents of the sphermatic cord. These constituents aggregate at the superficial inguinal ring and act as a plug for the superficial inguinal ring.
    e. Superficial inguinal ring is guarded by conjoint tendon and reflected part of inguinal ligament.
    f. Deep inguinal ring is guarded by fibers of internal oblique.
    g. Hormones play an important role in maintaining tone of inguinal musculature.

2. **Development:** The canal is (developmentally) formed by the descent of gubernaculum of testis or ovary.

3. **Applied Anatomy:**
   A. The inguinal canal is a region of potential weakness in the lower part of anterior abdominal wall. Therefore following an increased intra-abdominal pressure, the abdominal contents are pushed out through inguinal canal called inguinal hernia.
   B. If contents are pushed out indirectly through deep inguinal ring, inguinal canal and superficial inguinal ring into the scrotum, it is called indirect inguinal hernia. Indirect inguinal hernias enter the inguinal canal through the deep ring i.e. lateral to the inferior epigastric artery and lie within the spermatic cord.
   C. If the contents are pushed out directly forwards through posterior wall of inguinal canal and through the superficial inguinal ring into the scrotum, it is called 'direct inguinal hernia'. The direct inguinal hernias pass through the inguinal canal i.e. medial to the inferior epigastric artery and lie medial to the spermatic cord. The direct hernia are sub-classified as medial direct inguinal hernia and lateral direct inguinal hernia depending upon the relation to the obliterated umbilical artery.

D. Both indirect and direct inguinal hernias lie superior to the inguinal ligament and medial to the pubic tubercle. This is in contrast to the femoral hernias.

E. Direct inguinal herniae are more frequent in old individual person than in the young individuals: In the old age, muscles become lax due to loss of tone and power. The lax muscles yield easily following a heavy strain, as in chronic cough and constipation. Therefore the direct inguinal hernias are more common in young individuals.

SAQ-4 Superficial inguinal ring

1. **Location:** It is situated one cm above the pubic tubercle.

2. **Formation:** It is formed in the external oblique muscle.

3. **Shape:** It is triangular in shape.

4. **Axis:** It is oblique.

5. **Dimension:**
   A. Length: One inch.
   B. Breadth: Half an inch.

6. **Relations:**
   A. Anterior:
      a. Skin and
      b. Superficial fascia.
   B. Medial: Pubic tubercle.
   C. Lateral: Inferior crus of external oblique muscle which is attach to pubic tubercle.
   D. Posterior:
      a. Conjoint tendon.
      b. Reflected part of the inguinal ligament.

7. **Contents:**
   A. Ilioinguinal nerve.
   B. Spermatic cord or round ligament of uterus.

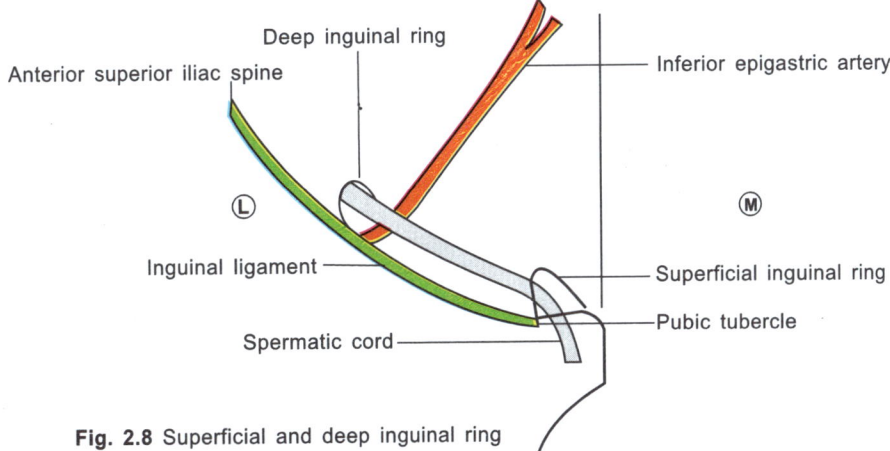

Fig. 2.8 Superficial and deep inguinal ring

SAQ-5 — Deep inguinal ring

1. **Location:** It is situated 1 cm above the mid-inguinal point.

2. **Formation:** It is present in the fascia transversalis.

3. **Shape:** It is oval in shape.

4. **Axis:** It is vertical.

5. **Relations:**
   A. Anterior: Arched fibers of transversus abdominis.
   B. Medial: Inferior epigastric artery.

Refer the Fig. 2.8 of superficial inguinal ring.

SAQ-6 — Coverings of spermatic cord

Coverings of spermatic cord: These are described from superficial to deep.

1. **External spermatic fascia** is formed by external oblique. It covers the cord below the superficial inguinal ring.

2. **Cremasteric fascia** is derived from internal oblique and transversus abdominis muscle. It covers the cord below the level of these muscles.

3. **Internal spermatic fascia** is derived from fascia transversalis. It covers the cord in whole extent.

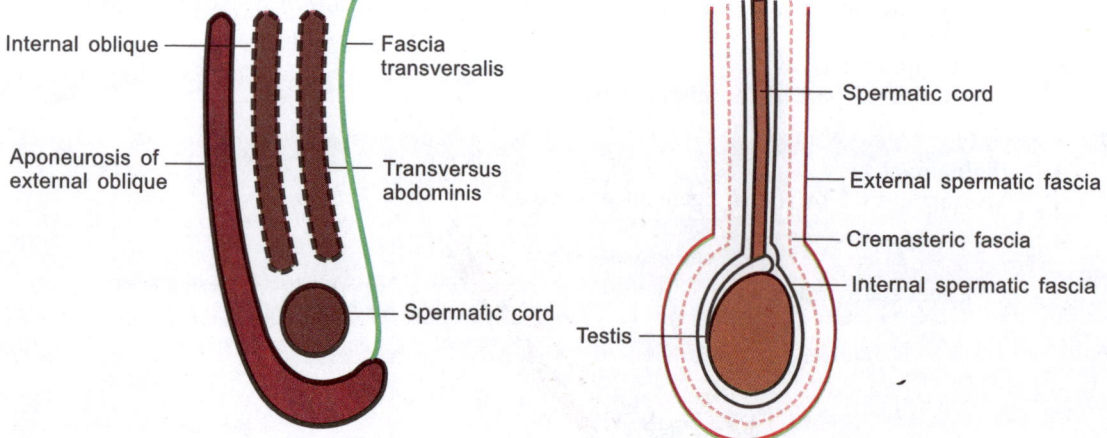

Fig. 2.9 Coverings of spermatic cord

SN-4 — Spermatic cord

1. **Introduction:** Each testis develops in the lower thoracic and upper lumbar region and migrates into the scrotum. During its descent it carries along with it vas deferens, its vessels, nerves etc It is one on each side.

2. **Gross:**
   A. Length: 7 cms.
   B. Extent: It extends from upper pole of testis to the deep inguinal ring.
   C. Course: It ascends in the scrotum and enters the inguinal canal to the superficial inguinal ring, passes through the inguinal canal and ends at the deep inguinal ring.

3. **Constituents:**
   A. Vas deferens: It starts at the tail of epididymis. At the upper pole of the testis it is accompanied by other constituents of the spermatic cord. At the deep inguinal ring it leaves all the structures and enters the abdomen.
   B. Artery to vas, branch of inferior or superior vesical artery, which is a branch of anterior division of internal iliac artery.
   C. Testicular artery, a branch of abdominal aorta.
   D. Testicular sympathetic plexus: It is formed by renal and aortic plexus.
   E. Testicular lymph vessels: They drain into the lateral aortic group of lymph nodes.
   F. Artery to cremaster, a branch of inferior epigastric artery.
   G. Nerve to cremaster, a branch of genital branch which is a branch of genitofemoral nerve.
   H. Extra peritoneal parietal tissue.
   I. Pampiniform plexus: It forms main bulk of the spermatic cord.

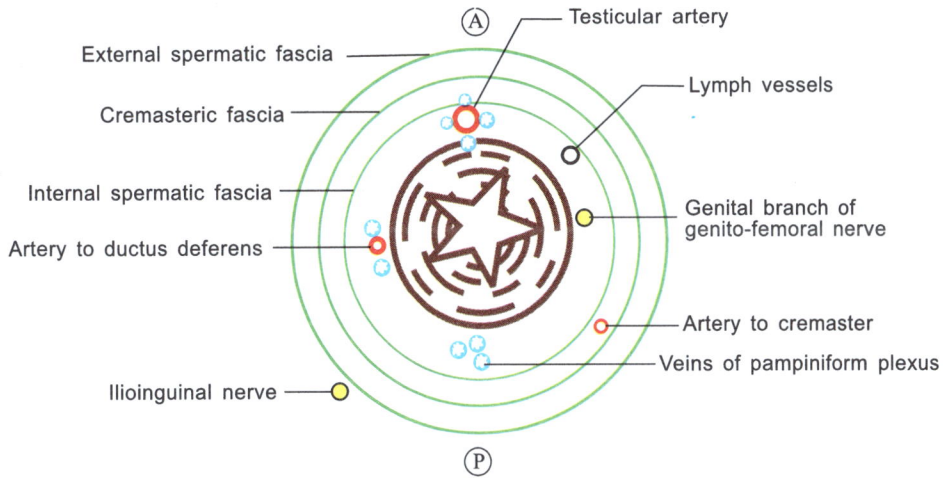

Fig. 2.10 Spermatic cord

Hesselbach's triangle
(Trigonum inguinale - Inguinal trigone)

1. **Introduction:** It is a triangular area present on the antero-inferior wall of abdomen. It is bounded.
   A. Medially by the lateral border of rectus abdominis muscle.
   B. Laterally by the inferior epigastric artery.
   C. Base by the inguinal ligament.
   D. Floor by the posterior wall of inguinal canal.

2. **Distribution:** Inguinal hernia is divided into two types depending upon the relation in the Hesselbach's triangle.
   A. If hernia is passing outside the Hesselbach's triangle, it is called indirect inguinal hernia.
   B. If hernia is passing through the Hesselbach's triangle, it is called direct inguinal hernia (i.e. medial to inferior epigastric artery). Direct inguinal hernia is again subdivided into
      a. Lateral direct inguinal hernia: Lies lateral to obliterated umbilical artery. The contents of the direct hernia enters through medial inguinal fossa.
      b. Medial direct inguinal hernia: It lies medial to obliterated umbilical artery. The contents of the hernia enters through the supravesical fossa.

3. **Characters:**
   A. It is acquired
   B. It is usually bilateral and occurs in old age

3. **Applied anatomy:** In long standing hernia inferior epigastric artery helps to differentiate between direct and indirect inguinal hernia.

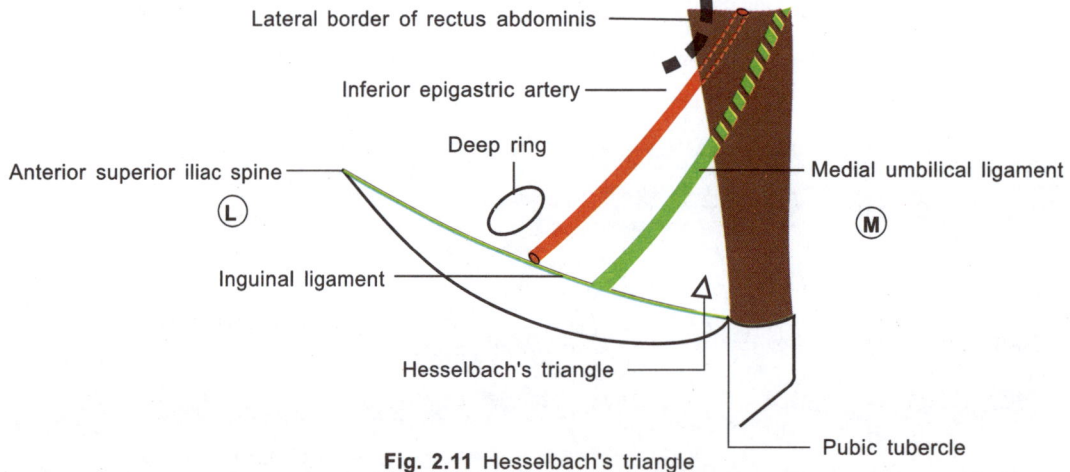

Fig. 2.11 Hesselbach's triangle

| SN-6 | **Inguinal hernia** |

1. **Introduction:** It is an abnormal protrusion of abdominal contents through the weak point of abdominal wall.

2. **Classification:**
   A. Based upon the situation of the contents of hernia.
      a. Direct (Old age): The contents of hernia are medial to inferior epigastric artery. These are subdivided into
         I. Medial: Contents of hernia are medial to obliterated umbilical artery.
         II. Lateral: Contents of hernia are lateral to obliterated umbilical artery.
      b. Indirect (oblique): The contents of hernia are lateral to inferior epigastric artery.
         I. Congenital.
         II. Acquired.

B. Difference between direct and indirect hernia.

Table 2.2 Showing difference between direct and indirect hernia

Particulars	Direct	Indirect (Oblique)
a. Direction	Directed almost straight & forward.	Directed forwards and medially.
b. Age	Occurs above the age of 40 years.	Occurs in young adult. It may be congenital.
c. Cause	Is due to acquired weakness of abdominal muscle.	Contents are passing through deep inguinal ring → inguinal canal → superficial inguinal ring.
d. Course	Contents are passing directly through superficial inguinal ring.	Is due to congenital weakness of muscle.
e. Relation	The neck of the hernial sac lies medial to the inferior epigastric artery.	The neck of the hernial sac lies lateral to the inferior epigastric artery.
f. Uniformity	Usually it is bilateral and appears in old age.	Usually it is unilateral and occurs in young subjects.

LAQ-3   Describe the testis under
1. Gross anatomy,   2. Histology,
3. Development and   4. Applied anatomy.

1. **Gross anatomy:**
   A. Introduction: Testis are pair of reproductive organs present in the scrotal bag. They are homologous to the ovary in female.
   B. Shape: Ellipsoid.
   C. Dimension:
      a. Length: 5 cm.
      b. Breadth: 2.5 cm.
      c. Antero-posterior dimension: 3 cm.
      d. Weight: 10 to 14 gms.
   D. External features:
      a. Poles: It has upper and lower pole.
         I. Upper pole is directed upwards and laterally and is connected to the head of epididymis by efferent ductules of the testis.
         II. Lower pole is directed downwards and medially. The tail of the epididymis is connected by fibrous tissue.
      b. Borders: It has 2 borders.
         I. Anterior border is convex.
         II. Posterior border is separated by a pouch of the tunica vaginalis called sinus of epididymis. Testicular vessels & nerves enter through the posterior border.
      c. Surfaces: It has two surfaces:
         I. Lateral and
         II. Medial.
      d. Position: It is suspended by the spermatic cord. Left testis is at lower level as compared to right testis.

e. Side determination: Sinus of epididymis is present on the posterior border of lateral surface.

f. Appendix of testis is fibrofatty tissue present on the upper end of testis. It is remnant of cephalic part of Mullerian duct.

g. Coverings of testis: The testis is covered by 3 coats.
   I. Tunica vaginalis (tunica coat, vaginalis sheath): It represents the lower persistent portion of processes vaginalis. It has
      i. Parietal layer, which is lined by serous epithelium.
      ii. Visceral layer, which allows free gliding movement of testis.
      It is deficient at its posterior border.
   II. Tunica albuginea (albuginea white): It is a white, dense fibrous coat covering the testis. It is covered by the visceral layer of tunica vaginalis. It is deficient posteriorly through which testicular vessels and nerves enter.
   III. Tunica vasculosa (vasculosa vessel): It is the innermost, vascular coat of the testis lining its lobules.

SN-7   Blood supply of testis

E. Blood supply
   a. Arterial Supply
      I. Testicular artery: It is main artery of testis. It is a lateral branch of abdominal aorta arising at the level of body of L_2 vertebra.
      II. Artery to the vas: It is a branch of superior or inferior vesicle artery and sometimes it supplies the testis.
   b. Venous Drainage: Veins emerging from the testis form the pampiniform plexus (*Pampiniform* like a vine or a tendril) They are arranged into three parts:

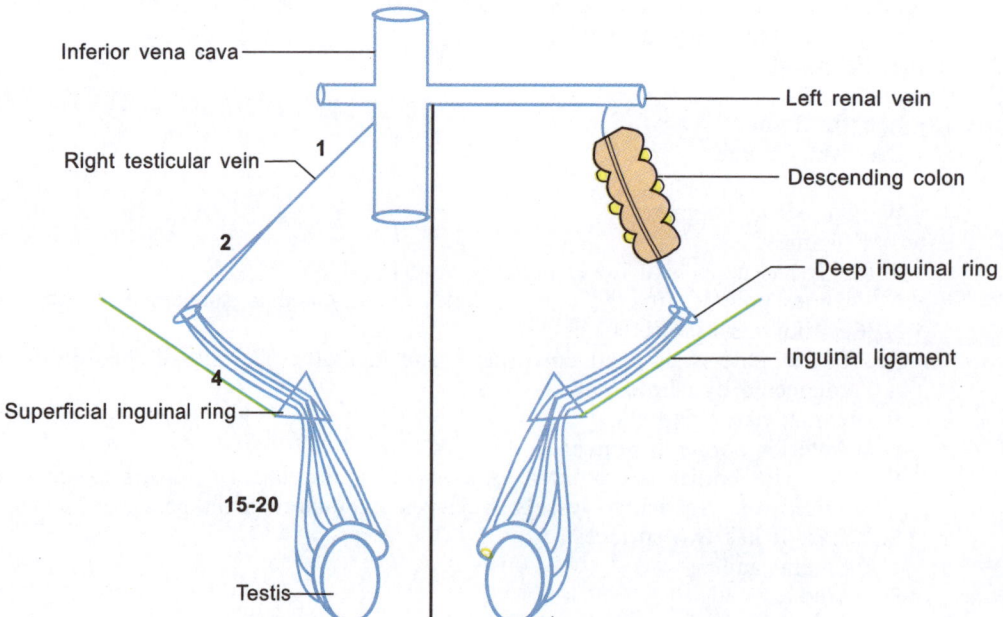

Fig. 2.12 Venous drainage of testis

I. Anterior part is present around the testicular artery.

II. Middle part is present around ductus deferens.

III. Posterior part is isolated.

Plexus condenses into :

i. 4 veins at superficial inguinal ring.

ii. 2 veins at deep inguinal ring.

iii. 1 vein at posterior abdominal wall.

These veins accompany the testicular artery. Right testicular vein drains into inferior vena cava and left testicular vein opens into left renal vein.

Counter current heat exchange mechanism. The temperature difference in the blood flowing through testis is 3° to 4° C. This is because of counter current heat exchange mechanism.

F. Nerve supply:

Sympathetic: The fibers arise from T_{10} segment of the spinal cord. They pass through the renal and aortic plexuses. The fibers carry testicular sensation and are vasomotor in nature.

G. Lymphatic drainage: Lymph vessels draining the testis run along the testicular artery and end in the lateral aortic group of the lymph node which is situated at the level of 1st lumbar vertebra i.e. at the transpyloric plane. Because it is developed in the lumbar region. This pathway explains why testicular seminoma disseminates widely and rapidly behind the peritoneum.

SN-8 Histology of testis

2. **Histology:**

A. Mediastinum: It is posterior thickened part of tunica albuginea. It sends fibrous septa to divide the interior into 200 to 250 pyramid shaped structures called testicular lobules.

B. Testicular lobule contains

a. Seminiferous tubules: They are tightly coiled and blind ended. They are one to three in each lobule.

b. Leydig cells are present between seminiferous tubules.

c. Germ cells: The details of the germ cell is shown in the following table.

Table 2.3 Showing details of spermatogenetic cells

Cells	Situation	Morphology of cell	Nucleus
I. Spermatogonium	Situated near basal lamina between cells of Sertoli	Cytoplasm is clear	Shows network
II. Primary spermatocyte	Situated next to spermatogonium	Large, spherical	Shows big nucleus
III. Secondary spermatocyte	Situated on inner side of primary spermatocyte	Smaller size	Shows division
IV. Spermatid	Near the lumen	Small cell	Rounded nucleus
V. Spermatozoa	In the lumen	Cell with tail	Forms head

d. Cells of Sertoli (Sustentacular cells or supporting cells)
    I.   They are pyramidal in shape.
    II. They have oval nucleus with prominent nucleolus.
    III. Outlines of cell are faint & irregular owing to pressure by neighbouring cells.

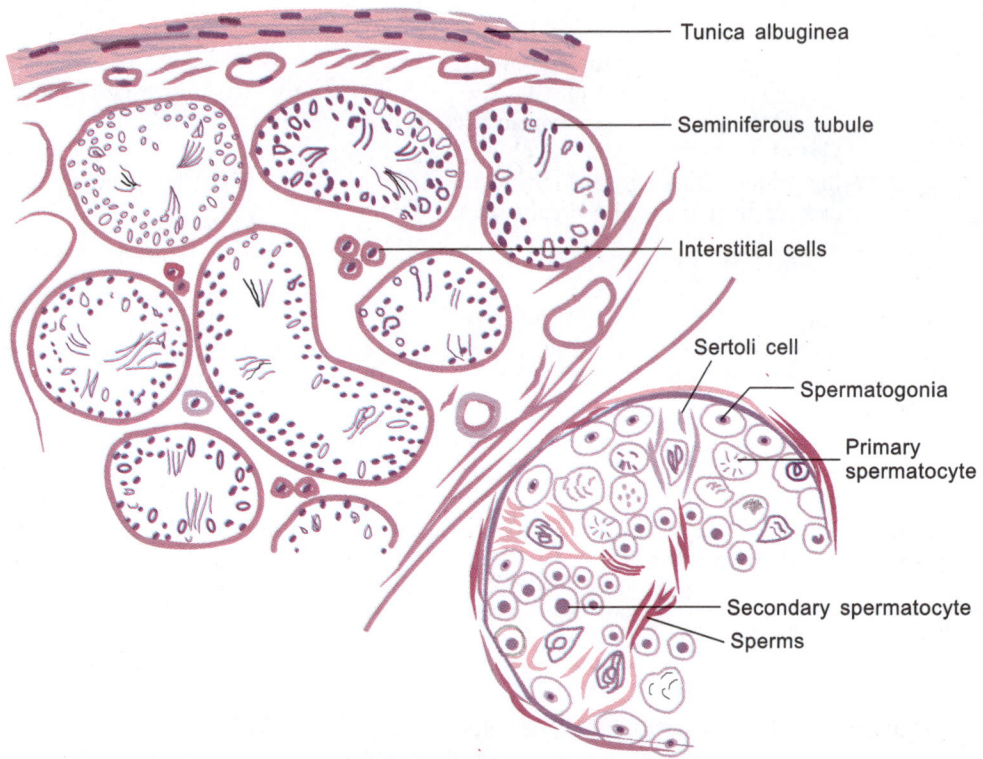

Fig. 2.13 Testis (On the right-seminiferous tubule under H. P.)

SAQ-7   Development of testis

3. **Development:**
    A. Chronological age: It develops in the seventh week of intrauterine life.

Table 2.4 Showing structures, their Germ layer and source of development of testis.

Particulars	B. Germinal layer	C. Source
a. Seminiferous tubules	Lateral plate mesoderm	Coelomic epithelium gets thickened which is called the genital ridge. This forms solid sex cords which gets canalized and forms seminiferous tubules.
b. Cells of Sertoli, sustentacular or supporting cells	Lateral plate mesoderm sex cords.	Non-canalized sex cords of coelomic epithelium forms the cells of Sertoli.

Particulars	B. Germinal layer	C. Source
c. Interstitial cell (cells of Leydig)	Intermediate mesoderm	Local mesoderm i.e. Intermediate mesoderm forms interstitial cells.
d. Germ cell	Endoderm	Migrate from dorsal wall of yolk sac through dorsal mesentery.
e. Tunica albuginea	Mesoderm	Mesenchyma surrounding developing testis.

D. Site: In the lateral plate mesoderm at the level of tenth thoracic vertebra.

E. Anomalies
   a. Monorchism: The testis may be absent on one of the side.
   b. Anorchism: The testis may be absent on both the sides.
   c. Undescended testis (cryptorchidism): The organ may lie in the lumbar, iliac, inguinal or upper scrotal region.
   d. Eptopic testis: The testis may occupy an abnormal position apart from the line of descent.
   e. Hermaphroditism (intersex): It is a condition in which an individual shows both testes and ovary.
   f. Hydrocele: The fluid accumulates in the processes vaginalis.
   g. Varicocele: It is dilatation of pampiniform plexus of veins.

4. **Applied anatomy:**
   A. *Testicular artery is tied away form the testis to establish communication between testicular artery and artery to vas and cremaster.*
   B. Hydrocele is a condition in which the fluid accumulates in the processus vaginalis. Following are different types of hydrocele:
      a. Vaginal: There is accumulation of fluid in tunica vaginalis.
      b. Congenital: The entire processus vaginalis is patent and communicates with the peritoneal cavity.
      c. Infantile: The processus vaginalis closes at the deep inguinal ring.
      d. Hydrocele of cord or encysted: The middle part of processus vaginalis is patent.
   C. Varicocele is produced by dilation of the pampiniform plexus of veins. It is usually present on the left side because of following facts of left testicular vein.
      a. It is clamped between root of superior mesenteric artery and descending abdominal aorta. Thus the left renal vein becomes pressed by superior mesenteric artery as it is dragged down by the loops of intestine.
      b. It is longer than right testicular vein.
      c. It opens in left venal vein at right angle.
      d. It is crossed by the loaded colon.
      e. It possesses less competent valves.
      f. The blood in the left testicular vein is rich in adrenaline and brings spasm of left testicular vein.
   D. The varicocele occurs in boys and young men and may be associated with reduced fertility, probably from increased venous pressure and elevated testicular temperature.

LAQ-4	**Describe the testis under**

Describe the testis under
1. **Chronological descent of the testis,**
2. **Factors responsible for descent of testis,**
3. **Anomalies of descent of testis and**
4. **Ectopic testis.**

1. **Chronological descent of the testis:**

Table 2.5 Showing chronological descent of the testis.

Month	Site
4	Iliac fossa
6	Deep inguinal ring
7	Inguinal canal
8	Superficial inguinal ring
9	Scrotum

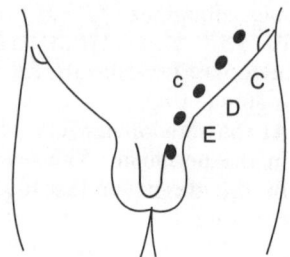

Fig. 2.14 Normal course of descent of testis

2. **Factors responsible for descent of testis:** Gonads develop retroperitoneally from the urogenital ridge in the region of the kidneys.

Factors for descent of testis: The exact cause for descent of testis is not known. However the factors can be grouped as

A. Factors which initiate the descent of testis.
   a. Abdominal temperature is not suitable for spermatogenesis
   b. Testicular hormone is the most important force and is the stimulus for the descent of testis.
   c. Gubernaculum of testis is a fibrous band, which extends from the testis to the scrotum. It helps in following ways
      I. The gubernaculum and the testis do not grow in the same proportion.
      II. It helps to dilate inguinal bursa
      III. It provides continuous pathway for the descent of testis.
   d. Formation of inguinal bursa It is formed by the out pouching of various layers of abdominal wall into the scrotum. The pouch progressively increases and various layers form the covering of testis.
   e. Processus vaginalis: This is a diverticulum of the peritoneal cavity. It actively grows into the peritoneal cavity. After the descent of testis, the processus vaginalis losses all its connections with the peritoneal cavity and becomes tunica vaginalis.
B. Factors which accelerate the descent of testis.
   a. Intra-abdominal pressure
   b. Squeezing action of inguinal muscles when testis enters the inguinal canal.

3. **Anomalies of descent of testis:** The testis may become arrested at any point along its normal journey from lumbar region to the base of the scrotum. Depending upon its location it is classified into following types.
   A. Lumbar i.e. located in the abdomen (entire failure to descent).
   B. Iliac i.e. situated at the entrance of inguinal canal.
   C. Inguinal i.e. situated within the inguinal canal.
   D. Pubic i.e. situated at the superficial inguinal ring.
   E. Scrotal i.e. situated high up in the scrotum.

4. **Ectopic testis (maldescent of testis):** The testis successfully completes its intra-abdominal descent, i.e. It has negotiated the inguinal canal and superficial inguinal ring but thereafter it deviates from its normal path and fail to reach the scrotum.

An ectopic testis is found at the following sites.

A. In the superficial fascia of the abdominal wall, above the superficial inguinal ring.
B. At the root of penis.
C. In the perineum.
D. In the thigh (in the region of femoral triangle).

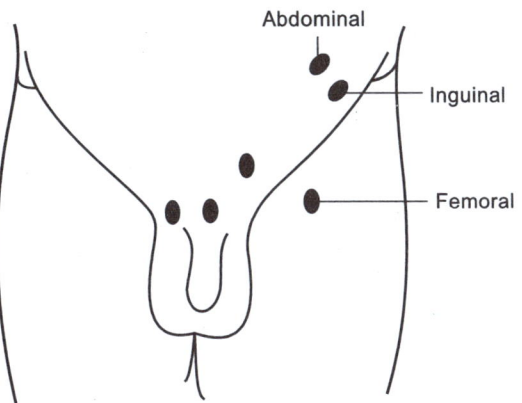

Fig. 2.15 Sites of ectopic testis

SAQ-8	**Epididymis**

It is a comma shaped body, situated along the lateral part of posterior border of testis.
It has head, body and tail.

1. **Head:** It is attached to the upper pole of testis and is composed of 10 to 15 efferent tubules.

2. **Body:** It is composed of single tubule coiled upon itself and lies on the posterior border of testis.

3. **Tail:** It is attached by fibrous tissue to the lower pole of testis. It continues as vas deferens.

SN-9	**Foramen of Winslow (Aditus to lesser sac, Epiploic foramen)**

1. **Introduction:** It is an opening communicating lesser sac to greater sac.

2. **Size:** 3 cm.

3. **Disposition:** It is vertically displayed.

4. **Boundaries:**
   A. Anterior: Right free margin of lesser omentum. It contains from left to right
      a. Hepatic artery.
      b. Portal vein (more posteriorly).
      c. Bile duct.
   B. Posterior: **S I T**
      a. **S**uprarenal gland (right).
      b. **I**nferior vena cava.
      c. **T**welfth thoracic vertebra.
   C. Superior: Caudate process of liver.

D.   Inferior:
    a.   Peritoneum extending from inferior vena cava to duodenum.
    b.   Horizontal part of hepatic artery.

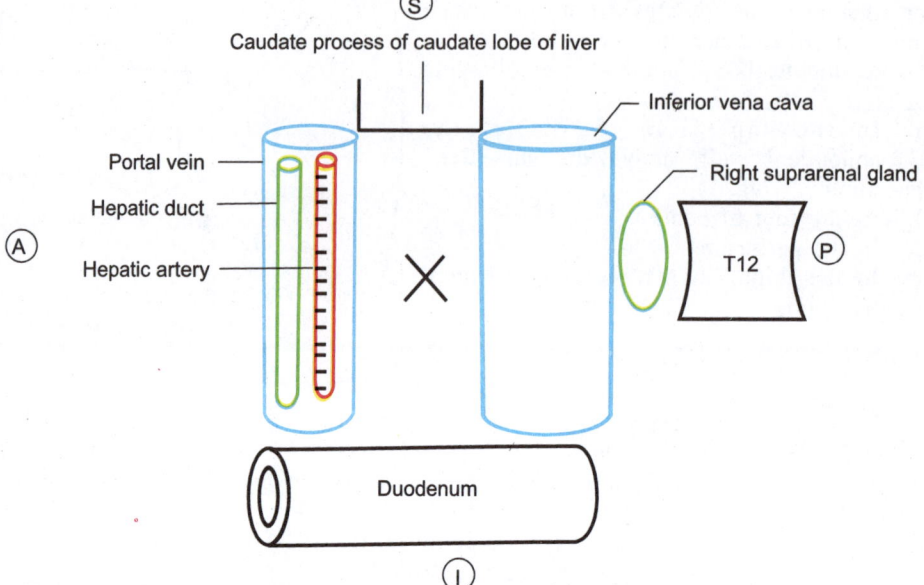

Fig. 2.16 Boundaries of foramen of Winslow

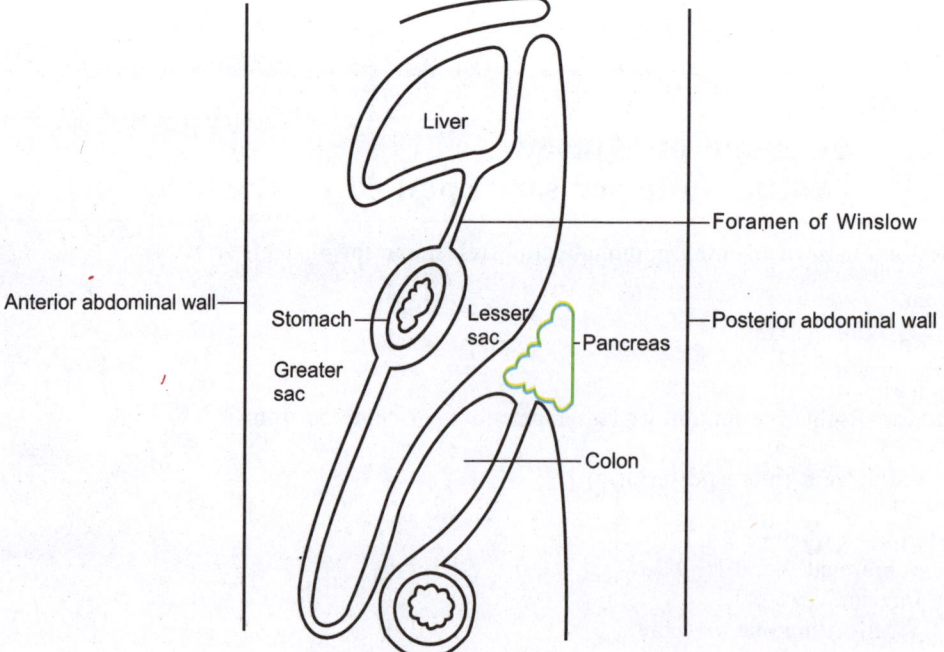

Fig. 2.17 Aditus to lesser sac

5. **Applied anatomy:**
   A. Foramen of Winslow cannot be enlarged since there are important structures situated in anterior wall.
   B. The intestines herniate through epiploic foramen.
   C. The infection spreads from greater sac to lesser sac or vice versa.

| SN-10 | **Lesser sac (Omental bursa)** |

1. **Gross:**
   A. Introduction: It is the large recess of peritoneal cavity present behind the stomach.
   B. Location: It lies behind the stomach and the lesser omentum.
   C. Extends: Into greater omentum.
   D. Communication: To greater sac through epiploic foramen.

2. **Boundaries:** Rule of three

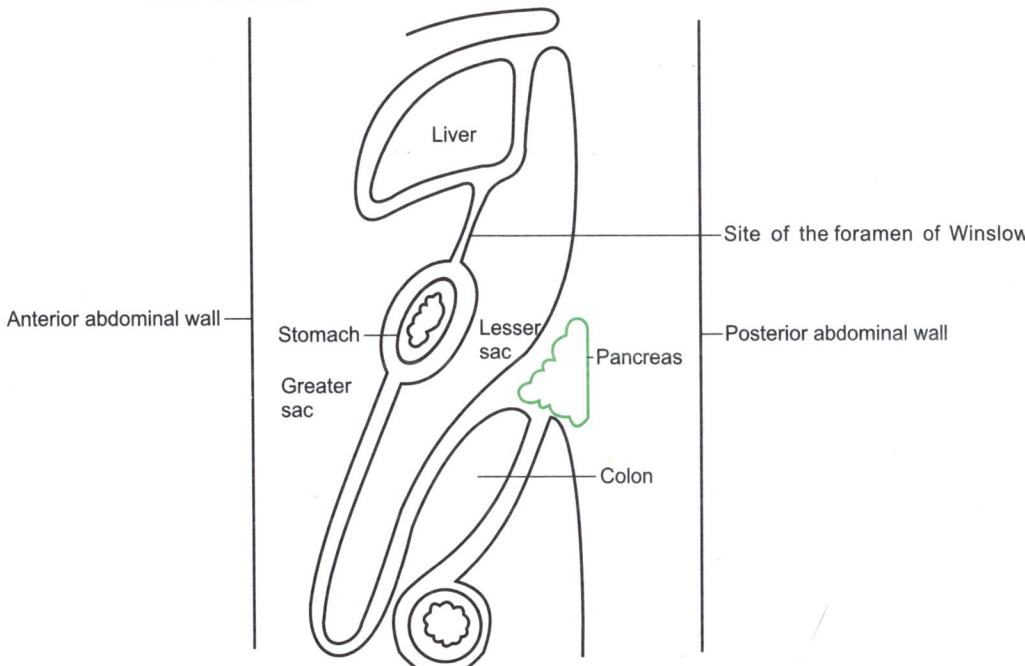

Fig. 2.18 Lesser sac

   A. Anterior wall
      a. Posterior layer of lesser omentum.
      b. Peritoneum on the posterior layer of stomach.
      c. Posterior of the anterior two layers of greater omentum.
   B. Posterior wall
      a. Below transverse colon: Anterior of the posterior two layers of greater omentum.
      b. Between transverse colon and pancreas: Posterior most layer of greater omentum fused with superior layer of transverse mesocolon.

c. Above pancreas: Anterior layer of posterior two layers continues as parietal peritoneum of posterior abdominal wall.

C. Inferior wall: Fusion of inner layer of greater omentum upto the level of transverse colon raises the inferior margin.

D. Superior wall
    a. Reflection of peritoneum from oesophagus to diaphragm.
    b. Upper end of fissure for ligamentum venosum.
    c. Upper border of caudate lobe of liver.

E. Right margin (from below upwards)
    a. Right margin of greater omentum.
    b. Right free margin of lesser omentum containing from left to right.
        I. Hepatic artery (left)
        II. Portal vein more posteriorly
        III. Bile duct
    c. Floor of aditus to lesser sac.

F. Left margin of lesser sac (from below upwards)
    a. Left margin of greater omentum
    b. Gastrosplenic and
    c. Lienorenal ligament

3. Functions:
A. Supports and facilitates the movements of stomach.
B. Acts as a bursa?
C. It is used by surgeon for operative procedures since it is bloodless area. The strangulated internal hernia is approached through greater omentum.

LAQ-5	**Describe stomach under**
	1. Gross anatomy, 2. Histology,
	3. Development and 4. Applied anatomy.

1. Gross anatomy:
A. Introduction:
Location: Stomach lies in the upper and left part of abdomen. It occupies
    a. Epigastrium,
    b. Umbilical and
    c. Left hypochondriac region.

B. External feature:
    a. Shape:
        I. Depends upon degree of distension.
        II. Physique of the individual.
        III. Position of adjacent organs.
        IV. It is a J shaped when stomach is empty.
        V. It is a pyriform shaped when partially distended.
        VI. It is steer horn in obese.

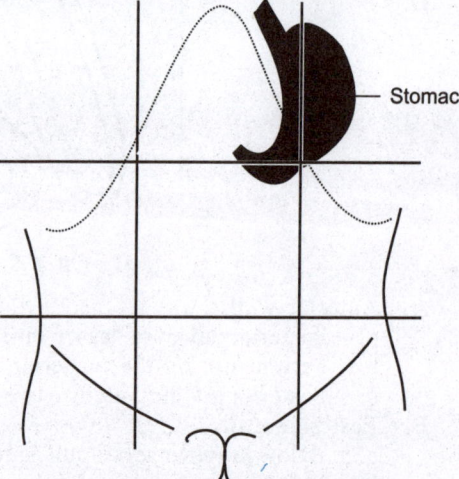

Fig. 2.19 Location of the stomach

    b.   Capacity: It varies with age.
        I.   At birth: 30 ml.
        II. At puberty: 1000 ml.
        III. In adult: 1.5 litre.
    c.   Curvatures: It has two curvatures.
        I.   Lesser curvature is concave and forms the right border of the stomach. It provides attachment to lesser omentum.
        II. Greater curvature is convex and forms the left border of the stomach. It provides the attachment to the
            i.   Greater omentum,
            ii. Gastro splenic ligament,
            iii. Gastro phrenic ligament.
    d.   Surfaces: It has two surfaces -
        I.   Anterosuperior and
        II. Posteroinferior.
    e.   Subdivision: It is divided into two parts by the line extending from angula incisura (junction of horizontal and vertical part at lesser curvature of stomach) to the greater curvature.
        I.   The larger part is called cardiac part & the smaller part is called pyloric area.
        II. Cardiac part is subdivided into fundus and the body.
            i.   Fundus: The area above the horizontal line extending form cardiac orifice to greater curvature.
            ii. Body of stomach: It lies between the fundus and pyloric antrum.
            iii. Pyloric antrum: It is 3 inches in length.
            iv. Pyloric canal: It is 1 inch long. It is narrow and tubular.

C. Internal features:
    Orifice: There are two orifices.
    a.   Cardiac orifice: It is present at the lower end of oesophagus. It is a physiological sphincter. It cannot be demonstrated anatomically.
    b.   Pyloric sphincter (*pylorus* gate): It is situated half an inch to the right of the median plane, at the lower border of L_1 vertebra.

D. Relations:
    a.   Peritoneal relations: The stomach is covered by the peritoneum everywhere except
        I.   The bare area: It is an area behind the cardiac end of the stomach, which is in contact with the diaphragm.
        II. At the lesser curvature along the attachment of lesser omentum.
        III. At the greater curvature along the attachment of
            i.   Gastrophrenic ligament,
            ii. Gastrosplenic ligament,
            iii. First and second layer of greater omentum.
    b.   Visceral relations:
        I.   Anterior:
            i.   Liver,
            ii. Diaphragm and
            iii. Anterior abdominal wall.
        II. Posterior surface of stomach is related to structures forming the stomach bed.
            i.   Left crus of diaphragm,
            ii. Splenic artery,
            iii. Transverse mesocolon,

iv. Left colic flexure,
v.   Anterior surface of the left kidney,
vi. Left suprarenal gland and
v.   Body of pancreas.

E. Blood supply:
   a. Arterial supply: It is supplied by
      I.   Left gastric artery, a branch of the coeliac trunk. It is principal artery of the
            stomach and supplies upper 2/3rd of the organ.
      II.   Right gastric, a branch of common hepatic artery. It anastomoses with the left
            gastric artery within the lesser omentum.
      III. Short gastric arteries: These are branches of splenic artery, and supply the
            fundus of the stomach.
      IV.   Left gastroepiploic: It is a branch of splenic artery and reaches the greater
            curvature.
      V.   Right gastroepiploic: It is a branch of gastroduodenal artery and anastomoses
            with the left gastroepiploic artery.

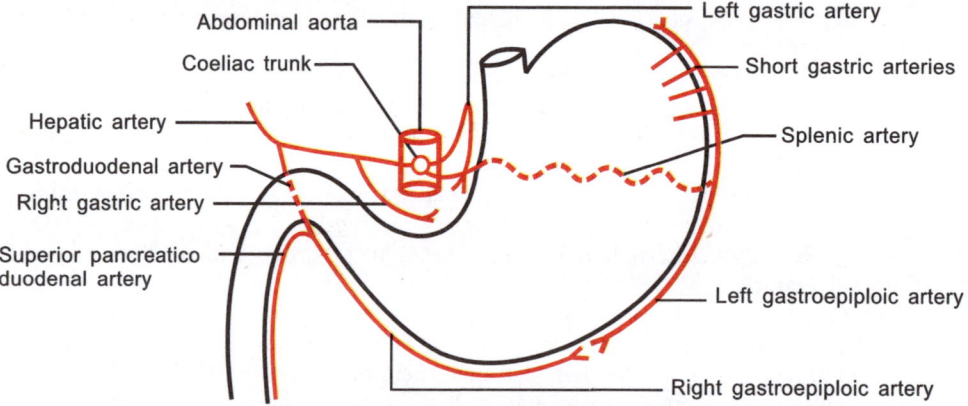

Fig. 2.20 Arterial supply of stomach

   b. Venous drainage:

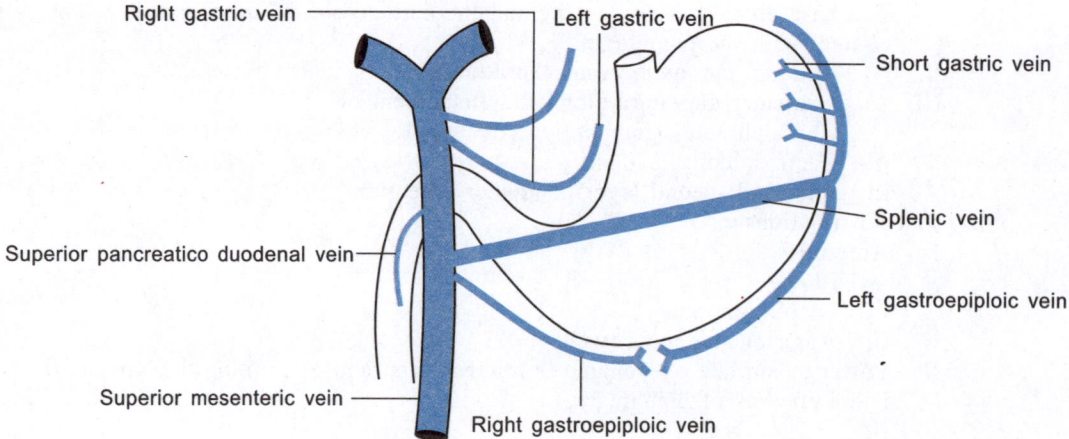

Fig. 2.21 Venous drainage of stomach

      I.   Right and left gastric veins drain into the trunk of portal vein.

      II. Short gastric and left gastroepiploic veins drain into splenic vein.

      III. Right gastroepiploic vein drains into superior mesenteric vein.

F.   Nerve supply: It is supplied by sympathetic and parasympathetic nerve.

    a.   Sympathetic fibers: They arise from coeliac plexus. The pre-ganglionic motor fibers arise from T_6 to T_9 segments of the spinal cord and the fibers reach via greater splanchnic nerves. The sympathetic fibers have following functions.

      I.   They are vasomotor in function.

      II. They stimulate the pyloric sphincter.

      III. They inhibit the rest of the gastric muscles.

      IV. Sensory sympathetic fibers convey painful sensations from the stomach.

    b.   Parasympathetic fibers: They are derived from both the vagus nerves in the form of anterior and posterior vagal trunks through esophageal plexus and gastric nerves. They consist of anterior and posterior gastric nerve.

      The stimulation of the parasympathetic nerve causes

      I.   Increased motility of the stomach.

      II. Secretion of gastric juice which is rich in pepsin and HCl.

      III. Inhibits pyloric sphincter.

G. Lymphatic drainage: All the lymphatics from the stomach ultimately drains into coeliac group of lymph node. It is divided into four regions.

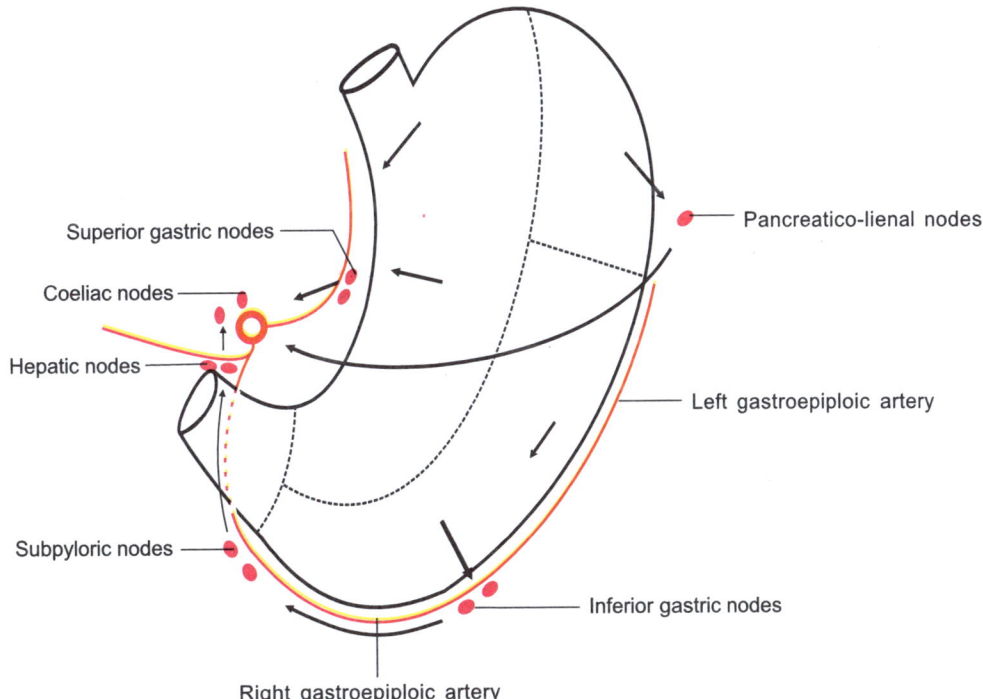

Fig. 2.22 Lymphatic drainage of stomach

Table 2.6 Showing the lymph nodes of the stomach and their afferent & efferent.

Lymph node	Situation of the lymph node	Afferent	Efferent
I. Pancreatico splenic.	Along splenic artery.	Pancreas & spleen	Coeliac nodes.
II. Left gastric nodes.	Along left gastric artery.	i. Right 2/3rd of the stomach. ii. Abdominal part of the esophagus.	Coeliac nodes.
III. Right gastro epiploic nodes.	Along the right and left gastro epiploic artery.	Lower 2/3rd of the left 1/3rd of the stomach.	Pyloric nodes } Hepatic nodes } →Coeliac nodes.
IV. Sub-pyloric nodes.	At the pyloric end of stomach.	Pylorus of stomach.	i. Pyloric, ii. Hepatic and iii. Left gastric. } →Coeliac nodes.

2. **Histology:** The wall of the stomach presents four coats from inside out.
   A. Mucous membrane: It consists of epithelium, lamina propria and muscularis mucosae.
      a. Simple columnar epithelium: It lies on the basement membrane.
      b. Lamina propria: It contains vessels, nerves and various types of gastric glands. The gastric glands are of three types.
         I. Cardiac glands: They are few in number. They are situated close to cardiac orifice. They secrete mucus.
         II. Pyloric glands: They are lined by mucous secreting cells. Some of the cells secrete the hormone, gastrin.

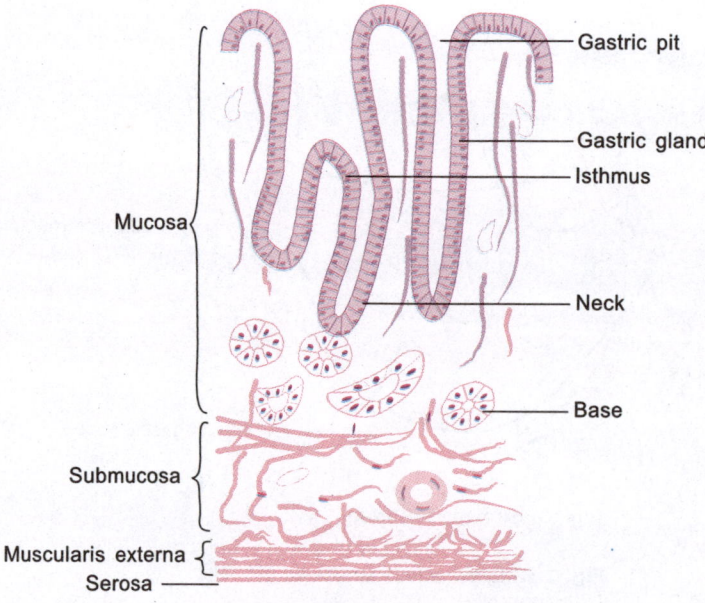

Fig. 2.23 Pylorus of stomach

III. Fundic glands: They are present in fundus and body. They contain three types of cells.
   i. Zymogenic or chief cells. These are cubical and possess basophilic cytoplasm.
   ii. Oxyntic cells: These are large polyhedral cells and possess acidophilic cytoplasm. They secrete HCl.
   iii. Mucous cells are found in the neck of the gland.

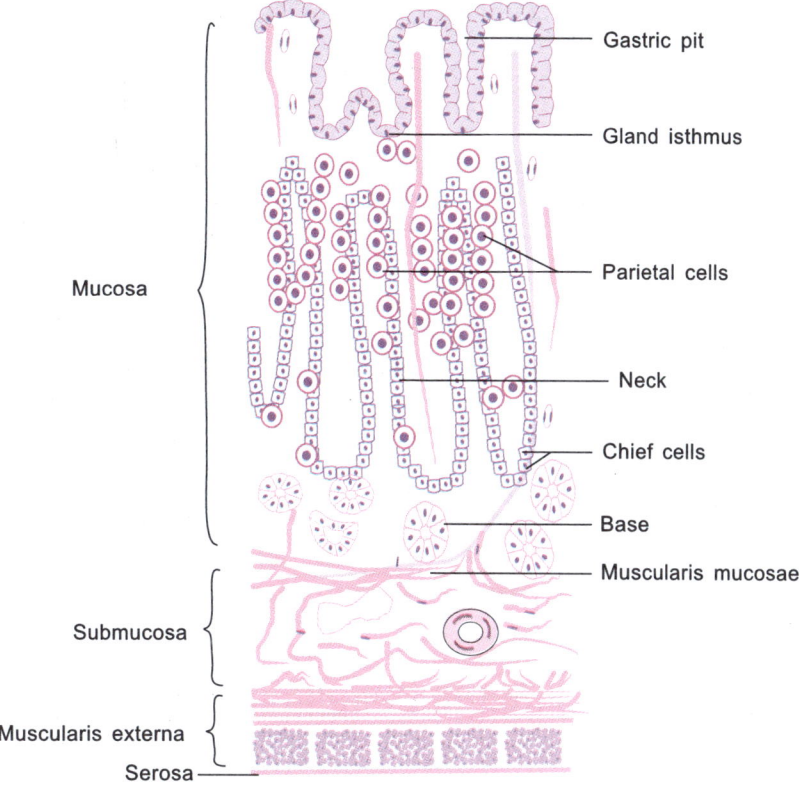

Fig. 2.24 Fundus of stomach

   c. Muscularis mucosae.
B. Submucosa:
C. Muscular coat: It consists of smooth muscles namely
   a. Outer longitudinal muscles.
   b. Inner circular muscles: They are thickened at the pylorus and forms a ring of muscle known as pyloric sphincter.
   c. Oblique muscles..
D. Serous coat: It is lined by simple squamous epithelium of peritoneum.

3. **Development:** It is described under
   A. Chronological age: It first becomes apparent at fourth week and rotation occurs in seventh week of intrauterine life.
   B. Germ layer: Endoderm and mesoderm.
   C. Site: Inferior to septum transversum.

D. Sources:
   a. The epithelium and the glands of stomach develops as a fusiform dilatation of foregut distal to the oesophagus.
   b. All the remaining layers of the stomach develop from intra embryonic splanchopleuric mesoderm.
E. Anomalies: Congenital hypertrophic pyloric stenosis. It is a congenital defect with a neuromuscular incoordination of the thickened pyloric sphincter. The infant suffers from progressive vomiting withing two weeks to two months of post natal life.

4. **Applied anatomy:**
   A. Gastric pain is felt in epigastrium because the stomach is supplied from segments T_6 to T_{10} of the spinal cord, which also supply the upper part of the abdominal wall. The pain is produced by spasm of muscle, or by overdistension.
   B. Gastric ulcers usually occur along the lesser curvature of stomach. This is because of following two factors.
      a. Gastric canal is formed along the lesser curvature of the stomach. During swallowing, the liquid or bolus of the food passes through this canal and thus the gastric mucosa is exposed to irritant liquids and spices in food. This results in gastritis and ulceration.
      b. The vessels to the gastric mucosa along the lesser curvature do not arise from a submucous plexus but directly arise from gastric arteries outside the gastric wall.
   C. Trunkal vagotomy involves section of the main trunks of both vagi. It should always be accompanied by either pyloroplasty or gastro-jejunostmy.
   D. Selective vagotomy is designed to section the nerves of Laterajet of both vagi.
   E. Highly selective vagotomy is the operation of choice because it denervates only those small branches on the left side of both nerves of Laterajet which supply acid bearing area of the stomach.

SN-11 **Stomach bed**

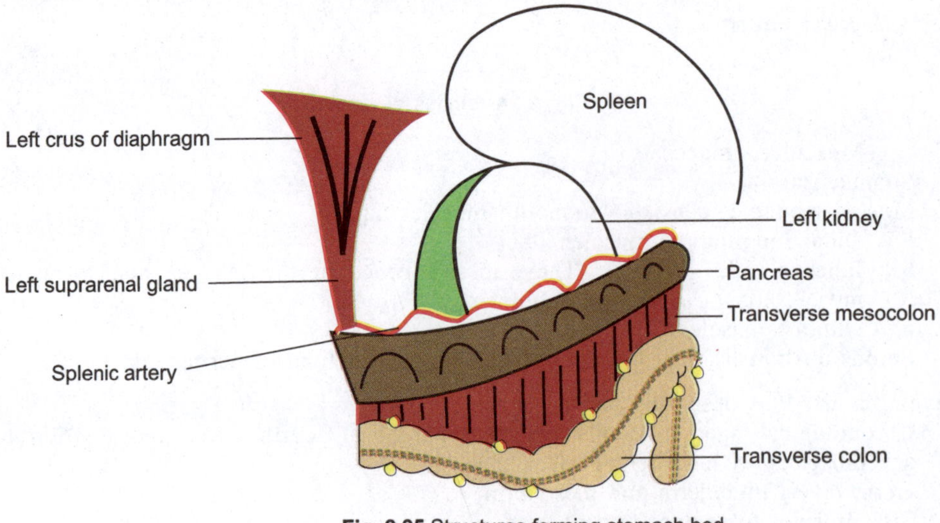

Fig. 2.25 Structures forming stomach bed

Left crus of diaphragm
Spleen
Left kidney
Left suprarenal gland
Pancreas
Transverse mesocolon
Splenic artery
Transverse colon

Posteroinferior surface of stomach is covered with peritoneum of lesser sac except bare area. It forms shallow fossa upon which the stomach rests in a recumbent supine position. The bed consists of the following structures.

1. The **m**ain structure is left crus of diaphragm.

2. **T**ortuous splenic artery.

First letter of week days
Mon, **T**ue, **W**ed, **T**hu, **F**ri, **S**at, **S**un

3. **W**hen stomach is distended, gastric surface of spleen also comes in contact. The spleen is separated from the stomach by a recess of greater sac.

4. **T**ransverse mesocolon.

5. Left colic **f**lexure.

6. Anterior **s**urface of the left kidney.

7. Anterior **s**urface of left suprarenal gland.

8. Body of the pancreas.

LAQ-6 **Describe second part of duodenum under**
1. **Gross anatomy,** 2. **Histology,**
3. **Development and** 4. **Applied anatomy.**

1. **Gross anatomy:**
   A. Introduction:
      a. General introduction: It is the junction of the foregut and midgut.
      b. Location: It is present in umbilical region on the right margin of second lumbar vertebra.
   B. Internal features:
      The interior of the second part of duodenum shows the following special features
      a. The major duodenal papilla, an elevation present posteromedially, 8 to 10 cm distal to the pylorus. The hepatopancreatic ampulla opens at the summit of the papilla.
      b. The minor duodenal papilla is present 6 to 8 cm distal to the pylorus, and presents the opening of the accessory pancreatic duct.
   C. Relations: It is described as
      a. Peritoneal relations: It is retroperitoneal and most fixed part of duodenum.
         I. Anterior surface is related to
            i. The transverse colon.
            ii. Above and below, the transverse colon, it is covered by peritoneum of greater sac.
         II. Posterior surface is non-peritoneal.
      b. Visceral relations
         I. Anterior surface: It is divided into
            i. Area above the transverse colon is related to
               - Inferior surface of the right lobe of liver.
               -. Body of the gall bladder.
            ii. Area below the transverse colon is related to coils of jejunum.
         II. Posterior surface
            i. Anterior surface of right kidney.

    ii. Structures at hilum of the right kidney (from anterior to posterior).
- Right renal vein.
- Right renal artery.
- Pelvis of right ureter.

  iii. Right margin of inferior vena cava.

  iv. Right psoas major.

  v. Right crus of diaphragm.

III. Right border is related to right colic flexure.

IV. Left border is related to head of pancreas in its entire course.

    i. Anastomosis between the superior and inferior pancreatico-duodenal vessels.

    ii. Pancreatico-duodenal lymph nodes. It is pierced by
- Bile duct,
- Pancreatic duct and
- Accessory pancreatic duct.

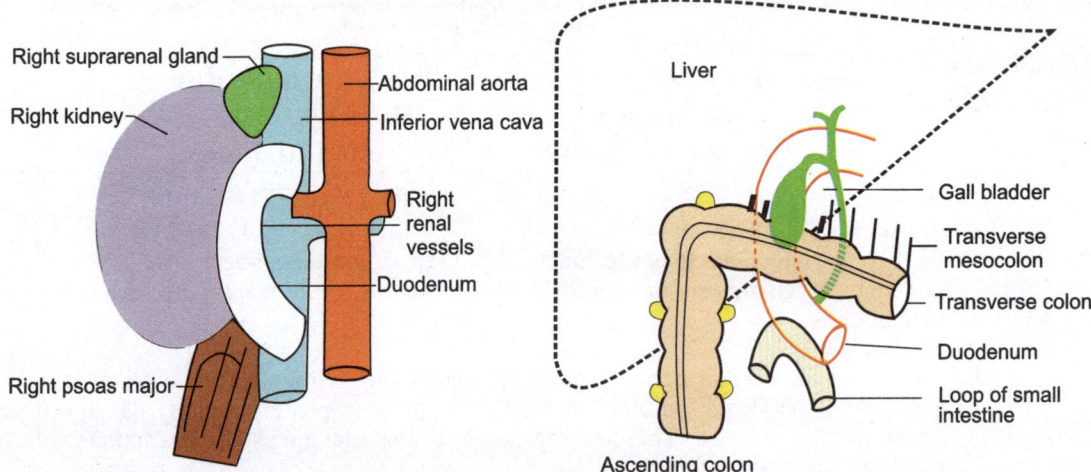

Fig. 2.26 Posterior relations of second part of duodenum   **Fig. 2.27** Anterior relations of second part of duodenum

D. Blood supply

  a. Arterial supply:

    I. Part of the duodenum above the opening of bile duct belongs to foregut. Hence supplied by branches of coeliac trunk which is the artery of foregut. The arteries supplying this area is superior pancreatico-duodenal artery branch of gastroduodenal artery.

    II. Part of the duodenum below the opening of bile duct belongs to midgut. Hence supplied by branches of artery of midgut namely inferior pancreatico duodenal artery, which is a branch of superior mesenteric artery.

  b. Venous drainage:

    I. Superior pancreatico-duodenal vein drains into portal vein.

    II. Inferior pancreatico-duodenal vein drains into superior mesenteric vein.

E. Nerve supply:

  a. Sympathetic nerves: They arise from spinal segments of T_9 and T_{10}.

  b. Parasympathetic nerves: They arise from vagus nerves.

F.   Lymphatic drainage: Lymph vessels drain into
   a.   Pancreatico-duodenal lymph nodes.
   b.   Pyloric lymph nodes: The efferent lymphatics go to
      I.   Coeliac group of lymph nodes.
      II. Superior mesenteric group of pre aortic lymph nodes.

2.   **Histology:** It consists of four coats
  A.   Mucous coat containing
    a.   Simple columnar epithelium with intestinal glands.
    b.   Lamina propria.
    c.   Muscularis mucosa.
  B.   Submucosa containing Brunner's glands (alkaline).
  C.   Muscularis externa containing smooth muscles namely
    a.   Inner circular and
    b.   Outer longitudinal.
  D.   Serous coat is lined by simple squamous epithelium or adventitia.

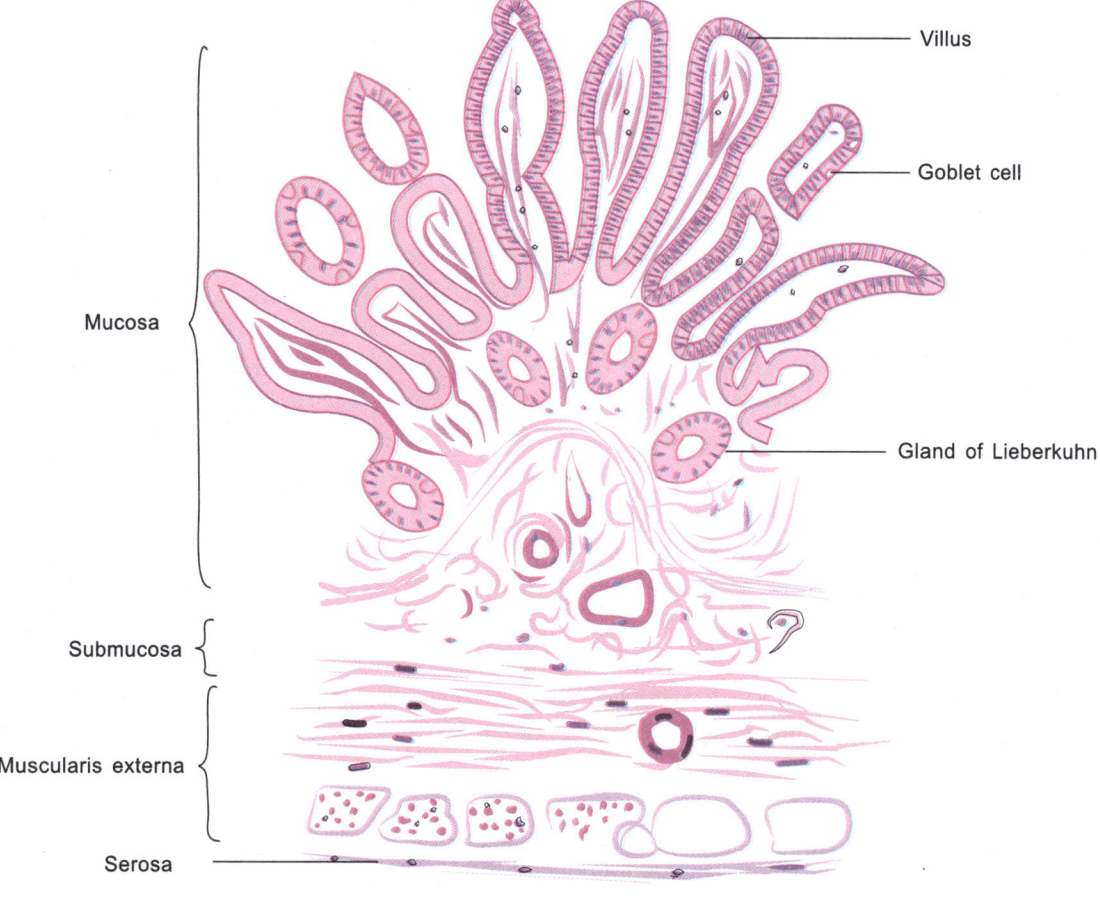

Fig. 2.28 Small intestine

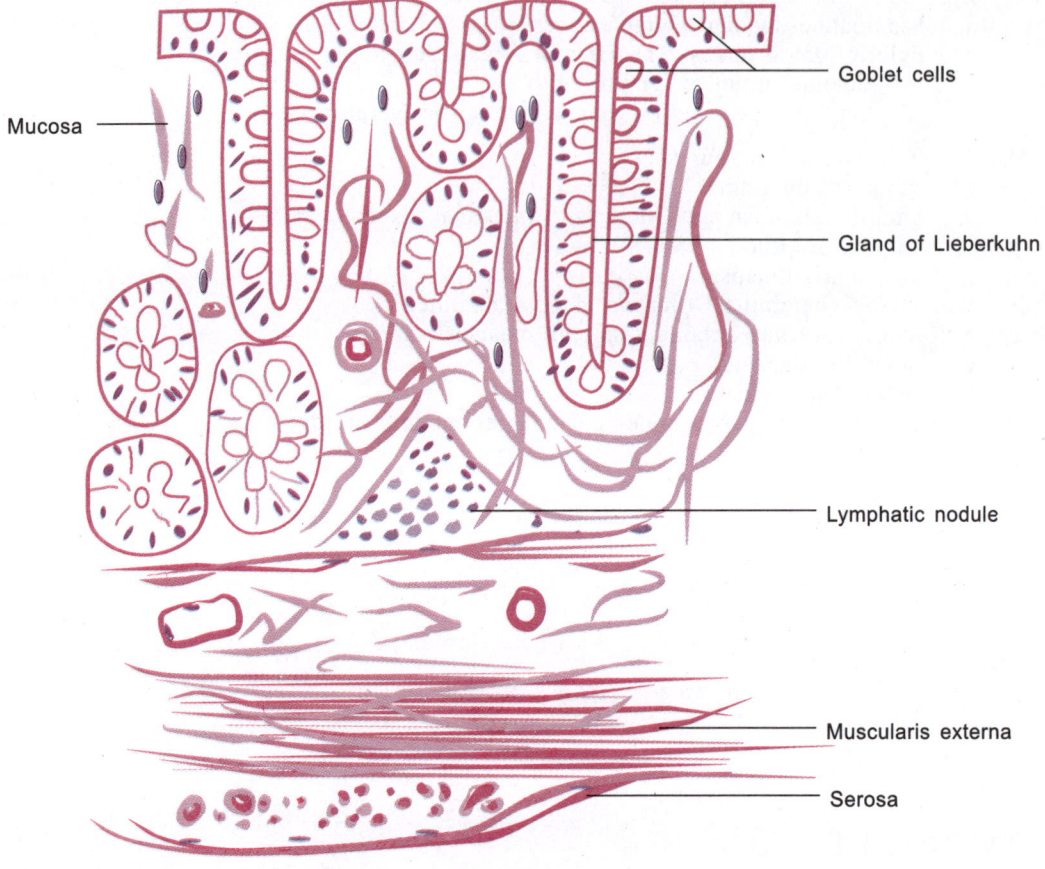

Mucosa

Goblet cells

Gland of Lieberkuhn

Lymphatic nodule

Muscularis externa

Serosa

Fig. 2.29 Large intestine

3. **Development:**
    A. Chronological age: It develops in the fourth week of intrauterine life.
    B. Germ layer: Endoderm and mesoderm.
    C. Site: Caudal part of foregut.
    D. Sources:
        a. The epithelium of the second part of duodenum
            I.   Above the opening of bile duct develops from endoderm of the foregut.
            II. Below the opening of the bile duct develops from endoderm of the midgut.
        b. All the coats of duodenum except epithelium and glands develop from intra-embryonic splanchnopleuric mesoderm.
        c. During rotation of the stomach, the duodenum also rotates to the right and forms a superior retention band, which fixes it at the junction of duodenum with jejunum. The superior retention band becomes suspensory ligament of duodenum.
        d. During rotation, the dorsal mesentery disappears except 1 inch near pyloric end and the duodenum become retroperitoneal organ.
        e. There is temporary blockage of duodenal lumen by proliferation of endoderm. The lumen is re-established after some time. The failure of the formation of the lumen leads to atresia.

E. Anomalies:
    a. Abnormal fixation: There is no functional disturbance.
    b. Excessive fixation may cause interference with mobility, kinks, and compression of the lower bowel.
    c. Failure of fixation may cause ptosis, torsion or volvulus.
    d. Abnormal rotation predisposes to volvulus, which causes internal obstruction. Such obstruction is particularly likely to occur within the first few days of life (volvulus neonatorum).

4. Applied anatomy:
A. Duodenal diverticula are fairly frequent. They are generally seen at the point of entry of arteries.
B. Congenital stenosis and obstruction may occur at the site of opening of the bile duct. Other causes of obstruction includes
    a. Annular pancreas.
    b. Pressure by superior mesenteric artery.
    c. Constriction of suspensory muscle of duodenum.
C. Second part is most protected from the external injury, since it is situated behind the forward curvature of the vertebral column in the paravertebral gutter. Sometimes small bile stones may be impacted on the summit of the major papilla producing obstructive jaundice.

SN-12   Duodenal cap

It is a smooth triangular shadow seen in the first part of duodenum in barium meal x-ray of the abdomen. It has a base and a apex. The base is below and apex is above.
The following anatomical factors appears to be responsible for it.
1. The first part of duodenum runs upward, backward & to the right to continue as second part

2. The knob like pylorus invaginates into the first part of duodenum which is thus kept open and filled with barium paste.

3. The mucus membrane of proximal half of duodenum is devoid of circular folds.

4. The proximal half of the first part of the duodenum is mobile. Because it has mesentery.

5. The viscosity of the barium sulphate coming out of a narrow pyloric canal gives a conical appearance.

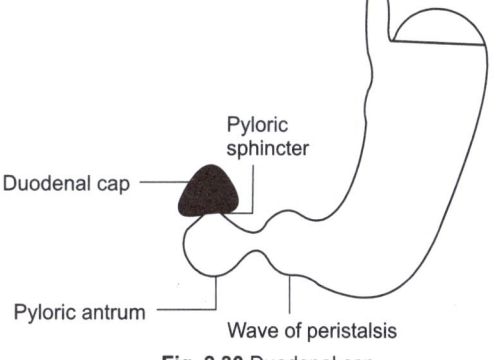

Fig. 2.30 Duodenal cap

SN-13   Ligaments of Treitz (Suspensory muscle of duodenum)

1. **Introduction:** It is the fibromuscular band extending from right crus of the diaphragm to the duodenojejunal flexure.

2.   **Formation:** It is formed by
     A.   In upper part by striped muscle fibers.
     B.   In middle part by elastic fibers.
     C.   In lower part by smooth muscle fibers.

3.   **Importance:**
     A.   It marks duodenojejunal junction.
     B.   If it is attached only to flexure, its contraction may narrow the angle of flexure, causing partial obstruction of gut.

SN-14   Meckel's diverticulum

1.   **Introduction:** This is the persistent proximal part of the vitellointestinal duct.

2.   **Gross anatomy:** Rule of two
     A.   Situation: It is located at the anti mesenteric border of the ileum.
     B.   Length: 2 inches.
     C.   Distance from the ileocaecal valve: 2 feet.
     D.   Incidence: 2% of population.
     E.   Its caliber is equal to that of ileum.
     F.   Its apex may be free or may be attached to the umbilicus or any other abdominal structure.

3.   **Content:** It contains
     A.   Pancreatic tissue and
     B.   Gastric mucosa.

4.   **Applied anatomy:**
     A.   It is one of the most common congenital anomaly of the gastro intestinal tract.
     B.   It is responsible for intestinal obstruction and intussusception.
     C.   It may enter into hernial sac.
     D.   It is the one of the differential diagnosis of appendicitis.
     E.   There may be discharge from the umbilicus. It may present as bulging umbilicus or cystic umbilical tumour.

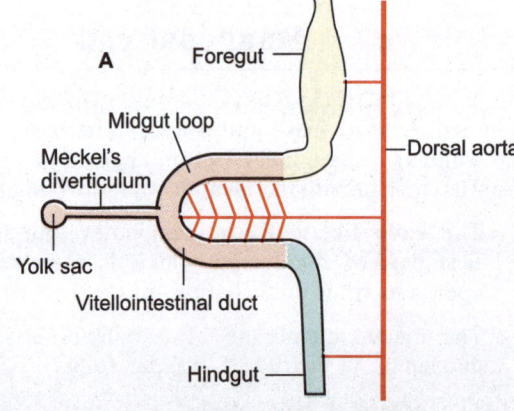

Fig. 2.31 Meckel's diverticulum

LAQ-7   Describe caecum under
1.   Gross anatomy,   2.   Applied anatomy.

1.   **Gross anatomy:**
     A.   Introduction:
          a.   General introduction: It is the proximal end of the large intestine where the large and small intestine meet.
          b.   Location: It is situated in right iliac fossa above the lateral half of inguinal ligament.

c. Size: Length 6 cm x breadth 7.5 cm
   (It has greater width than length similar to prostrate)
d. Shape: Usually asymmetrical cul - de - sac.

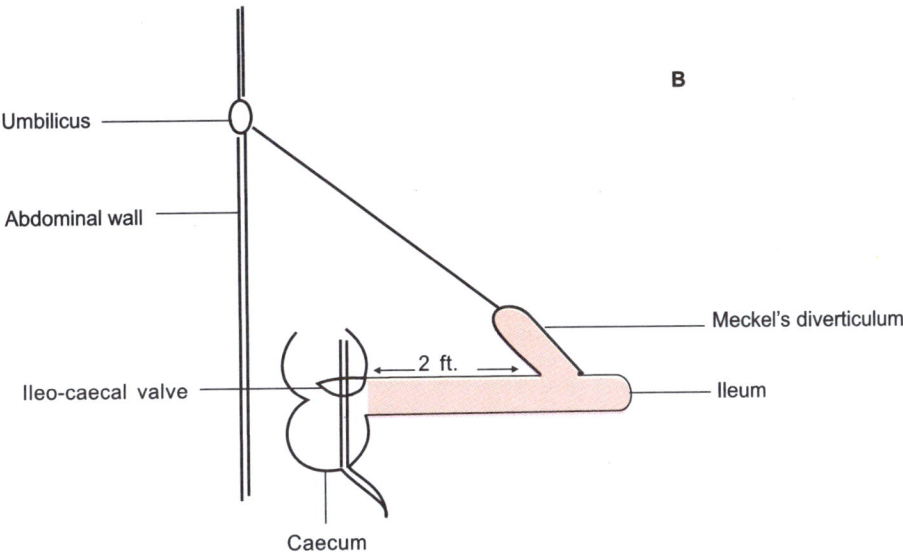

Fig. 2.32 Position of caecum

B. Internal structure: It shows two orifices.
   A. Ileo - caecal orifice.
   b. Appendicular orifice.

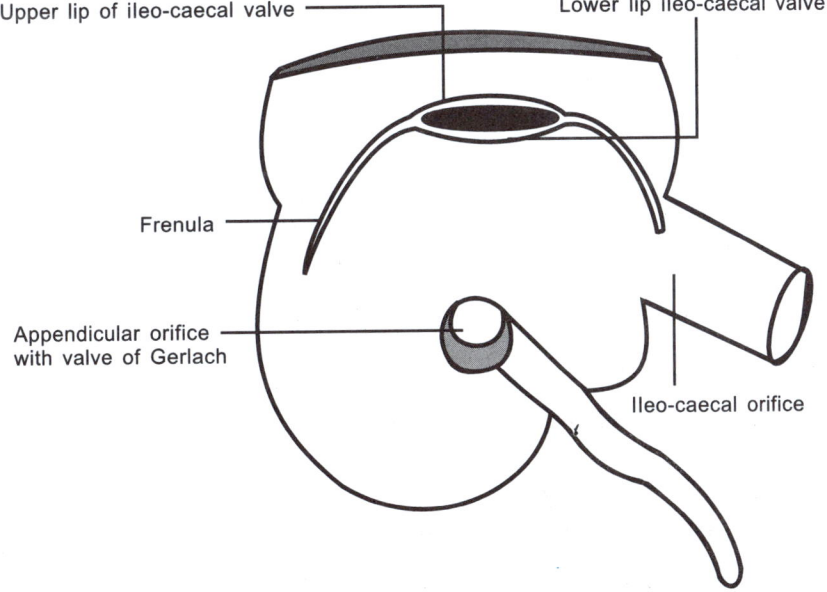

Fig. 2.33 Interior of caecum.

Table 2.7 Showing orifices in the caecum

Features	Ileocaecal orifice	Appendicular orifice
Situation	Present at the junction of caecum & ascending colon.	Situated 2 cm below ileo-caecal orifice
Guarded by	Valve having upper horizontal & lower concave lip	A semicircular mucous fold called valve of Gerlach
Shape	Slit like having 2.5 cm transverse diameter	Small circular opening.

C.   Relations:
    a.   Peritoneal relations:
        I.   It is covered by peritoneum on all sides except posterior surface.
        II.   It has no mesentery.
        III.   It is movable & bound to the lateral abdominal wall by one or more caecal fold of peritoneum.
    b.   Visceral relations:
        I.   Anterior relations: ·
            i.   Coils of the intestine.
            ii.   Anterior abdominal wall.
        II.   Posterior relations:
            i.   Appendix in retrocaecal recess.
            ii.   Right psoas & iliacus muscle.
            iii.   Genitofemoral, femoral & lateral cutaneous nerve of thigh.
            iv.   Right gonadal & right external iliac vessels.

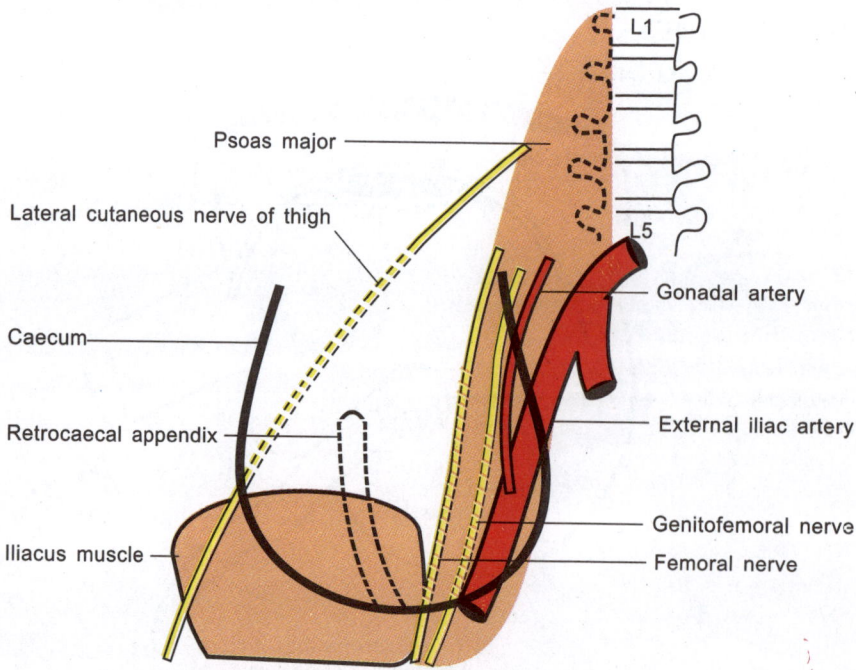

Fig. 2.34 Posterior relations of the caecum

      III. Medial:
         i.   Appendix.
         ii. Terminal part of ileum.
         iii. Inferior ileo - caecal recess.

D. Blood Supply:
    a. Arterial supply: Anterior & posterior caecal arteries (branches of ileocaecal artery which is a terminal branch of superior mesenteric artery).
    b. Venous drainage: Ileocolic vein drains into superior mesenteric vein which drains into portal vein.

E. Nerve supply: From superior mesenteric plexus
    a. Sympathetic fibers arise from T_{10} to L_1 segments of spinal cord.
    b. Parasympathetic fibers arise from vagus nerve.

F. Lymphatic drainage: Ileocolic lymph nodes, which drain into superior mesenteric lymph nodes.

2. Applied Anatomy:
A. If distended with faeces or gas, the caecum may be palpable through anterior abdominal wall.
B. The caecum acts as a guide line for localization of obstruction.
    a. If the caecum is distended, the obstruction is in the large intestine.
    b. If the caecum is empty, the obstruction is in the small intestine.
C. Intussusception: sometimes terminal part of ileum is telescopically invaginated into caecum and ascending colon at ileocaecal junction. This phenomenon is known as intussusception.
D. The tuberculosis of intestine is common at ileocaecal junction.

LAQ-8   **Describe appendix under**
        1. Gross anatomy,   **2. Histology,**
        3. Development and   **4. Applied anatomy.**

1. Gross anatomy:
A. Introduction:
    a. General introduction: It is a narrow worm like tubular diverticulum, arises from posteromedial wall of the caecum. It resembles round worm, hence called vermiform appendix.
    b. Location: It is situated in the right iliac fossa about 2 cm below the intersection of transtubercular (upper part of fifth lumbar vertebra) and right lateral plane.
    c. Length is 2 cm to 20 cm, (average is 9 cm). Length increases in young adults and diminishes after mid adult life.
    d. Peculiarities: Although appendix is the part of large intestine it is devoid of
        I.   Sacculations,
        II. Appendices epiploicae and
        III. Taenia coli.

B. External feature: Position of appendix
    a. The base is fixed and is attached to posteromedial wall of the caecum about 2 cm below the ileocaceal (junction). All taenia of the caecum converge to the base of the appendix.

b. Body is narrow and tubular and it contains a canal, which opens into caecum, it is guarded by incomplete mucosal fold called the valve of Gerlach.

c. The tip is least vascular. According to the direction of the tip of the appendix, it is classified as

    I.   Retrocaecal appendix
        i.   12 O'clock position.
        ii. It is most common position of appendix.
        iii. The appendix passes retro-peritoneally behind the caecum and ascending colon.
        iv. It presents as pain and tenderness at McBurney's point.
        v. Patient experiences pain in extension of hip joint.

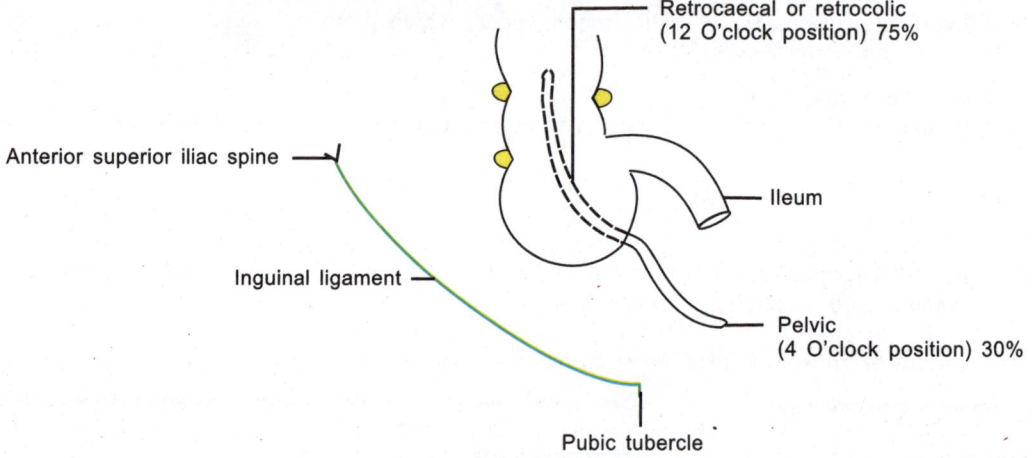

Fig. 2.35 Commonest positions of appendix

    II. Pelvic appendix
        i.   4 O'clock position.
        ii. It is second common position of appendix.
        iii. It presents as pain & tenderness at McBurney's point and haematuria due to pressure of inflamed appendix on the right ureter.
        iv. Patient experiences pain in flexion and medial rotation of hip joint.

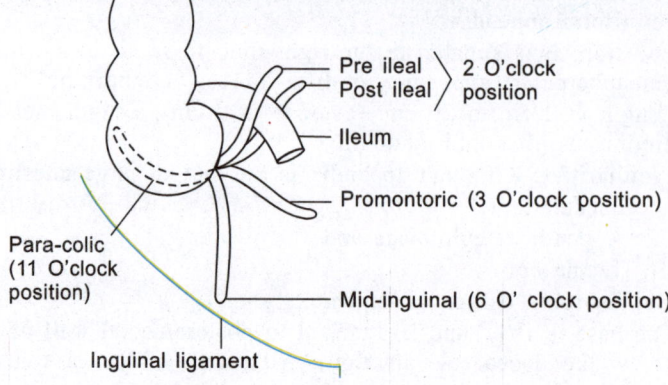

Fig. 2.36 Less common positions of appendix

III. Splenic appendix
    i.   2 O'clock position.
    ii. It is rare position of appendix.
    iii. It presents as pain and tenderness at McBurney's point and haematuria.
    iv. It is most dangerous because infection spreads to the general peritoneal cavity.

C. Internal features:
Appendicular orifice
    a. It is situated on the postero-medial aspect of the caecum 2 cm below the ileocaecal orifice.
    b. It is occasionally guarded by semilunar fold of mucous membrane, known as valve of Gerlach.

D. Relations: Peritoneal relation
Mesoappendix: It is a small triangular fold of peritoneum suspending appendix.

E. Blood Supply:
    a. Arterial: Appendicular artery, a branch of inferior division of ileocolic artery. It gives a recurrent branch, which anastomoses with the posterior caecal artery. It is an end artery, & hence the tip is least vascular.
    b. Venous: Appendicular vein drains into superior mesenteric vein which joins with splenic vein and forms the portal vein.

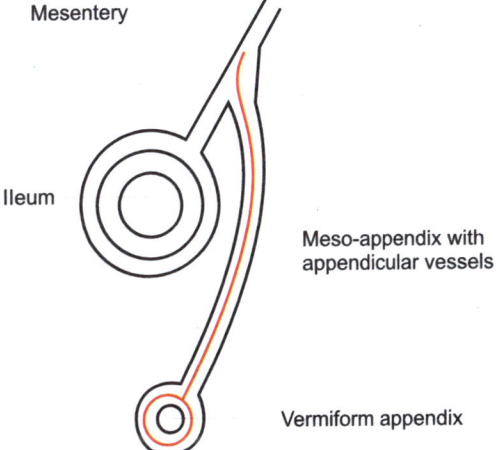

Fig. 2.37 Meso-appendix with appendicular artery

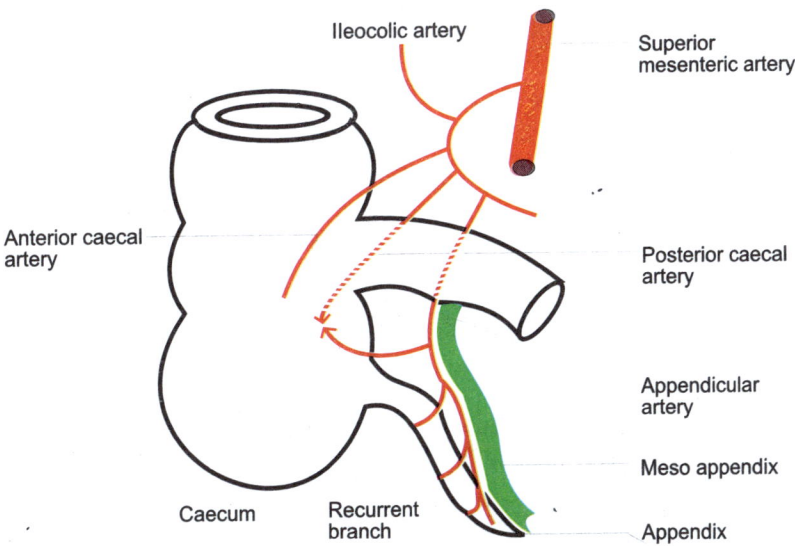

Fig. 2.38 Arteries supplying caecum and appendix

F. · Nerve supply:
    a. Sympathetic nerves are derived from superior mesenteric plexus. Preganglionic fibers come from T_{10} segment. Therefore pain is referred to umbilical region.
    b. Parasympathetic nerve: Vagus.
G. Lymphatic: Superior mesenteric lymph nodes via ileo-colic nodes.

2. **Histology:** Appendix shows four coats from inside to outside which are as follows:
A. Mucosa
    a. Simple columnar epithelium with numerous goblet cells.
    b. Occasional enterochromaffin cells are present.
    c. Absence of villi.
    d. Muscularis mucosae & lamina propria is present. Lamina propria shows lymphatic follicle.
    e. Presence of glands.

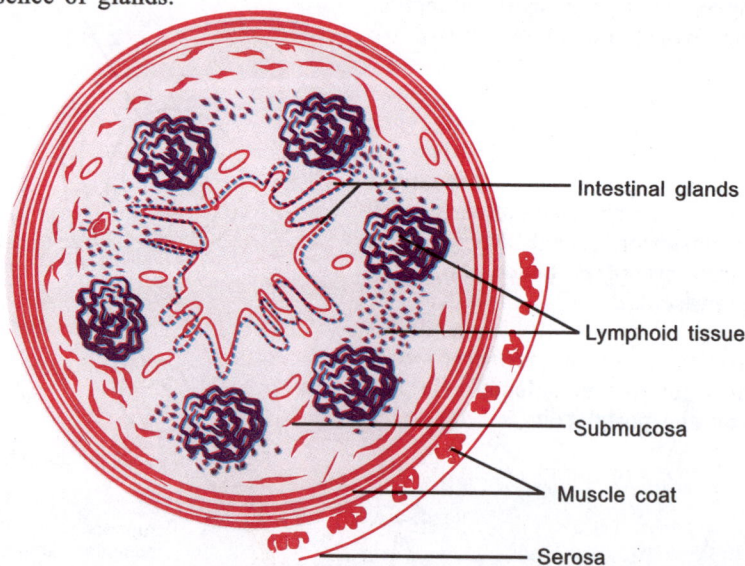

Fig. 2.39 Histology of appendix

B. Submucosa: It shows lymphatic follicle, which are in ring form.
C. Muscularis externa -
    a. Inner circular muscle.
    b. Outer longitudinal muscle.
    Hiatus muscularis is deficient area in muscularis externa.
D. Serosa is derived from peritoneum & covers the entire tube - except the border where mesoappendix is attached. It is lined by simple squamous epithelium.

3. **Development:**
A. Chronological age: It develops in the early eighth week of intrauterine life.
B. Germ layer: Endoderm and mesoderm.
C. Source:
    a. Epithelium and glands develop from lower narrow part of caecal diverticulum, which arise from midgut and is enodermal in origin.
    b. Remaining coats develop from splanchnopleuric mesoderm.

D. Anomalies:

Subhepatic appendix: It creates a problem in diagnosis of subhepatic appendicitis and during the surgical removal of the appendix.

4. **Applied anatomy:**

A. Inflammation of appendix is known as appendicits. It is manifested by Murphy's triad

   a. Pain is first felt at umbilical region because appendix and the skin of the umbilicus are supplies by tenth thoracic segment of spinal cord. It then localizes at right iliac fossa due to local peritonitis. It is associated with the tenderness and rigidity at McBurney's point.

   b. Vomiting.

   c. Temperature because of the infection.

B. Anatomical factors for appendicitis

   a. Appendix is a blind tube. A faecolith may obstruct the lumen and precipitate the attack of appendicitis.

   b. It is supplied by an end artery.

   c. It shows presence of hiatus muscularis.

   d. It shows numerous lymphatic follicle in sub mucosa.

C. In retrocaecal appendix, patient experiences pain on extension of right hip joint due to irritation of right psoas major muscle.

D. In pelvic appendix patient experiences.

   a. Pain on flexion & medial rotation of right hip joint because of the irritation of obturator internus muscle.

   b. Haematuria is due to pressure of inflamed appendix on right ureter.

E. During appendicectomy, appendix can be located by tracing taenia coli, which converges at the base of the appendix.

F. Obstruction of the appendicular artery results into gangrenous appendix.

G. Ilio inguinal nerve supplies lower most fibers of the internal oblique and transversus abdominus muscle. During split muscle incision of appendix operation, ilio inguinal nerve may be damaged resulting into direct inguinal hernia. This is due to paralysis of internal oblique and transversus abdominus muscle.

H. The damage to the ilio inguinal nerve in the inguinal canal does not paralyse the internal oblique and transversus abdominus muscle because the nerve is purely sensory at this site.

I. Appendicitis is less likely in extreme ages. In children, the lumen of the appendix is wide and in old age the lumen gets obliterated.

LAQ-9	**Describe coeliac trunk under**
	1. **Origin,** 2. **Relations,**
	3. **Branches and** 4. **Applied anatomy.**

Introduction: It is the artery of the foregut. It supplies alimentary canal up to the opening of bile duct and its derivatives namely liver, spleen and pancreas.

1. **Origin:** It arises from the front of abdominal aorta just below the aortic opening of the diaphragm. It arises at the level of intervertebral disc present between T_{12} & L_1 vertebra.

2. **Relations:**
   A. Anterior:
      a. Lesser sac and
      b. Lesser omentum.
   B. Right:
      a. Right crus of diaphragm,
      b. Right coeliac ganglion and
      c. The caudate process of liver.
   C. Left:
      a. Left crus of diaphragm,
      b. Left coeliac ganglion and
      c. Cardiac end of the stomach.
   D. Inferior:
      a. Tuber omentale of the pancreas and
      b. Splenic vein.
   E. It is surrounded by coeliac plexus.

3. **Branches:**

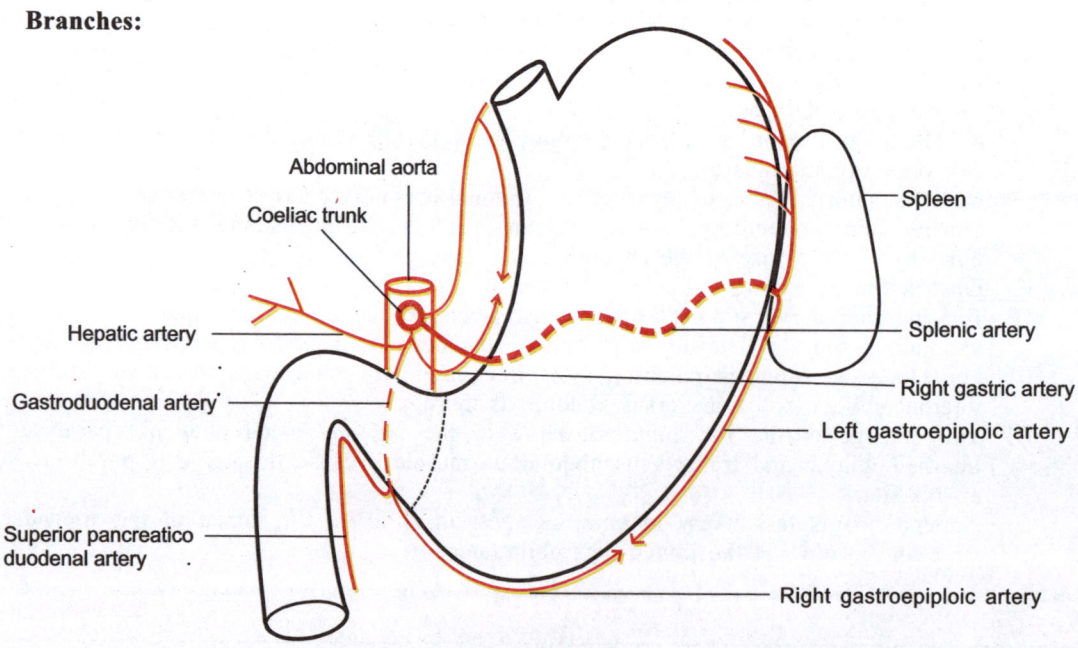

Fig. 2.40 Coeliac trunk & its branches

A. Left gastric artery: *It is the smallest branch of coeliac trunk and supplies the largest area of stomach.* It runs in opposite direction of the hepatic artery. It lies behind the peritoneum and gives an esophageal branch and supplies the lower end of the oesophagus. It runs between two layers of lesser omentum and breaks into two parallel branches, which anastomose with two branches of right gastric artery and distribute the lesser curvature of the stomach.

B. Splenic artery: *It is a largest, very tortuous branch of coeliac trunk.* It lies behind the peritoneum and enters the hilum of the spleen through lieno renal ligament and breaks into five to seven splenic branches. *It is the main source of arterial supply to pancreas.* It gives following branches:

a. Left gastroepiploic artery which runs on the greater curvature and anastomosis with the right gastroepiploic artery. It supplies blood to the greater curvature of the stomach.

b. Short gastric arteries run upward and supply fundus of the stomach.

C. Hepatic artery: It passes over the upper border of pancreas. It runs forward at the opening into the lesser sac. It reaches porta hepatis and divides into right and left branches to supply left and right halves of the liver. It gives following branches.

a. Right gastric artery: It passes between two layers of lesser omentum and divides into two branches, which anastomose with the branches of left gastric artery.

b. Gastro duodenal artery: It passes behind the first part of duodenum and divides into two branches.

I. The right gastroepiploic artery, which runs in the gastrocolic omentum and anastomose with left gastroepiploic artery. It gives branches to the anterior and posterior wall of the stomach along greater curvature.

II. Superior pancreatico duodenal artery: It divides into two branches which encircle the head of pancreas. They anastomose with the inferior pancreatico duodenal artery, a branch of superior mesenteric artery.

4. **Applied anatomy:** obstruction of the common hepatic artery proximal to the right gastric artery may save the liver from necrosis due to an establishment of collateral circulation between the gastric and gastroepiploic arteries. But when the occlusion affects the hepatic artery proper, the liver necrosis is invariable.

LAQ-10	**Describe portal vein under** **1. Formation, 2. Course and relations, 3. Branches,** **4. Tributaries, 5. Porto systemic anastomosis,** **6. Development, 7. Applied anatomy.**

1. **Formation:**

A. General introduction: The portal system consists of all the veins which carry blood from the abdominal part of the alimentary canal except the lower part of the rectum and the whole of the anal canal. It also drains blood from the pancreas, spleen and gall bladder. From all these viscera, blood is carried to the liver via one channel called the portal vein. The blood of the portal system traverses two sets of capillaries. They are as follows:

a. Capillaries in the wall of the gut and other viscera.

b. In the liver it ends in the sinusoids. The blood is collected by central vein and open into hepatic vein which drains into the inferior vena cava.

B. Length: 8 cm.

C. Formation: By the union of

a. Superior mesenteric vein and   ⎱ Behind the neck of pancreas, infront of inferior
b. Splenic vein.   ⎰ vena cava at the level of L_2 vertebra.

2. **Course and relation:**

A. Course: It runs upward and a little to the right, first behind the neck of pancreas, next behind the first part of the duodenum and lastly in the right free margin of lesser omentum.

B. Relations: Relations are described in three parts

Table 2.8 Showing relations of portal vein

	Parts	Anterior	Posterior
a.	Infra duodenal	Neck of pancreas	
b.	Retro duodenal	I. First part of duodenum II. Common bile duct III. Gastro duodenal artery	
c.	Supra duodenal I. Within the lesser omentum.	i. Anterior and to the right: Bile duct. ii. Anterior and to the left: - Hepatic artery. - Hepatic plexus of nerves. - Lymphatics.	Inferior vena cava
	II. At porta hepatic.	i. Right and left hepatic ducts. ii. Right and left branches of hepatic artery. iii. Right and left branches of portal vein.	

3. **Branches:**
   A. Right branch is shorter and wider. It enters the right lobe of liver after receiving cystic vein.
   B. Left branch is longer and narrower than the right. It traverses the porta hepatis from its right end to the left end and gives branches to caudate and quadrate lobes. It receives paraumbilical vein in following ligament.
      a. Ligamentum teres and
      b. Ligamentum venosum.

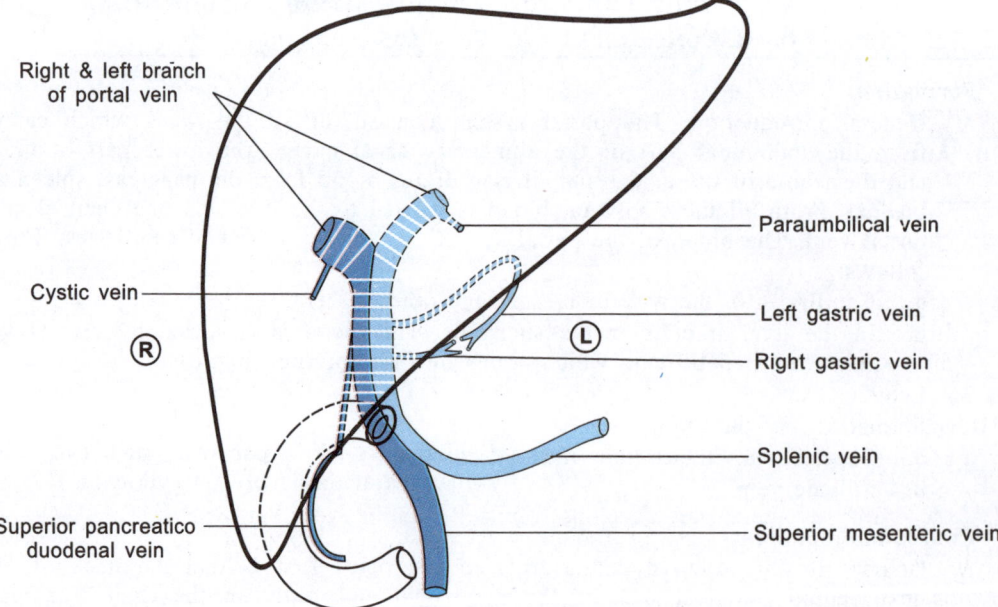

Fig. 2.41 Portal vein and its tributaries

4. **Tributaries:** It receives following veins
   A. At origin
      a. Splenic vein and
      b. Superior mesenteric vein.
   B. From main stem:
      a. Left gastric vein,
      b. Right gastric vein and
      c. Superior pancreatico duodenal vein.
   C. From the right branch: Cystic vein.
   D. From the left branch: Paraumbilical vein.

5. **Porto systemic anastomosis:**

Table 2.9 Showing porto systemic anastomosis.

Site	Branch of portal vein	Branch of systemic vein	Clinical features
A. Abdominal wall a. Anterior (umbilicus)	Left branch of portal vein	Paraumbilical vein.	Caput medusae.

b. Posterior	Veins of the retro peritoneal organs like
	I. Superior mesenteric vein of
	   i. Duodenum,
	   ii. Ascending colon,
	
	II. Inferior mesenteric vein.
	III. Veins of the descending colon.
		Retro peritoneal vein of the abdominal wall, Renal vein.	------

B. Gastro intestinal tract a. Lower end of oesophagus.	Oesophageal tributaries of left gastric vein.	Oesophageal tributaries of accessory hemi azygos vein.	Oesophageal varices and haematemesis.
b. Anal canal	Superior rectal vein.	Middle and inferior rectal vein.	Haemorrhoids or piles
C. Liver a. Bare area of liver.	Hepatic venules	Phrenic and inter costal vein.	------
b. In case of patent ductus venosus	Left branch of portal Vein.	Directly to the inferior vena cava.	------

6. **Development:**
   A. Chronological age: It develops in the second and third month of intrauterine life.
   B. Sources:
      a. Infra duodenal part develops from left vitelline vein between
         I. Joining of splenic vein and superior mesenteric vein.
         II. Dorsal intervitelline anastomosis.
      b. Retro duodenal part develops from dorsal anastomosis between right and left vitelline veins.

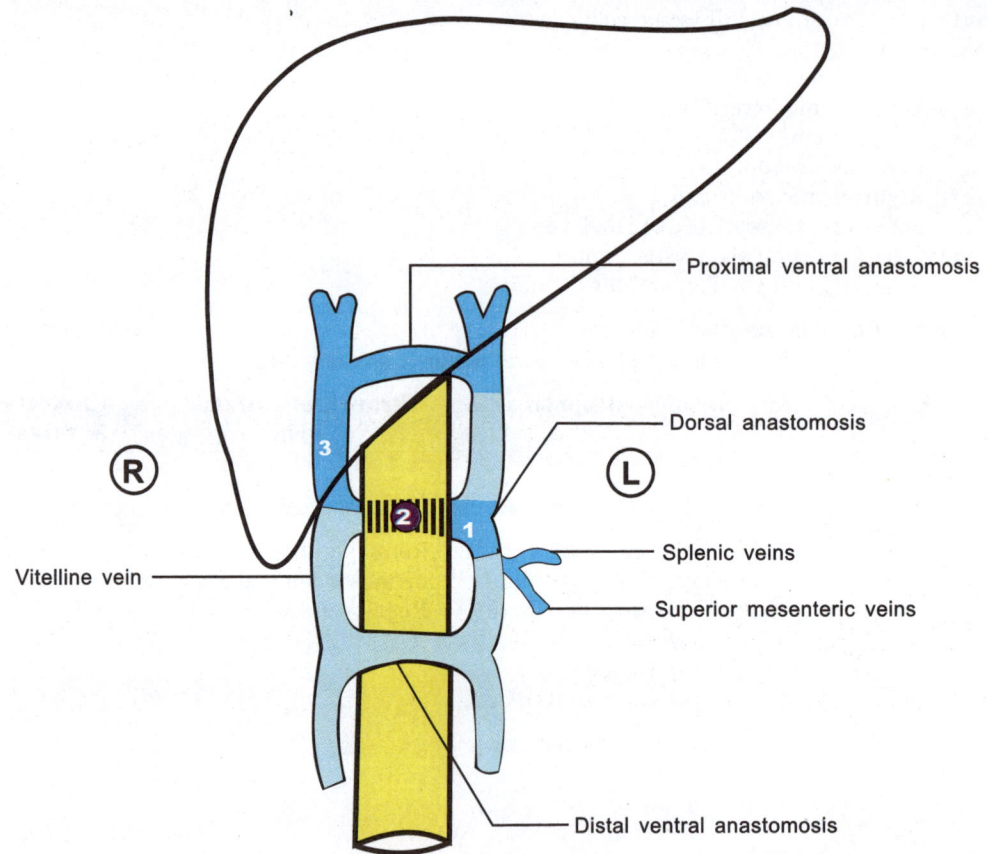

Fig. 2.42 Development of portal vein

    c.   Supra duodenal part develops from right vitelline vein between the cephalic ventral anastomosis and dorsal anastomosis.

    d.   Right branch: From the part of right vitelline vein cephalic to the ventral anastomosis.

    e.   Left branch: From

        I.   Cephalic ventral anastomosis,

       II. Part of the left vitelline vein cephalic to the ventral anastomosis.

7. Applied anatomy:

    A. Portal pressure: Normal pressure in the portal vein about 5 to 15 ml of Hg. It is usually measured by splenic puncture and recording the intra splenic pressure.

    B. Portal hypertension: It is caused by

       a.   Cirrhosis of liver,

       b.   Thrombosis of portal vein.

    C. The effect of portal hypertension are

       a.   Congestive splenomegaly,

       b.   Ascites and

       C.   Collateral circulation through portosystemic anastomosis.

LAQ-11 Describe extrahepatic biliary apparatus under
1. Gross anatomy, 2. Histology of gall bladder & 3. Applied anatomy.

1. Gross anatomy:

A. Introduction:

Parts: Extra hepatic biliary apparatus consists of

a. Right and left hepatic ducts arise from the respective lobes of liver. The arrangement of the structures at porta from posterior to anterior

I. Branches of portal vein,

II. Branches of hepatic artery,

III. Branches of hepatic duct.

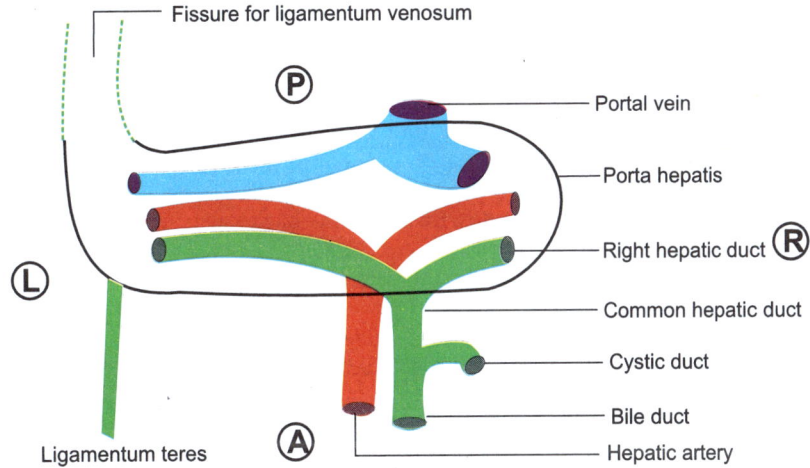

Fig. 2.43 Arrangement of structures in the porta hepatis.

b. Common hepatic duct: It is formed by the union of right and left hepatic ducts near the right end of porta hepatis. It joins the cystic duct and forms the bile duct.

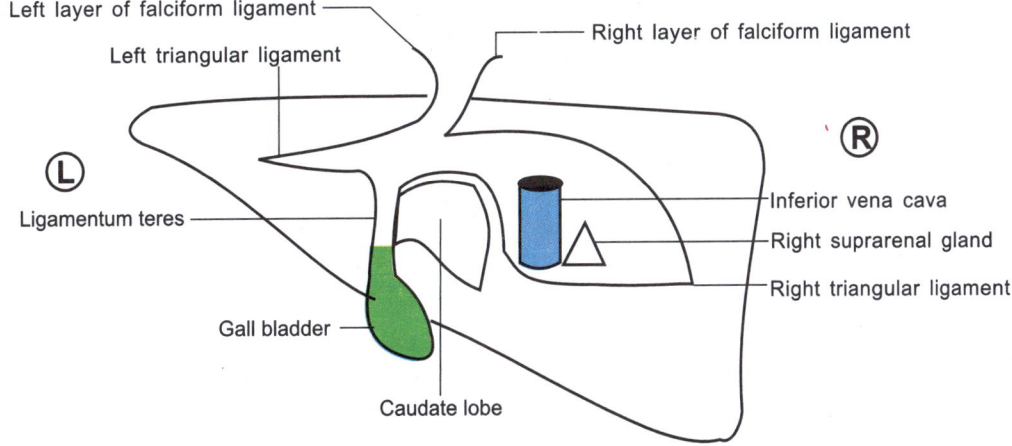

Fig. 2.44 Peritoneal reflection on the inferior surface of liver

c. Gall bladder:
   I. Situation: It is situated on the inferior surface of right lobe of liver.
   II. Shape: Pear shaped.
   III. Measurement:
      i. Length: 7 to 10 cm.
      ii. Breadth is 3 cm at the widest part.
      iii. Capacity is 30 to 50 ml.
   IV. External features
      i. Fundus: Part of the gall bladder below the inferior border of liver.
      ii. Body: Lies in the fossa of the gall bladder of the liver.
      iii. Hartmann's pouch: It is dilated part of gall bladder present in the posteromedial wall of the neck.

d. Cystic duct:
   I. Length: 3 to 4 cm.
   II. Features: Mucous membrane of the cystic duct forms a series of 5 to 12 crescentic folds, arranged spirally to form the spiral valve of Heister. This is not a true valve.

e. Bile duct: It is formed by the union and cystic and common hepatic duct.
   I. Length is 8 cm.
   II. Diameter is 6 mm.
   III. Course : It runs downward and backward in the free margin of lesser omentum.
      i. Comes in contact with pancreatic duct in the middle of second part of duodenum.
      ii. Course of the duct in duodenum is oblique.
      iii. Within the wall, the two ducts unite and form hepatopancreatic ampulla.

B. Relations:
   a. Relations of the parts of gall bladder.

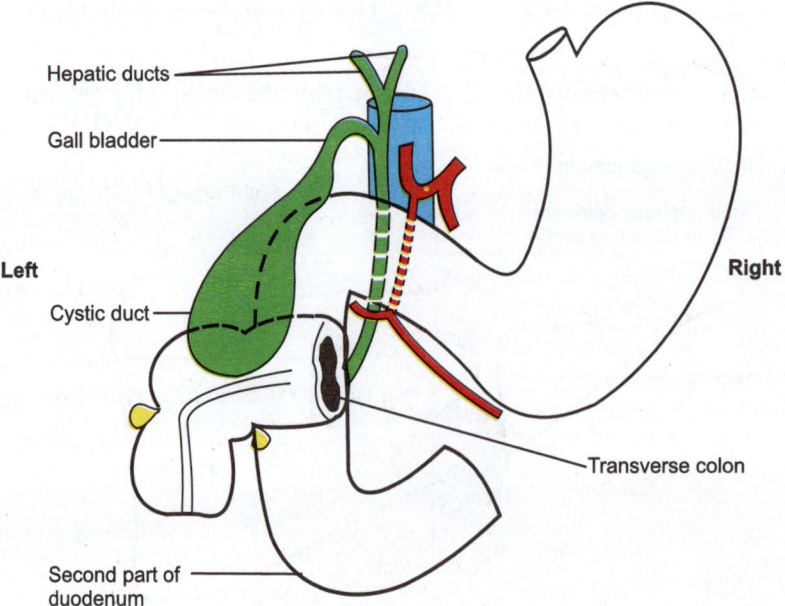

Fig. 2.45 Extrahepatic biliary apparatus

Table 2.10 Showing relations of the parts of gall bladder

Parts	Superior	Inferior	Right	Left	Peritoneum
I. Fundus	Anterior abdominal wall	Transverse colon	Rectus abdominis	9th costal cartilage	Entirely surrounded by peritoneum.
II. Body of gall bladder	Liver	Transverse colon and second part of duodenum.	-	-	Superior surface is devoid of peritoneum. Inferior surface is covered by peritoneum.
III. Neck	Liver with cystic vessels.	1st part of duodenum	-	-	-

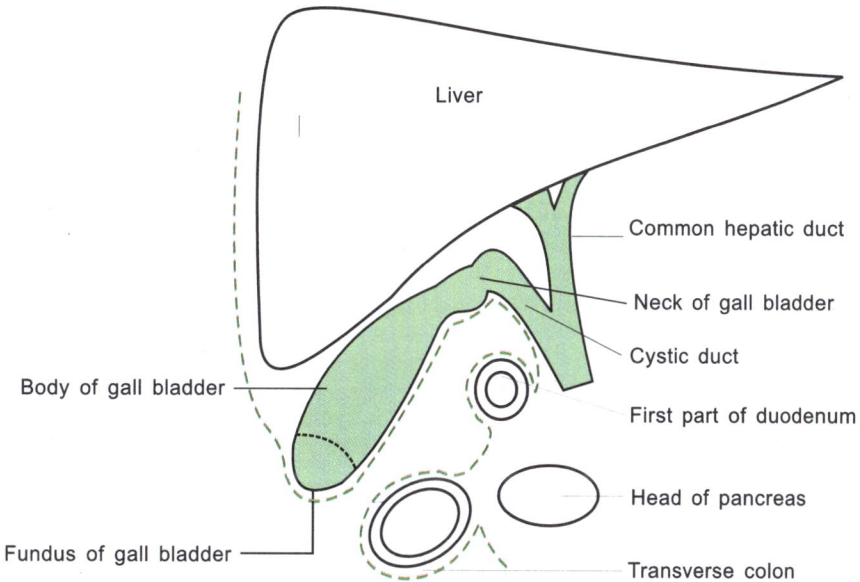

Fig. 6.46 Relations of extrahepatic biliary apparatus

b. Relations of the bile duct

Table 2.11 Showing relations of the bile duct

Part	Anterior	Posterior	Left
Supraduodenal	Liver	Inferior vena cava	Hepatic artery
Retroduodenal	1st part of duodenum	------"------	Gastro duodenal artery.
Infraduodenal	Head of pancreas	------"------	-

C. Blood supply: It is divided into
   a. Arterial supply: It is divided into
      I. Arterial supply of biliary apparatus except lower part of bile duct.
         i.   Cystic artery branch of hepatic artery.
         ii. Artery supplying right hepatic duct.
         iii. An accessory cystic artery branch of common hepatic artery.

    II. Arterial supply of lower part of bile duct: Several branches from superior pancreatico duodenal artery.

b. Venous drainage:It is divided into

    I. Venous drainage of biliary apparatus except lower part of bile duct.

        i. Superior surface of gall bladder drains into hepatic vein, which drains into inferior vena cava.

        ii. Inferior surface of gall bladder drains into veins of hepatic duct, which drains into inferior vena cava.

    II. Lower part of bile duct drains into portal vein.

D. Lymphatic drainage: It is divided into

a. Lymphatic drainage of the biliary apparatus except lower part of bile duct drains into cystic lymph nodes.

b. Lower part of bile duct drains into hepatic and upper pancreatico splenic lymph nodes.

E. Nerve supply:It is divided into

a. Part of the biliary apparatus except lower part of bile duct is by cystic plexus, which is formed by

    I. Vagi,

    II. Phrenic nerve and

    III. Branch from coeliac plexus.

b. Lower part of bile duct is by plexus over superior pancreatico duodenal artery.

    I. Parasympathetic is motor to musculature of gall bladder and bile duct and inhibitory to the sphincters.

    II. Sympathetic nerve is vasomotor and inhibitory to sphincter.

    III. Pain is referred to

        i. The stomach by vagi,

        ii. The right scapular region through sympathetic and

        iii. The right shoulder through right phrenic nerve.

2. Histology of gall bladder:

A. The mucous membrane of the gall bladder is lined by tall columnar epithelium.

B. The mucosa is highly folded.

C. It is characterized by absence of goblet cells and muscularis mucosa.

D. The muscle coat is poorly developed.

E. The serosa is lined by simple squamous epithelium.

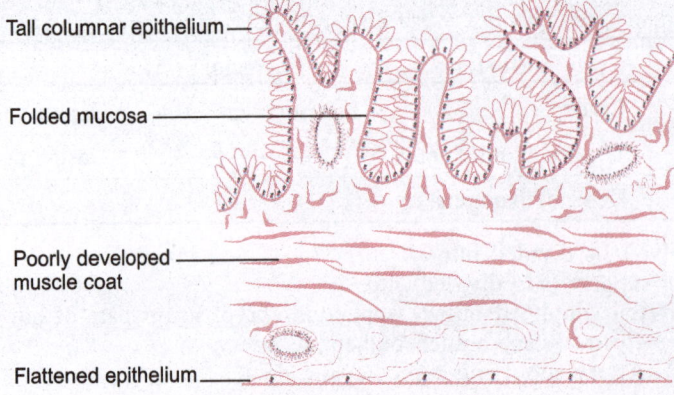

Fig. 2.47 Histology of gall bladder

3. **Applied anatomy:**
   A. Functions of gall bladder can be investigated by cholecystography.
   B. Inflammation of gall bladder is called cholecystitis. This can be diagnosed by the history of pain in the right hypochondrium associated with tenderness during inspiration at the tip of ninth costal cartilage. This is called Murphy's sign.
   C. Presence of gall stones in the gall bladder is called cholelithiasis.
   D. The operation for removal of gall bladder is called cholecystectomy.

LAQ-12	**Describe spleen under**
	1. Gross anatomy, 2. Histology,
	3. Development and 4. Applied anatomy.

1. **Gross anatomy:**
   A. Introduction:
      a. Location: It occupies
         I. Mainly in the left hypochondrium.
         II. Partly in the epigastrium.
      b. Shape: Wedge shaped.
      c. Dimension:
         I. 1″ thick.
         II. 3″ width.
         III. 5″ length.
         IV. 7 ounce (1 ounce = 30gms.) weight.
         V. 9th to 11th ribs are related to the spleen.
      d. Axis: Oblique, downward, forward and laterally.

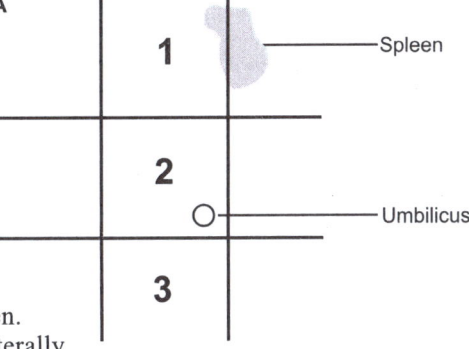

Fig. 2.48 Location of the spleen

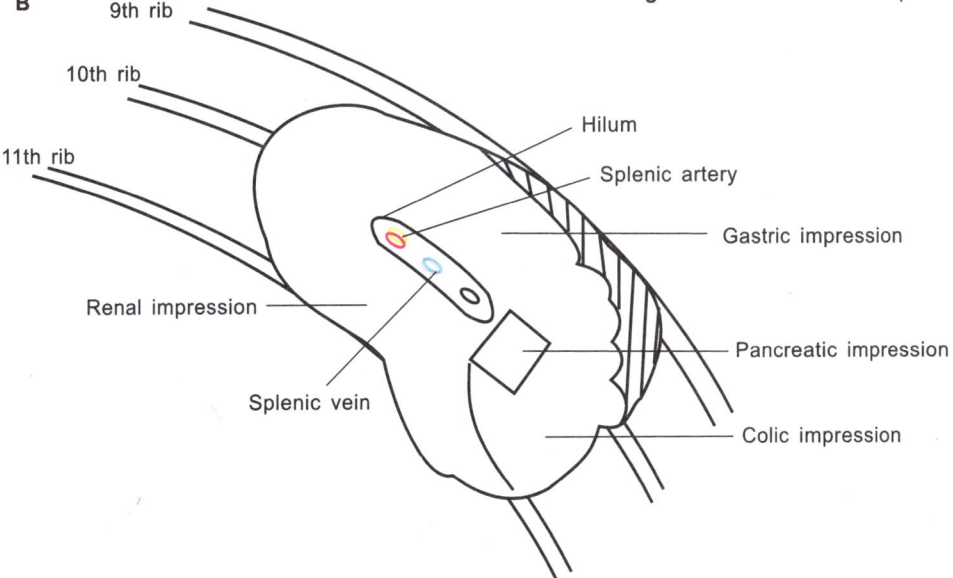

Fig. 2.49 External features of spleen

B. External features:
    a. Two ends.
        I. Anterior end is expanded and reaches mid axillary line.
        II. Posterior end is rounded and rests on the upper pole of left kidney.
    b. Three borders:
        I. Superior border in characteristically notched near the anterior end.
        II. Inferior border is rounded.
        III. Intermediate border is also rounded.
    c. Two surfaces:
        I. Diaphragmatic surface is convex and smooth.
        II. Visceral surface is concave and irregular. It is occupied by many impressions.
            i. Gastric impression for the fundus of the stomach which is largest.
            ii. Renal impression for the left kidney. It lies between inferior and intermediate border.
            iii. Colic impression for the splenic flexure.
            iv. Tail of pancreas.
        III. Hilum: It lies on the inferomedial part of gastric impression along the long axis of the spleen.
C. Relations:
    a. Peritoneal relations: Spleen is surrounded by peritoneum and is suspended by following ligaments -
        I. Gastro splenic ligament,
        II. Lieno renal ligament and
        III. Phrenico colic ligament.
    b. Visceral relations:
        I. Diaphragmatic surface.
        II. Visceral surface is related to
            i. Fundus of the stomach,
            ii. Anterior surface of the left kidney,
            iii. Splenic flexure of the colon and
            iv. Tail of the pancreas.
D. Blood supply:
    a. Arterial supply: Splenic artery is a largest tortuous artery which breaks into 5 to 7 branches and passes through the lieno renal ligament to supply vascular segment of the spleen.
    b. Venous drainage: It is drained by splenic vein which is formed at the hilum of the spleen. It joins the superior mesenteric vein behind the neck of pancreas and forms the portal vein.
E. Nerve supply: They are derived from coeliac plexus. They are mainly sympathetic in nature and are vasomotor in function. They also supply smooth muscle present in the capsule.
F. Lymphatic drainage: The splenic tissue has no lymphatics. A few lymphatics arise from the connective tissue of the capsule and trabeculae and drain into the pancreatico splenic group of lymph nodes, situated along the splenic artery.

2. **Histology:** The section of the spleen shows:
A. Serous coat, which is lined by simple squamous epithelium.
B. Fibro-elastic coat consists of
    a. Fibrous coat: It sends trabeculae projecting into the substance of the spleen and branches to form a network.

b. Elastic fibers are present in the capsule and trabeculae. These fibers bring contraction and relaxation of the spleen.

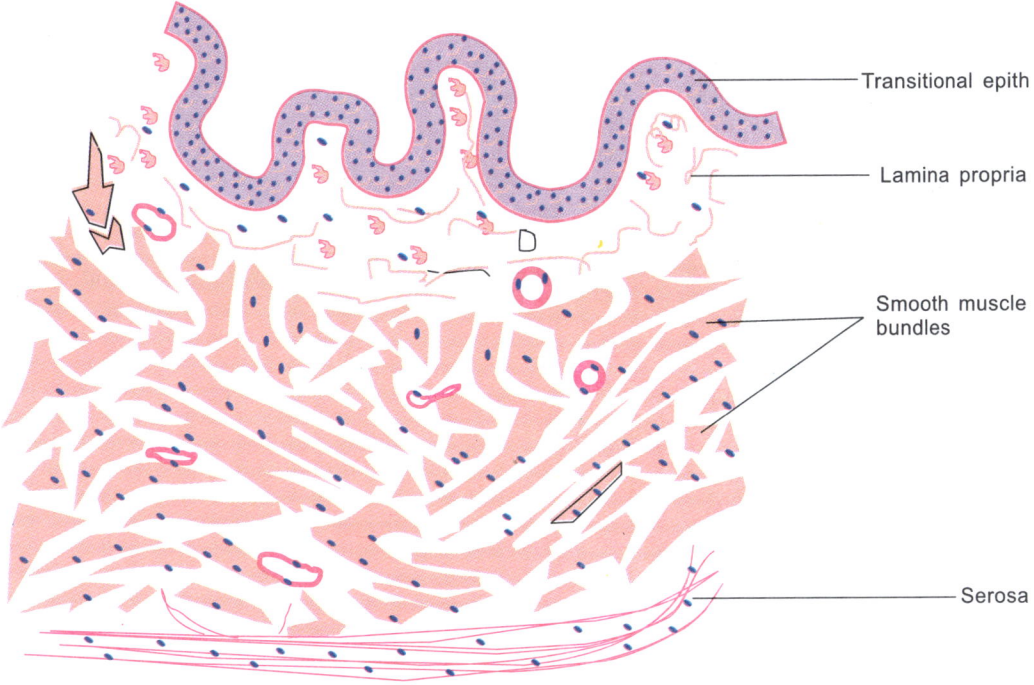

Transitional epith

Lamina propria

Smooth muscle bundles

Serosa

Fig. 2.50 Urinary bladder

C. Splenic pulp: It is of two types depending upon the type of blood cells.
   a. Red pulp
      I. It is scattered through out the organ.
      II. It is supported by reticular network.
      III. It is composed of
         i. Element of blood,
         ii. Debris of RBC,
         iii. Macrophages and
         iv. Reticulo endothelial cells.
   b. White pulp:
      I. These are collection of lymphoid tissue, which are precursors of lymphocytes in the blood.
      II. The very striking point is an eccenteric arteriole, a branch of trabecular artery surrounded by lymphocytes.
      III. Germinal center may be seen.

3. Development:
   A. Chronological age: It develops in the fifth week of intrauterine life.
   B. Germ layer: Mesoderm.
   C. Site: Dorsal mesogastrium near the posterior wall.
   D. Sources: Spleen is derived from the dorsal mesogastrium, <u>not from the gut tube endoderm</u>.

            a.   Mesencymal cells,
            b.   Cells of the coelomic epithelium.
       E.   Anomalies:
            a.   Abnormal formation: Accessory spleen.
            b.   Abnormal site:
                 I.   In the derivatives of the dorsal mesogastrium
                      i.   Gastrophrenic ligament,
                      ii.   Lienorenal ligaments,
                      iii. Greater omentum.
                 II. In the broad ligament
                 III. In the spermatic cord.
            c.   Spleen develop as splenic lobules, which combine together and form adult spleen.
                 However the superior border fails to fuse, hence it demonstrates notch of the
                 superior border.

4.   **Applied anatomy:**
     A.   Palpation of the spleen: Normally spleen is not palpable. It is palpable when it is
          enlarged to about twice its normal size. The slightly enlarged spleen can be palpated in
          the left lateral position.
     B.   Splenomegaly: Enlargement of spleen is called splenomegaly. It projects towards the
          right iliac fossa in the direction of the axis of the 10th rib.
     C.   Splenectomy: The surgical removal of the spleen is called splenectomy.
     D.   Splenic laceration: The spleen can be lacerated by a fractured rib. The laceration of this
          vascular organ is a fatal condition. Immediately splenectomy is sometimes indicated.
     E.   During splenectomy, tail of the pancreas should be sought first, before putting ligatures
          to the pedicles of the spleen.

LAQ-13 Describe liver under
1. Gross anatomy,   2. Histology,
3. Development and   4. Applied anatomy.

1.   **Gross anatomy:**
     A.   Introduction:
          a.   General introduction: It is the largest mixed
               gland in the body.
          b.   Location: It is situated in the right upper
               quadrant of the abdominal cavity. It
               occupies
               I.   Whole of the right hypochondrium.
               II.   Greater part of epigastrium.
               III. Left hypochondrium.
          c.   Shape: Wedge shaped.
          d.   Dimension:
               Weight: About 1500 gms.
     B.   External features: 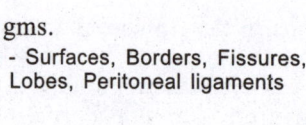 **5** - Surfaces, Borders, Fissures,
          a.   **Five** surfaces: Lobes, Peritoneal ligaments
               I.   Superior,
               II.   Inferior,

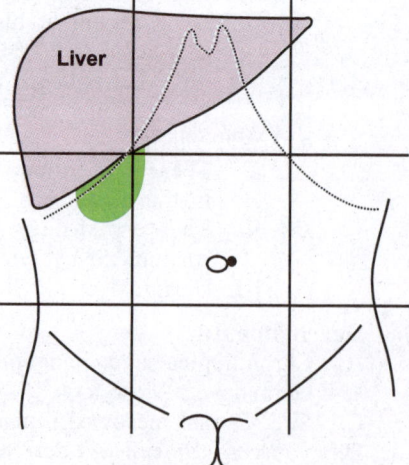

Fig. 2.51 Location of the liver

    III. Anterior,

    IV. Posterior and

    V. Right lateral.

b. **Five** borders: They are ill defined except inferior border which is well defined.

c. **Five** fissures:

    I. Fissure for ligamentum teres,

    II. Fissure for ligamentum venosum,

    III. Groove for inferior vena cava,

    IV. Fossa for gall bladder and

    V. Porta hepatis.

d. **Five** lobes: ,

    I. Anatomical right and left lobes: The liver is divided by a line extending from falciform ligament to the ligamentum teres, which divides into anatomical right and left lobe.

    II. **P**hysiological right and left lobes: It is separated by the **c**holecysto **v**enacaval line into physiological right and left lobe. **PVC**

    III. Caudate lobe.

    IV. Quadrate lobe.

    V. Riedel's lobe: Sometimes a tongue like projection arises from the lower border of liver called as Riedel's lobe. It extends below the right costal margin.

e. **Five** peritoneal ligaments:

    I. Falciform ligament.

    II. Coronary ligament.

    III. Right triangular ligament.

    IV. Left triangular ligament.

    V. Lesser omentum.

C. Relations:

a. Peritoneal relation: Most of the liver is covered by peritoneum except bare areas.

    Bare area: There are five bare areas.

    I. The bare area,

    II. Groove for inferior vena cava,

    III. Porta hepatis,

    IV. Fossa for gall bladder and

    V. Triangular area on the superior surface between two layers of falciform ligaments.

b. Visceral relation:

    I. Anterior surface: It is related to

        i. Xiphoid process,

        ii. Anterior abdominal wall and

        iii. The diaphragm.

    II. Posterior surface: It is triangular. It is related to

        i. Vertebral column,

        ii. The diaphragm,

        iii. Right suprarenal gland,

        iv. Inferior vena cava and

        v. Oesophagus.

III. Superior surface: It is quadrilateral and is related to
  i. Heart and
  ii. The dome of the diaphragm.
IV. Inferior surface:
  i. It is occupied by porta hepatis which is H shaped.
  ii. Right limb of the H is formed by inferior vena cava and gall bladder. Left limb of the H is formed by ligamentum venosum and ligamentum teres.
  iii. Cross piece of H is formed by portal vein and hepatic artery.
  iv. In porta hepatis the relations are (from posterior to anterior) as follows:
    - Portal vein,
    - Hepatic artery and 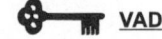 VAD
    - Hepatic duct.
    The other structures related to inferior surface are
    - Lesser omentum,
    - Impression for gall bladder,
    - Right suprarenal gland,
    - Right colic flexure.
V. Right lateral surface:
  i. Lower 1/3rd: Ribs and the diaphragm.
  ii. Middle 1/3rd: Ribs, pleura and the diaphragm. } separated from rib & pleura by diaphragm
  iii. Upper 1/3rd: Ribs, pleura, lung and the diaphragm.
D. Blood supply:
  A. Arterial supply: The liver receives blood from two sources.
    I. The oxygenated blood or arterial blood is received by hepatic artery which divides into right and left branches in the porta hepatis. The division is Y shaped in contrast to the T shaped division of portal vein.
    II. Venous blood is carried to the liver by portal vein which is divided in the porta hepatis into right and left branches which in turn gives segmental branches like the arteries. This portal vein carries the products of digestion which are absorbed from the alimentary canal which gets metabolized in the liver.
        There is no communication between right and left halves of the liver. Even the arteries are end arteries within the each half of the liver. Hence the left lobe shows toxic changes in ingested liver poison. The left lobe shows cirrhotic changes.
  b. Venous drainage: It is different from the arterial supply, there is mixing of the venous blood of right and left halves of the liver. Three main hepatic veins drain into the inferior vena cava. The veins have no extra hepatic course.
E. Nerve supply:
  a. Sympathetic fibers arise from the coeliac ganglion. They run with the vessels in the free edge of lesser omentum and enter the porta hepatis.
  b. Parasympathetic fibers arise from vagus nerve.
  The above nerves form hepatic plexus in porta hepatis.
F. Lymph drainage: Lymphatics of the liver drain into 3 or 4 hepatic nodes in the porta hepatis. They drain downwards along the hepatic artery to the retro pyloric nodes and to the coeliac nodes. The lymphatics from the bare area drain into extra peritoneal lymphatics which perforate the diaphragm and drain to the nodes in the posterior mediastinum.

2. **Histology:**
   A. The liver is made up of liver cells (hepatocytes) arranged in the form of hexagonal areas called hepatic lobules.
   B. The lobules are separated by the connective tissue.
   C. Each lobule has a central vein and shows numerous sinusoids between the cords of hepatocytes.
   D. Between the lobules there are areas filled by connective tissue which contain
      a. A branch of portal vein,
      b. A branch of hepatic artery and
      c. Inter lobular bile duct.
   E. There are phagocytic cells called Kuffer cells in the walls of sinosoids.

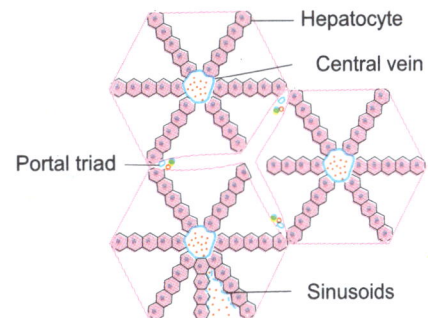

Fig. 2.52 Hepatic lobule

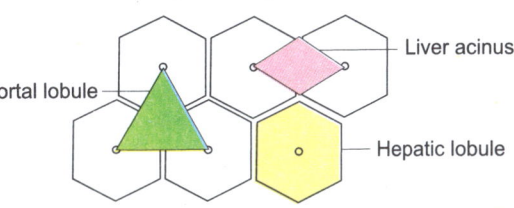

Fig. 2.53 Liver lobule & liver acinus

3. **Development:**
   A. Chronological age: It develops in the fourth week of intra uterine life.
   B. Germ layer: Epithelium develops from endoderm and remaining structure develops from mesoderm.
   C. Site: It develops in the ventral mesogastrium and septum transversum.
   D. Source:
      a. It arises as hepatic bud at the junction of foregut and midgut.
      b. It develops from an endodermal bud which arises from the ventral aspect of the gut, (at the junction of foregut and midgut).
      c. It grows into the ventral mesogastrium and passes through it into the septum transversum.

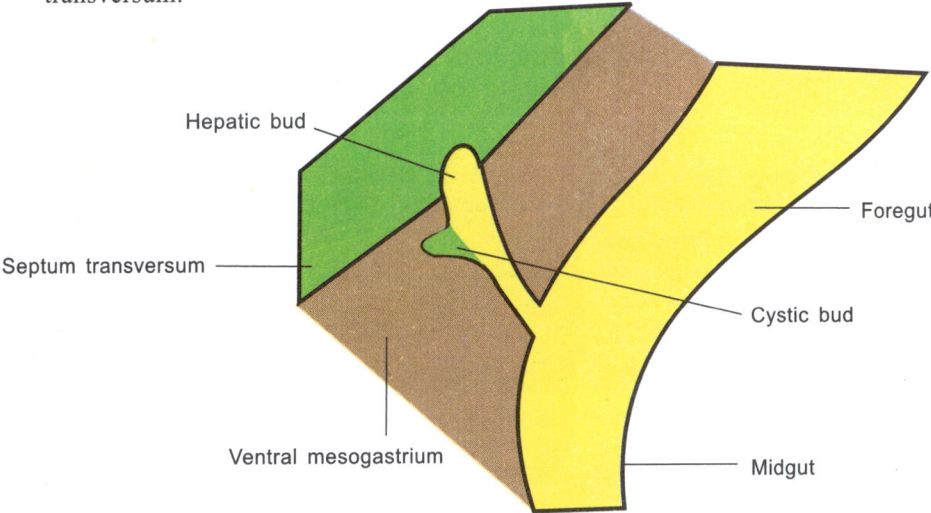

Fig. 2.54 Development of liver

d. The endodermal cells of the hepatic bud give rise to parenchyma of the liver and to bile capillaries.

e. The mesoderm of the septum transversum forms the capsule and fibrous tissue of the liver.

E. Anomalies:

    a. Rudimentary left lobe,   b. Anomalous lobulation,   c. Reidel's lobe,

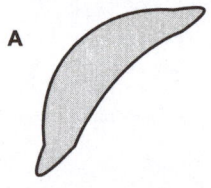 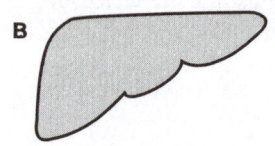 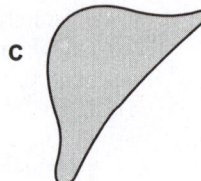

    d. Absence of quadrate lobe with absence of gall bladder.   E. Accessory liver in falciform ligament.

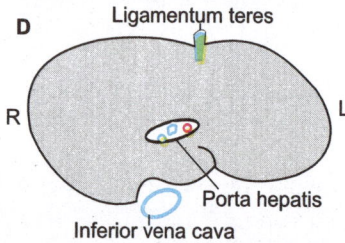

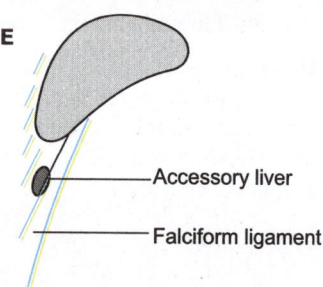

Fig. 2.55 (A, B, C, D & E) Anomalies of liver

4. Applied anatomy:

A. The ligation of right and left hepatic artery does not usually lead to infarction of the liver. This is because about 75% of total hepatic blood flow is derived from portal vein and only remaining 25% comes form hepatic artery.

B. The right lobe of liver is susceptible for toxic changed in cases of ingested liver poisons and left lobe for cirrhosis in deficiencies of substances like choline and methionine.

C. Inflammation of the liver is referred to as hepatitis.

D. Under certain conditions liver tissue undergoes fibrosis and shrinks. This is called cirrhosis of the liver.

SAQ-9   The bare area

It is a largest non peritoneal area on the posterior surface of the right lobe. It is triangular and presents following boundaries.

1. **Apex:** Right triangular ligament.

2. **Base:** Groove for inferior vena cava.

3. **Upper** and lower limits are formed by superior and inferior layers of coronary ligaments.

LAQ-14   Describe head of pancreas under
1. Gross anatomy,   2. Histology,
3. Development and   4. Applied anatomy.

1. **Gross anatomy:**
   A. Introduction:

   Situation: It is situated in the C shaped curvature formed by 1st, 2nd, and 3rd part of duodenum.

   B. External features:
   - a. One Process: Uncinate process.
   - b. Two Surfaces:
     - I. Anterior and
     - II. Posterior.
   - c. Three Borders:
     - I. Superior,
     - II. Inferior and
     - III. Right lateral.

   C. Relations:
   - a. Peritoneal:
     - I. Upper part of the anterior surface is nonperitoneal and related with transverse colon.
     - II. Lower part is covered with peritoneum which is derived from the inferior layer of transverse mesocolon and is related with coils of jejunum.
     - III. Posterior surface is nonperitoneal.
   - b. Visceral:
     - I. Uncinate process:
       - i. Anteriorly: Superior mesenteric vessels.
       - ii. Posteriorly: Abdominal aorta.
     - II. Surfaces:
       - i. Anterior surface
         - Near the middle: Transverse colon separated by areolar tissue.
         - Above transverse colon: Overlapped by first part of duodenum.
         - Below transverse colon: Coils of jejunum.
       - ii. Posterior surface
         - Inferior vena cava.
         - Bile duct: Runs downwards and to the right, embedded in the substance of pancreas.
         - Right crus of diaphragm.
         - Terminal part of renal veins.
         - Right middle suprarenal artery.
         - Right sympathetic trunk.
         - Bodies of L_1, L_2 vertebrae with intervertebral discs.
     - III. Borders:
       - i. Superior border:
         - First part of duodenum and
         - Superior pancreatico duodenal vessels.
       - ii. Inferior border
         - Third part of duodenum and
         - Inferior pancreatico duodenal vessels.

   iii. Right lateral border
- Second part of duodenum,
- Terminal part of bile duct,
- Anastomosis between superior and inferior pancreatico duodenal vessels and
- Pancreatico duodenal lymph nodes.

D. Blood supply:
  a. Arterial supply
    I. Superior pancreaticoduodenal artery, one of the terminal branch division of the gastroduodenal artery.
    II. Inferior pancreaticoduodenal artery, a branch of the superior mesenteric artery.

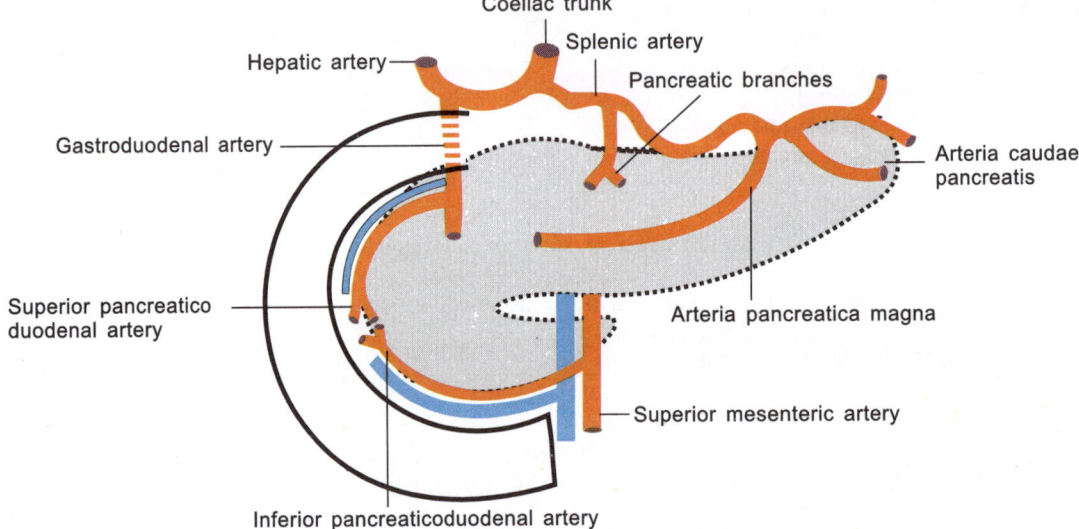

Fig. 2.56 Arterial supply of the pancreas.

  b. Venous drainage:
    I. Superior pancreatico duodenal vein drains into the portal vein.
    II. Inferior pancreatico duodenal vein drains into the superior mesenteric vein.

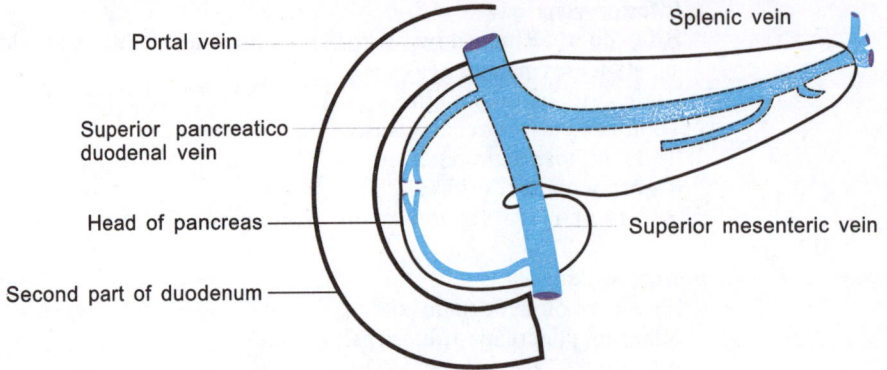

Fig. 2.57 Venous drainage of head of pancreas

E. Nerve supply:
    a. Sympathetic nerve: They are derived from coeliac and superior mesenteric plexus. They are vasomotor in function.
    b. Parasympathetic: They are derived from vagus nerve. They control pancreatic secretion.
F. Lymphatic Drainage:
    a. The lymphatic of the upper part of the head drains into coeliac group of lymph node.
    b. The lower part of the head and the uncinate process drains into the superior mesenteric group of pre-aortic lymph nodes.

2. **Histology:** It is lobulated gland, composed of endocrine and exocrine parts.
    A. The exocrine part shows:
        a. Very few ducts.
        b. The basal part of the cell of the alveolus is deeply stained and basophilic.
        c. The area near the lumen of the cell is stained less heavily and is acidophilic.
        d. The nuclei are large, deeply stained situated in the basal part of each cell.
        e. The ducts are lined by simple columnar epithelium.

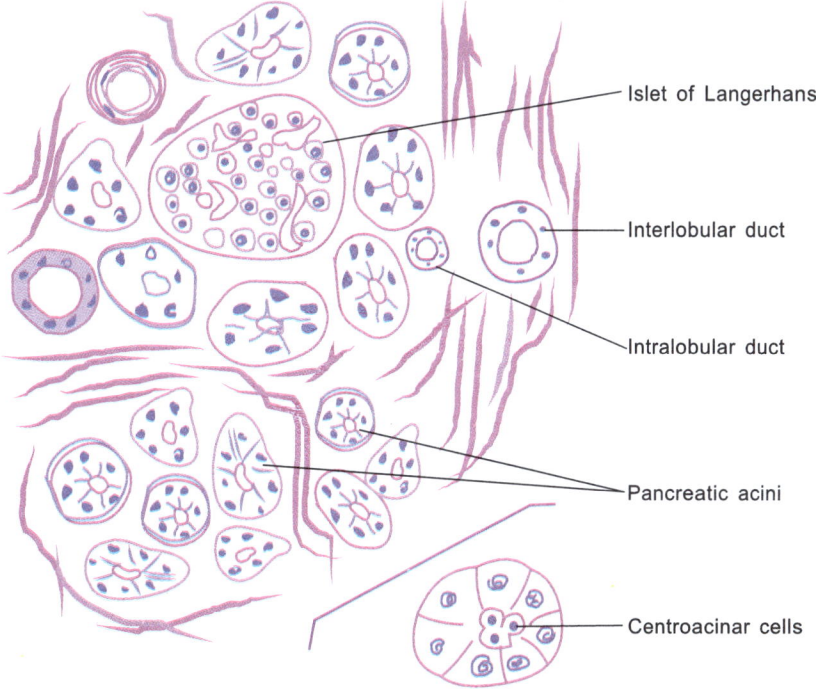

Islet of Langerhans

Interlobular duct

Intralobular duct

Pancreatic acini

Centroacinar cells

Fig. 2.58 Histology of the pancreas.

B. The endocrine part shows:
    a. The islets of Langerhans are scattered in the deeply stained pancreatic tissue.
    b. They vary in size, and diameter.
    c. They are composed of tightly packed mixture of acidophilic and basophilic small round cells.
    d. β cells of the islets of Langerhan produce insulin and a cells produce glucagon.

3. **Development:**
   A. Chronological age: It develops in the fourth to eighth week of intrauterine life.
   B. Germ layer: Endoderm and mesoderm.
   C. Site: It develops as ventral and dorsal pancreatic bud, at the junction of foregut and midgut.
   D. Sources:
      a. The ventral pancreatic bud forms
         I.   The main pancreatic duct.
         II. The uncinate process.
         III. Lower part of the head of pancreas.
      b. The dorsal pancreatic bud forms
         I. Accessory pancreatic duct and
         II. The remaining part of head of pancreas not formed by ventral bud.
   E. Anomalies:
      a. Annular pancreas: Encircles the 2nd part of duodenum (may cause duodenal obstruction). The right part of the ventral bud migrates along the normal route but the left part migrates in an opposite direction. In this manner the duodenum becomes completely surrounded by pancreatic tissue, and an annular pancreas is formed.
      b. Accessory pancreatic tissue: It is formed in the walls of the stomach, small intestine, gall bladder or spleen. This is a common finding.
      c. Inversion of the pancreatic duct: The accessory pancreatic duct is larger than main duct.

4. **Applied anatomy:**
   A. The carcinoma of the head of pancreas is common. The 80% of the pancreatic carcinoma are located in the head. The prognosis for recovery is usually poor because metastases may spread widely along the retro peritoneal lymph channels. It presents as the obstructive jaundice. It is due to the obstruction of bile duct or hepato pancreatic ampulla.
   B. The acute pancreatitis is secondary to complication of mumps.
   C. Pain of pancreatic origin is referred to T_6 - T_{10} dermatomes. However involvement of the local parietal peritoneum causes a severe intense pain in the middle of the back.

LAQ-15 — Describe kidney under following head
1. Gross anatomy, 2. Histology,
3. Development and 4. Applied anatomy.

1. **Gross anatomy:**
   A. Introduction:
      a. General introduction: Kidneys are the paired of excretory organs present behind the peritoneum in lumbar region.
      b. Shape: Bean shape.
      c. Location: Kidneys are present in the epigastric, hypogastric, lumbar and umbilical region.
      d. Extent: They extend from upper border of vertebra T_{12} to the center of vertebra L_3. Left kidney is slightly higher level than the right kidney.

e. Dimension: 1, 2, 3, 4, 5
  I. Thickness: **1**".
  II. Width: **2**".
  III. Length: **4**".
  IV. Weight: **5** ounce i.e.150 gm.

B. **External features:**
  Coverings: There are three coverings.
  a. Fibrous capsule (true capsule): The fibrous capsule is a thin membrane, which closely invests the kidney and lines the renal sinus. Normally it can be easily stripped off from the kidney, but in certain diseases it becomes adherent and cannot be stripped.
  b. Fatty layer: Perirenal (perinephric) fat. This is a layer of adipose tissue lying outside the fibrous capsule. It is thickest at the borders.
  c. Fascial layer (false capsule): Renal fascia has anterior and posterior layer. Anterior layer is called fascia of Toldt and posterior layer is called fascia of Zukerkandl. Following is the fate of these layers.

Fig. 2.59 Superior reflection of renal fascia

Table 2.12 Fate of renal fascia of the kidney

Particulars	Anterior	Posterior
Medially	Merges with connective tissue around aorta and inferior vena cava.	I. Fascia covering quadratus lumborum & psoas major. II. Vertebrae. III. Intervertebral disc.
Inferiorly	Extra peritoneal connective tissue.	Fascia iliacus.
Laterally	Merges with fascia transversalis.	
Superiorly	Fuses and splits to enclose suprarenal gland & continues as diaphragmatic fascia.	

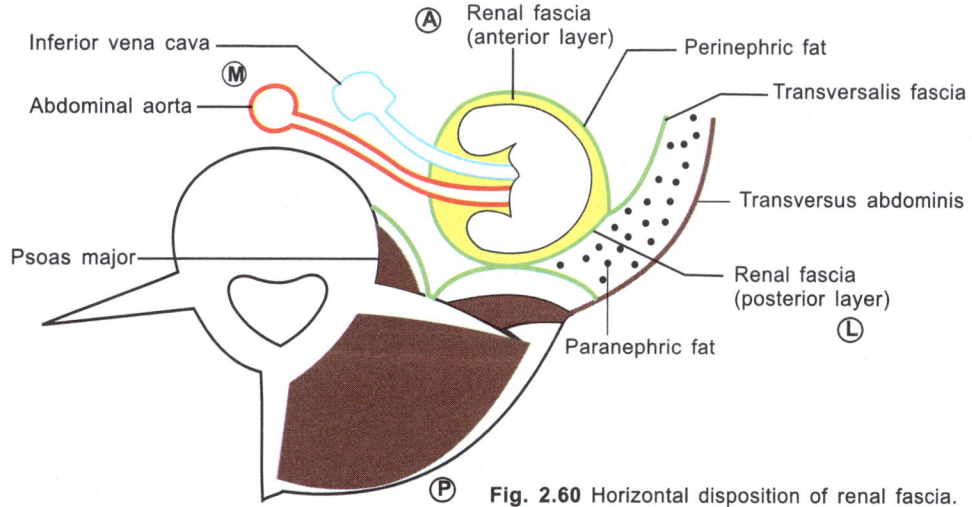

Fig. 2.60 Horizontal disposition of renal fascia.

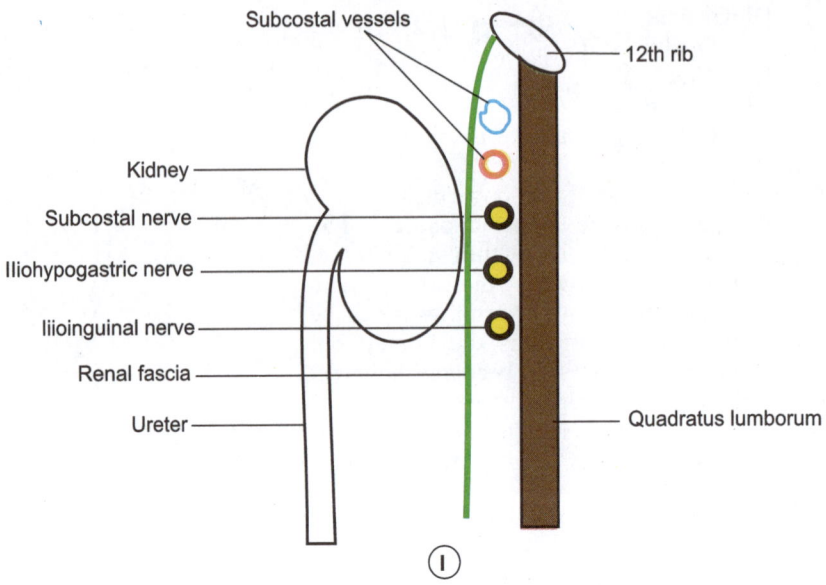

Fig. 2.61 Vertical disposition of renal fascia.

C. Relations of right kidney:
    a. Peritoneal relations:
        I.   Anterior surface is partially covered with peritoneum.
        II. Posterior surface is entirely non-peritoneal.
    b. Visceral relations:
        I.   Anterior surface:
            i.   Right adrenal gland,
            ii. Liver,
            iii. Hepatic flexure,
            iv. Second part of duodenum and
            v. Jejunum.

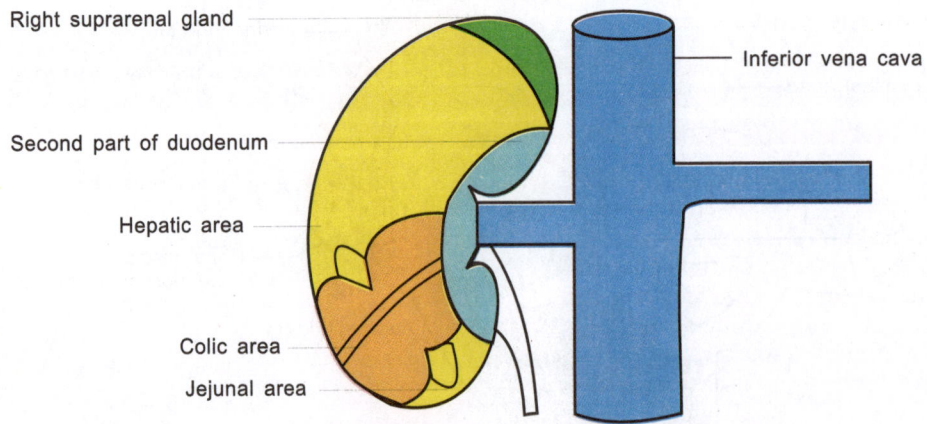

Fig. 2.62 Anterior relations of right kidney

II. Posterior surface: Costo diaphragmatic recess of the pleura is most important relation on the posterior surface.

i. **1** bone: 12th rib. 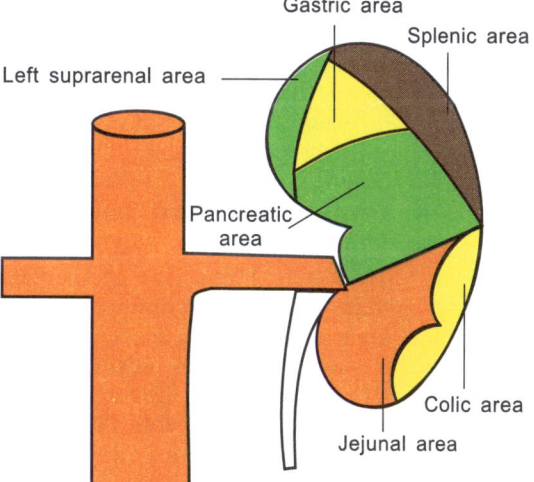 **1**, **2**, **3**, **4**

ii. **2** vessels:
- Subcostal vessels and
- Fourth lumbar artery.

iii. **3** nerves:
- Ilio hypogastric,
- Ilio inguinal and
- Subcostal.

iv. **4** muscles:
- Psoas major,
- Quadrtus lumborum,
- Transversus abdominis and
- The diaphragm.

III. Medial border:
i. Inferior vena cava and
ii. Ureter.

IV. Lateral border:
i. Liver and
ii. Ascending colon.

D. Relations of left kidney:
a. Peritoneal relations:
I. Anterior surface is partially covered with peritoneum.
II. Posterior surface is entirely non-peritoneal.

b. Visceral relations:
I Anterior surface:
i. Adrenal gland,
ii. Splenic flexure,
iii. Pancreas,
iv. Stomach and
v. Jejunum.

II. Posterior surface: Costo diaphragmatic recess of the pleura is most important relation on the posterior surfac surface.
i. 1 Artery: Subcostal.
ii. 2 bones:
- Eleventh rib and
- Twelfth ribs.
iii. 3 nerves:
- Ilio hypogastric,
- Ilio inguinal and
- Subcostal.
iv. 4 muscles:
- Psoas major,
- Quadratus lumborum,
- Transversus abdominis and
- The diaphragm.

Fig. 2.63 Anterior relations of left kidney

III. Medial border: Duodenojejunal flexure, inferior mesenteric vein, adrenal gland and ureter.

IV. Lateral border:
  i.   Descending colon.
  ii. Spleen.

E. Blood Supply:
  a. Arterial supply: The wide bored renal arteries supply the arterial blood to the kidney at a flow of 1 liter per minute.

   I. Renal artery: It is a branch of abdominal aorta which arises at the level of inter vertebral disc between L_1, L_2. It enters the hilum and divides into

      i. Anterior trunk which sub-divides into four segmental arteries
         - Apical,
         - Upper,
         - Anterior upper &
         - Lower.

      ii. Posterior trunk continues as posterior segmental artery. Segmental artery divides into lobar branches.
         - Interlobar arteries,
         - Arcuate arteries and
         - Interlobular arteries.
      There is no collateral circulation between the segmental arteries.

   II. Sometimes an accessory renal artery arises from the abdominal aorta and supplies upper or lower pole of the kidney.

  b. Venous drainage: Veins form the renal segments and communicate with one another unlike the arteries.

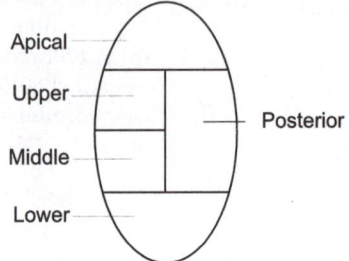

Fig. 2.64 The vascular segments of kidney as seen in a sagittal section.

Apical
Upper
Posterior
Middle
Lower

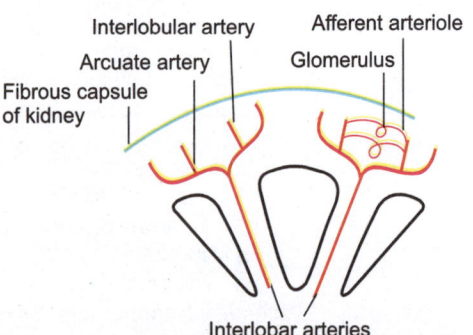

Interlobular artery
Arcuate artery
Afferent arteriole
Glomerulus
Fibrous capsule of kidney
Interlobar arteries

Fig. 2.65 Arrangement of the arteries in the kidney.

Ultimately forms five or six vessels that unite at the hilum to form a single renal vein. Renal veins drain into inferior vena cava. Left renal vein is longer than the right renal vein. It receives left gonadal and left suprarenal veins.

F. Nerve supply: By renal plexus. This is formed by
  a. The sympathetic fibers take origin from last three thoracic and first lumbar segment of spinal cord (T_{10} L_1). The sympathetic fibers are vasomotor in function.
  b. Parasympathetics are derived from vagus nerve. The functions are not clearly understood.
  c. The pain arising due to calculus present in the ureter or renal pelvic passes to the coeliac plexus - splanchnic nerve - to the sympathetic trunk - spinal cord. The pain is thus referred to the back and the lumbar region, and radiate to the anterior abdominal wall and down to the external genitalia.

G. Lymphatic drainage: The lymphatics of the kidney drain into para-aortic lymph nodes which are present at the level of origin of the renal arteries.

2. **Histology:** It consists of inner medulla and outer cortex.
   A. Inner medulla: It presents about 8 to 18 renal pyramids which are striated, pale conical masses. The base of the pyramid is directed to the cortex and apex projects into the wall of the renal sinus as renal papillae. It contains 15 to 16 ducts of Bellini, project into the calyces minors. Each minor calyx receives 2 or 3 renal papillae.
   B. Outer cortex: It consists of two portions
      a. An outer part towards the capsule and
      b. Inner part near the medulla called juxtamedullary cortex. Cortex lying between two adjacent pyramids is called renal columns. Cortex over the base of the pyramids is called cortical arch. The cortex consists of
         I. Light colored areas called the medullary rays, which are formed by the traversing collecting tubules.
         II. Dark colored areas are called convoluted part.

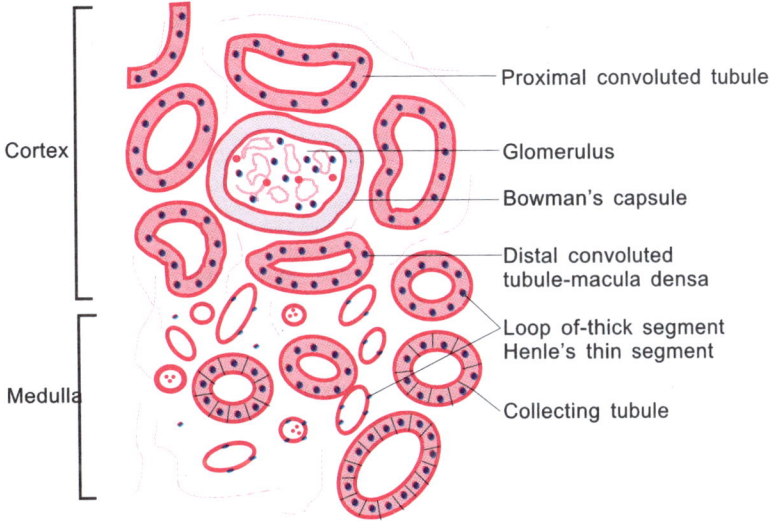

Fig. 2.66 Histology of kidney

3. **Development:**
   A. Chronological age: It develops in the fifth week and starts functioning at ninth week of intrauterine life.
   B. Germ layer: Intermediate mesoderm.
   C. Site: In the pelvis.
   D. Source:
      a. *Secretory part (nephron and renal corpuscle) develops from metanephric blastema.*
      b. *Collecting part (minor calyx, major calyx, pelvis of kidney and ureter) develops from uretric bud which arises from mesonephric duct.*
   E. Anomalies:
      a. Depending upon incidence:
         I. Horseshoe kidney: Inferior poles are usually fused (1/500).
         II. Unilateral agenesis of kidney is relatively common (1/1000).
         III. Bilateral agenesis (1/3000).
         IV. Congenital polycystic: There is a failure of fusion of the collecting and the secreting part. It may be autosomal dominant polycystic kidney disease (1/500 to 1/1000) or autosomal recessive polycystic kidney disease (1/5000).

b.   Depending upon the position shape and rotation.
I.   Anomalies of position.
    i.   Failure to ascent: The kidney lies in the sacral region.
    ii. Incomplete ascent: Kidney lies in the region of lower lumbar vertebrae.
    iii. Over ascent: Kidney lies in the thoracic cavity.
II. Anomalies of the shape
    i.   Horseshoe kidney: Lower or upper poles   may be fused.
    ii. Pancake kidney: The two kidneys form one mass.
    iii. Lobulated kidney normally lobulated and this lobulation may persist.

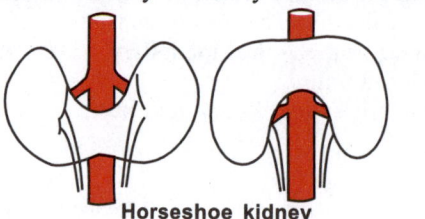 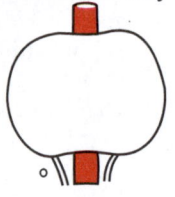

Horseshoe kidney   **Pancake kidney**

Fig. 2.67 Anomalies of the kidney

III. Abnormal rotation
    i.   Reverse rotation and
    ii. Non rotation of kidney.

4. Applied anatomy:
A. The angle between lower border of 12th rib and outer border of erector spinae is known as the 'renal angle'. The tenderness of the kidney is elicited over this angle.
B. The danger of opening the pleural sac must be kept in mind while exposing the kidney from back.
C. The hypermobile kidney can be moved vertically but not horizontally. Kidney lies in the abundant fat present in the renal fascia. In chronic debilitating patient, the kidney becomes hypermobile and produce symptoms of renal colic.

LAQ-16   **Describe ureter under**
              1. Gross anatomy,   2. Histology,
              3. Development and   4. Applied anatomy.

1. Gross anatomy:
A. Introduction:
    a.   Measurements:
       I.   Length: 25 cm (10″), of which 5″ lies in the abdomen and 5″ lies in the pelvis.
       II. Diameter: 3 mm
    b.   Constrictions: There are three normal constrictions
       I.   At the pelvi-ureteral junction.
       II. At the brim of the lesser pelvis and
       III. At its passage through the bladder wall.
B. Course:
    a.   It begins in the renal sinus as a funnel shaped dilation, called the renal pelvis. It gradually narrows till the lower end of the kidney and becomes ureter proper.

    b.   The ureter passes downwards and lies medial to the tips of transverse processes of the lumbar vertebrae.

    c.   It crosses the pelvic brim at the sacroiliac joint.

    d.   It passes to the ischial spine and enters the urinary bladder obliquely to open into the trigone of the bladder.

C. Relations of ureter

    a.   In abdominal part: This is described as in the

        I.   Renal pelvis: The structures are arranged from anterior to posterior as follows

            i.   Renal **v**ein most anteriorly. **VAU**

            ii.   Renal **a**rtery in the middle.

           iii.   **U**reter most posteriorly.

      II.   In the abdomen proper

            i.   Anteriorly and on the right side

              -   Peritoneum

              -   Right colic vessels.

              -   Root of mesentery.

              -   Ileo colic vessels.

              -   Gonadal vessels.

              -   Third part of duodenum.

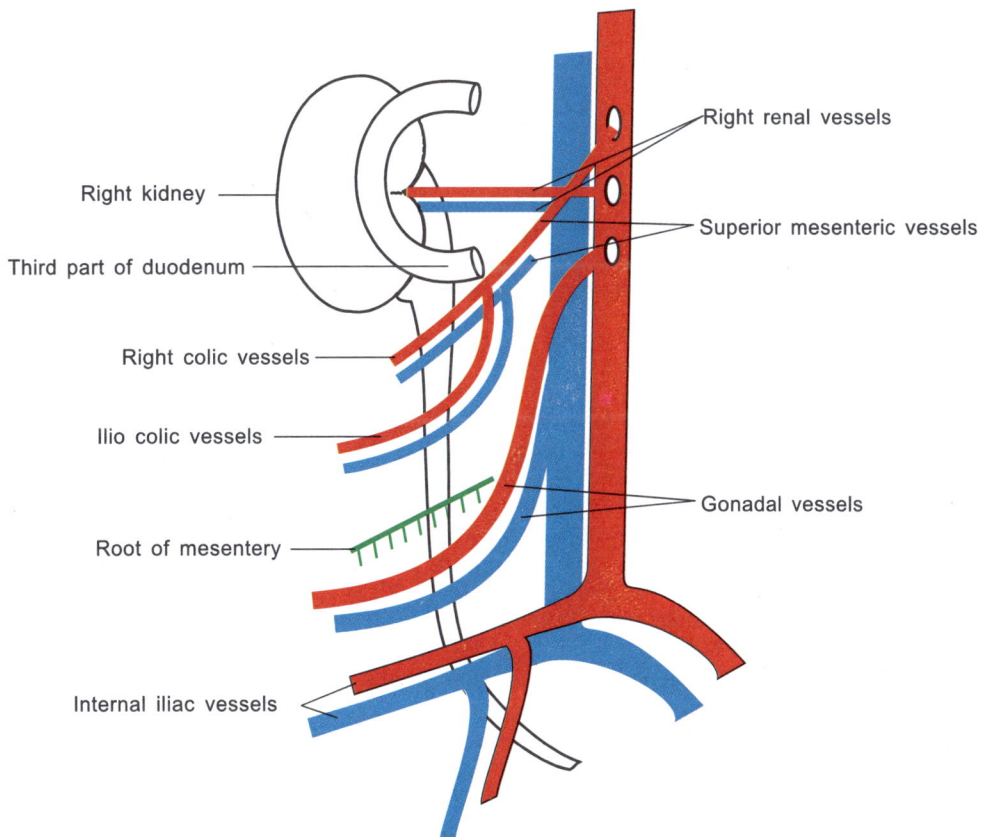

Fig. 2.68 Relations of right ureter in abdomen

ii.   Anteriorly and on the left side
     -   Peritoneum
     -   Left colic vessels.
     -   Sigmoid colon.
     -   Sigmoid mesocolon.
     -   Gonadal vessels.

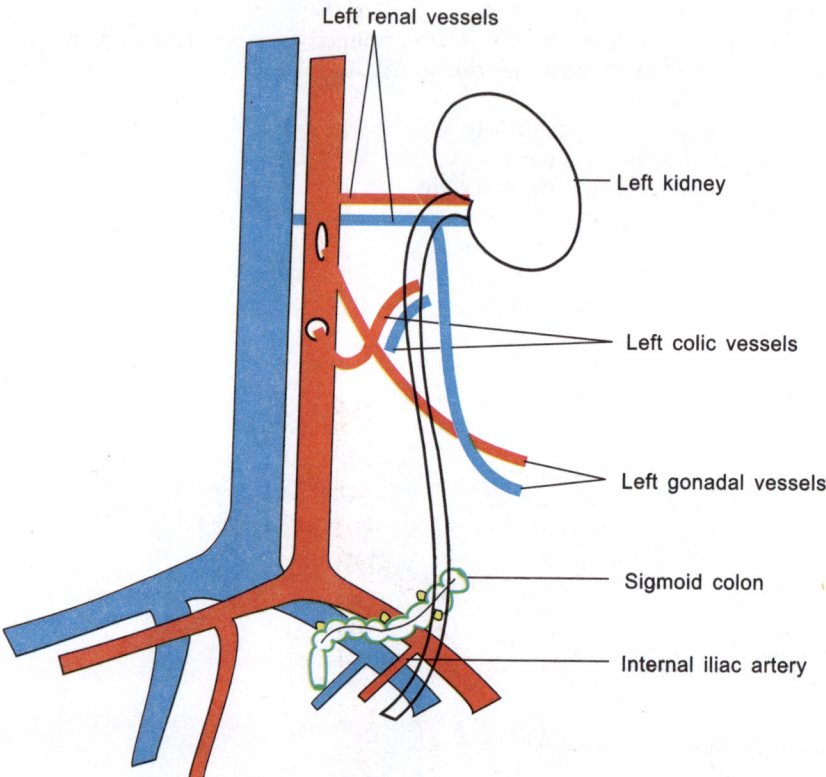

Fig. 2.69 Relations of left ureter in the abdomen

III. Posteriorly:
     i.   Psoas major,
     ii. Tips of the transverse processes and
     iii. Genitofemoral nerve.
IV. Medially:
     i.   On the right side: Inferior vena cava.
     ii. On the left side:
         -   Left gonadal vein and
         -   Inferior mesenteric vein.
b.   Relations of ureter in the pelvis
     I.   In its downward course
          i.   Posteriorly:
              -   Internal iliac artery,
              -   Anterior trunk of internal iliac artery,
              -   Internal iliac vein,

- Lumbosacral trunk and
- Sacroiliac joint.

ii. Laterally: It crosses the following structures (VAN from down above)
- Obturator **n**erve,
- Obliterated umbilical **a**rtery,   **VAN**
- Obturator **a**rtery,
- Obturator **v**ein,

Note: In female ureter forms the posterior boundary of ovarian fossa.

II. In its forward course
   i. Male
   - The ductus deferens: It crosses ureter from above and medially.
   - Seminal vesicle.

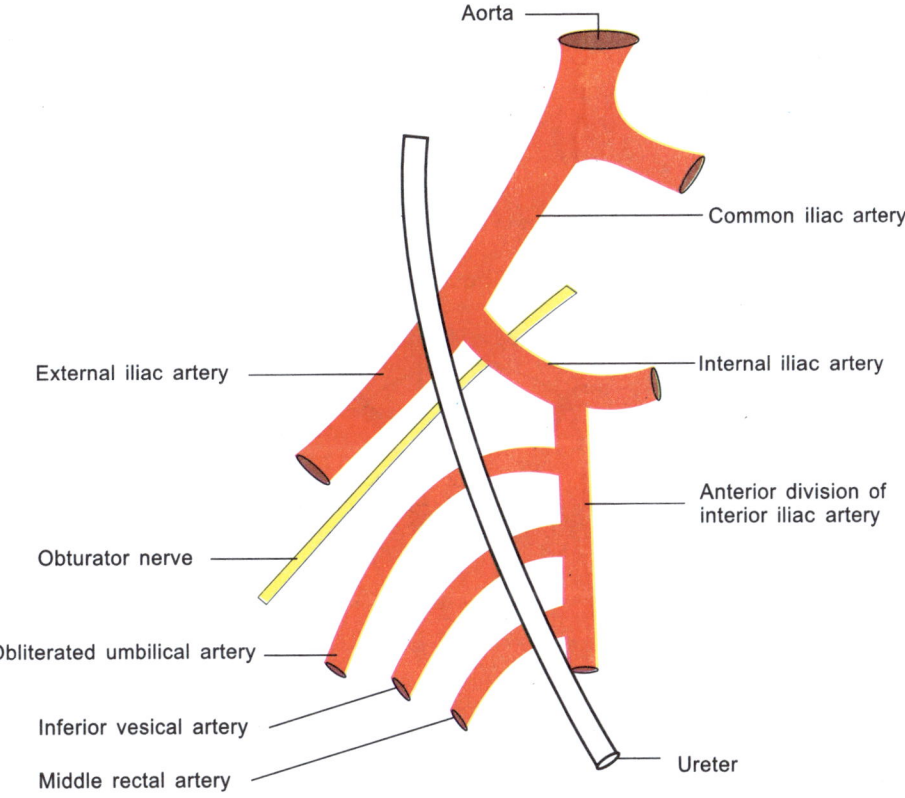

Aorta

Common iliac artery

External iliac artery

Internal iliac artery

Anterior division of interior iliac artery

Obturator nerve

Obliterated umbilical artery

Inferior vesical artery

Middle rectal artery

Ureter

Fig. 2.70 Relations of right ureter in pelvic part in male

ii. Female:
   - The broad ligament of uterus.
   - Uterine artery: It crosses above and infront of the ureter from lateral to medial side, and then passes upwards to enter between the two layers of the broad ligament.
   - Ureter lies 2 cm lateral to supravaginal part of the cervix.
   - It lies posterior to vagina.

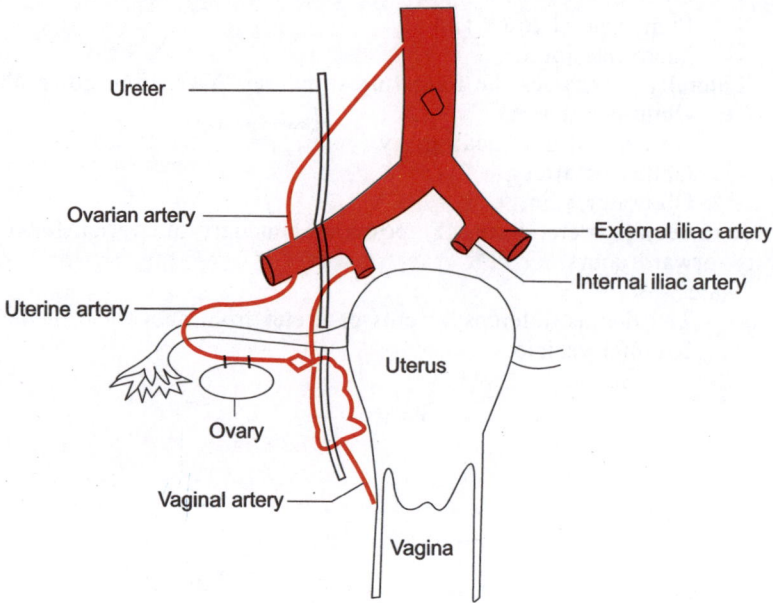

Fig. 2.71 Relations of the pelvic part of ureter in female

III. Intra vesical part: It is oblique and acts as a valve. It prevents regurgitation of urine.

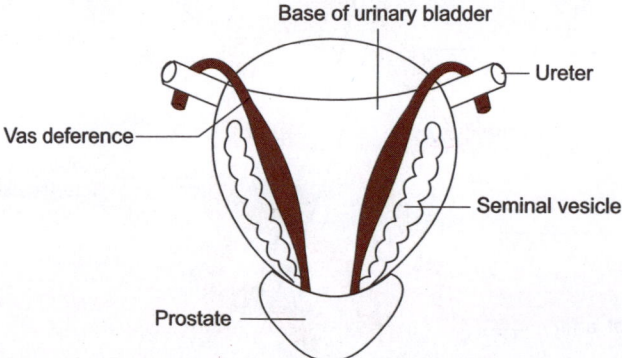

Fig. 2.72 Urinary bladder and prostate (from behind)

D. Blood supply:
   a. Arterial: It is supplied by the different arteries in three different parts.
       I.   Upper part: Receives branches from the
            i.   Renal artery, a branch of abdominal aorta.
            ii.   Gonadal artery, a branch of abdominal aorta and
            iii. Colic arteries, branches of superior and inferior mesenteric arteries.
       II. Middle part:
            i.   Branches from the abdominal aorta,
            ii.   Gonadal arteries and
            iii. Iliac arteries, terminal branches of abdominal aorta.

III. Pelvic part:
   i.   Vesical arteries, branches of internal iliac artery.
   ii. Middle rectal, branches of internal iliac artery.
   iii. Uterine artery, a branch of internal iliac artery.
The arteries of the ureter lie close to peritoneum. They divide into ascending and descending branches which first form a plexus on the surface of the ureter and then supply it.
  b. Venous drainage: Veins correspond to the arteries and drain into inferior vena cava.
E. Nerve supply: The ureter is supplied by sympathetic (T_{10}-L_1) and parasympathetic (S_2-S_4) nerves. They reach the ureter through the renal, aortic and hypogastric plexuses. All the nerves appear to be sensory in function. Parasympathetic nerves are motor in function.

2. **Histology:** It is lined by

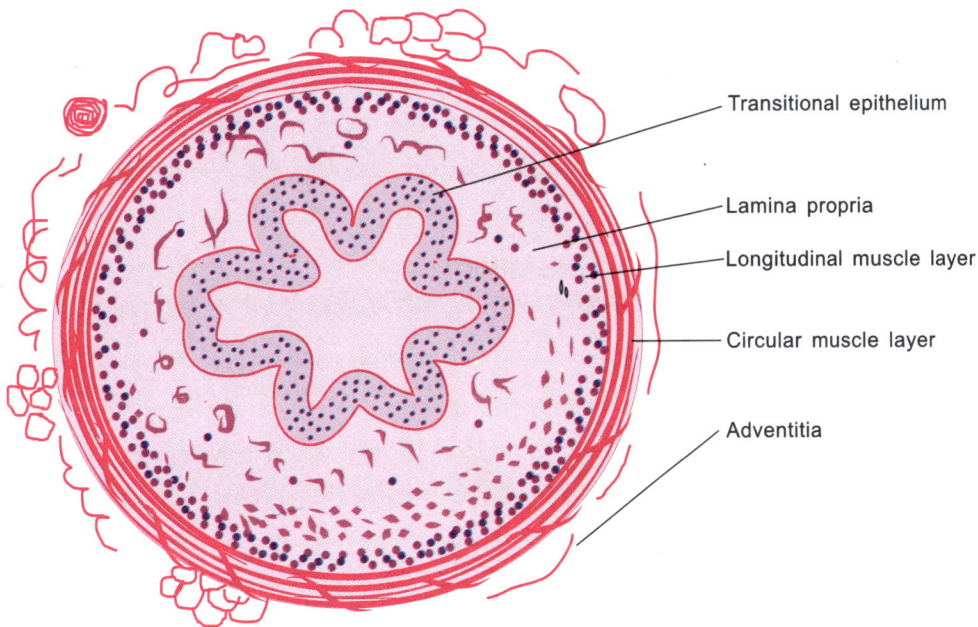

Transitional epithelium

Lamina propria

Longitudinal muscle layer

Circular muscle layer

Adventitia

Fig. 2.73 Histology of the ureter

A. Fibrous coat: It is composed mainly of elastic fibers and is continuous with the capsule of the kidney and adventitia of the urinary bladder.
B. Muscle coat:
  a. *In upper part of the ureter,*
     I. *Outer coat is circular and*
     II. *Inner coat is longitudinal.*
  b. *In the lower part of the ureter,*
     I.   *Outer coat is longitudinal,*
     II. *Intermediate is circular and*
     III. *Innermost is longitudinal.*
C. No submucous coat.

D. Mucous membrane:
a. It is lined by transitional epithelium. No distinct basal lamina. The cells of the epithelium rest on a fibrous tissue containing many elastic fibers. The plasma membrane of the surface epithelium are unusual. It encloses special glycoproteins. It is believed that these glycoproteins make the membrane impervious and resistant to toxic effects of substances present in urine and thus afford protection to adjacent tissue.
b. Lamina propria: It is thrown into 6 longitudinal folds when ureter is empty.
c. No muscularis mucosa.

3. **Development:**
A. Chronological age: It develops in the fifth week to ninth week of the intrauterine life.
B. Germ layer: Mesoderm.
C. Source: It is developed from uretreic bud which arises from caudal end of mesonephric duct. The upper part of the ureteric bud forms major and minor calyces of the renal pelvis and lower part forms ureter.
D. Anomalies:
a. Ureter may be partially or completely duplicated. It is usually associated with duplication of kidney.
b. Abnormal sites of opening of the ureter. The ureter may open in the
I. Prostatic urethra,
II. Ductus deferens,
III. Seminal vesicles or
IV. Rectum.
c. Upper end of the ureter may be blind.
d. Ureter may be dilated (hydroureter) because of the obstruction of the urine flow.

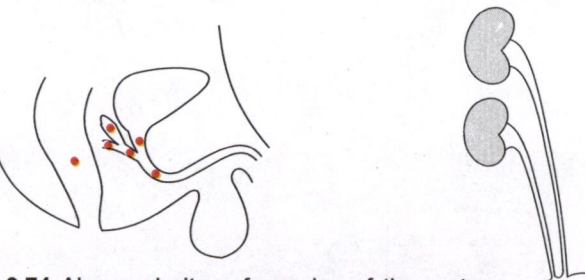

Fig. 2.74 Abnormal sites of opening of the ureter.

4. **Applied anatomy:**
A. During hysterectomy or surgical removal of the uterus, the ureter may by injured at the following points.
a. During ligation of the ovarian vessels in the infundibulo-pelvic ligament.
b. At the site of crossing of the uterine artery by the side of the cervix. The left ureter is more likely to be damaged due to the close relation with the cervix.
B. Renal colic: It is the severe pain arising from ureter due to the ureteric stone(s). It causes spasm of the ureter. It starts in the loin and radiates down to the groin, scrotum (or the labium majora), and the inner side of thigh. Because of the common innervation of the ureter and the skin of the above organ, the pain is referred to the above said regions.
C. The ureteric stone is liable to become impacted at one of the sites of the normal constriction of the ureter.

D. The ureteric stone lodged in the lower part of ureter in female can be felt by per vaginal examination because of close relationship of the ureter to the lateral fornix of vagina.

E. *The abdominal part of ureter receives blood supply from the medial side, therefore the surgery of ureter of abdominal part is done by approaching from lateral side.*

F. *The pelvic part of the ureter receives its blood supply from lateral side, hence the pelvic part of ureter is approached from the medial side.*

LAQ-17 Describe suprarenal gland under
1.   Gross anatomy,   2.   Histology,
3.   Development and   4.   Applied anatomy.

1. **Gross anatomy:**
   A. Introduction:
      a. Shape:
         I. Right suprarenal gland is triangular or irregular tetrahedron.
         II. Left suprarenal gland is semilunar.
      b. Dimensions:
         I. Right suprarenal gland is $4 \times 4 \times 1$ cm
         II. Left suprarenal gland $5 \times 3 \times 1$ cm
      c. Weight: 5 gm
      d. Situation:
         I. Right suprarenal gland is situated at upper pole of the right kidney. It encroaches the anterior surface.
         II. Left suprarenal gland is situated at the medial border of the left kidney.
   B. External features:

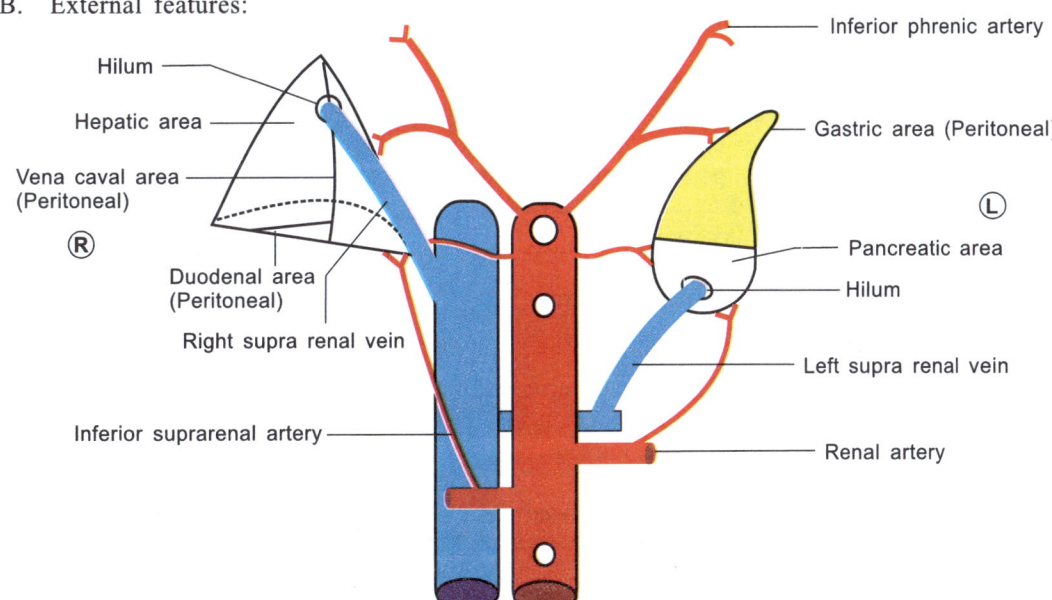

Fig. 2.75 Arterial supply and venous drainage of suprarenal gland

    a. Right suprarenal gland has
        I.   Apex,
        II. Base,
        III. Two surfaces and
        IV. Three borders.
    b. Left suprarenal gland has
        I.   Two ends,
        II. Two borders and
        III. Two surfaces.
    c. Hilum of the suprarenal gland:
        I.   Right hilum is situated on the anterior surface, near the upper pole of the right kidney and right suprarenal vein and lymph vessels leave the hilum.
        II. Left hilum situated on the anterior surface and near the lower pole of the left suprarenal gland. Left suprarenal vein and lymph vessels leave the hilum. *Arteries do not enter through the hilum.* **L** for **l**

C. Relations:
    a. Right suprarenal gland:
        I.   Anterior surface:
            i.   Medial part: Inferior vena cava (non peritoneal).
            ii. Lateral part:
                -   The bare area of the liver (non peritoneal). **L** for **l**
                -   Inferior surface of the liver (peritoneal).
        II. Posterior surface: Divided into lateral and medial part by crest
            i.   Lateral part: Anterior surface of the right kidney.
            ii. Medial part: Right crus of the diaphragm.
        III. Medial border:
            i.   Right inferior phrenic artery and
            ii. Right coeliac ganglion.
    b. Left suprarenal gland:
        I.   Anterior surface:
            i.   Upper part is covered with the peritoneum and related to the posterior surface of stomach.
            ii. Lower part is non peritoneal overlapped by the body of pancreas and crossed by tortuous splenic artery.
        II. Posterior surface:
            i.   Left kidney and
            ii. Left crus of diaphragm.
        III. Medial border:
            i.   Left coeliac ganglion,
            ii. Left inferior phrenic artery and
            iii. Left gastric artery.
        IV. Lateral border: Left kidney.

D. Blood supply:
    a. Arterial: It receives blood from following arteries. *All arteries enters through peripheral part of gland i.e. cortex not through the hilum.*
        I.   Superior suprarenal artery, a branch of inferior phrenic artery.
        II. Middle suprarenal artery, a branch of abdominal aorta.
        III. Inferior suprarenal artery, a branch of renal artery.

b. Venous drainage:
   The veins of the suprarenal gland drain in following veins.
   I.   Right suprarenal vein drains inferior vena cava.
   II.   Left suprarenal vein drains into left renal vein.
   Peculiarities of the veins draining supra-renal gland.
   I.   There is only one thick vein like the lead pencil which is present to have the uniform distribution of the hormone.
   II.   The vein draining the suprarenal gland leave through the hilum.
   III. Left suprarenal vein is longer as compared to right suprarenal vein.
E. Nerve supply:
   a. Cortex: Nerve supply of cortex is not known.
   b. Medulla is supplied by sympathetic i.e. thoracic splanchnic nerve as pre-ganglionic fibers, which go directly to the cells of medulla.
   c. It is also supplied by phrenic and vagus nerve but the exact function is not known.
F. Lymphatic: The lymphatics of the suprarenal glands may accompany any vessel reaching the adrenal gland. The lymphatics drain into para aortic nodes.
   a. The right para aortic nodes are situated near the right crus of the diaphragm.
   b. The left para aortic nodes are situated near the origin of the left renal artery.

2. **Histology:** Divided into cortex and medulla.
    A. Cortex is divided into three zones

Table 2.13 Zones of cortex of the suprarenal gland

Cortex	Zona glomerulosa	Zona fasciculata	Zona reticularis
a. Arrangement of cells	In the form of curved columns	In the form of straight columns, long bands of large cells	In the form of branching column.
b. Hormones secreted	Mineralo corticoids e.g. Aldosterone	Glucocorticoids e.g. Hydrocortisone	Sex hormones e.g. I. Androgen II. Oestrogen
c. Functions	Promote resorption of sodium ions by distal convoluted tubules of kidney	Participate in carbohydrate, fat and protein metabolism	Reproductive function.

B. Adrenal medulla: Cells of medulla exhibit chromaffin reaction i.e. when treated with potassium dichromate solution the cytoplasmic granules are oxidized & the medulla turns brown. It shows:
   a. Cords with pheochromocytes (pheo-dusky or brown, chroma - colors, cytes - cell). They are of two types.
      I.   Secreting adrenaline.
      II. Secreting noradrenaline.
   b. Few sympathetic ganglion cells show prominent vesicular nucleoli.
   c. Sinusoidal capillaries present between cell groups.

3. **Development:**
    A. Chronological age: Adrenal cortex develops in the sixth week of intrauterine life.
    B. Germ layer:
       a. *Cortex develops from mesoderm.*
       b. *Medulla develops from ectoderm.*
    C. Site: Between dorsal mesentery and developing gonad.

    D. Sources: In foetus, the suprarenal is 20 times larger than the adult because of large foetal cortex which regresses after birth.
        a. Cortex develops from coelomic epithelium.
        b. *Medulla develops from neural crest (Neuro-ectoderm).*
    E. Anomalies: Congenital adrenal hyperplasia. An abnormal increase in the cells of suprarenal cortex results in excessive androgen production during the foetal period. It results masculinization of female.

4. **Applied anatomy:**
    A. Addisons disease: It is caused by atrophy of the suprarenal cortex. It is mainly due to tuberculosis infection. It presents as muscular weakness, low blood pressure cutaneous pigmentation and change in electrolyte balance.
    B. Pheochromocytoma (*pheo* grey, *chroma* colour, *cytoma* tumour): It is a tumor of adrenal medulla, produces paroxysmal hypertension due to secretion of large amount of catecholamine. It produces palpitation, excessive sweating, pallor, hypertension and headache of long duration.
    C. Adrenal medulla can be sacrificed and the secretions are replaced by the medicines.

LAQ-18   Describe the diaphragm under
1. Gross anatomy,   2. Openings in the diaphragm,
3. Development and   4. Applied anatomy.

1. **Gross anatomy:**
    A. Introduction: It is the musculotendinous partition which separates thoracic cavity from abdominal cavity. It is described as a muscle under origin, insertion, nerve supply and action.
    B. Origin: 🔑 CVS
        a. **C**ostal fibers arise from inner surface of lower six costal cartilages and adjacent parts of the ribs.
        b. **V**ertebral fibers arise from
            I. Upper lumber vertebrae by two crura.
               i. The right crus arises from front of right surface of bodies of upper three lumbar vertebrae.
               ii. The left crus arises from front of left surface of bodies of upper two lumbar vertebrae.
            II. Fibrotendinous arches, called the medial and lateral arcuate ligaments.
        c. **S**ternal fibers arise from posterior surface of the xiphoid process.
    C. Insertion: The muscles insert into trilobed central tendon.
    D. Relations:
        a. Superiorly:
            I. Pleurae &
            II. Pericardium.
        b. Inferiorly:
            I. Peritoneum,
            II. Liver,
            III. Fundus of stomach,
            IV. Spleen,
            V. Kidneys &
            VI. Suprarenals.

E. Action: The actions of the diaphragm are
  a. Inspiration: Diaphragm is the principal muscle of the inspiration.
  b. It acts in all expulsive act, e.g. Sneezing, coughing, laughing, crying, vomiting, micturition, defecation and parturition.
  c. It acts as a partition between thoracic and abdominal cavity.
F. Blood supply: 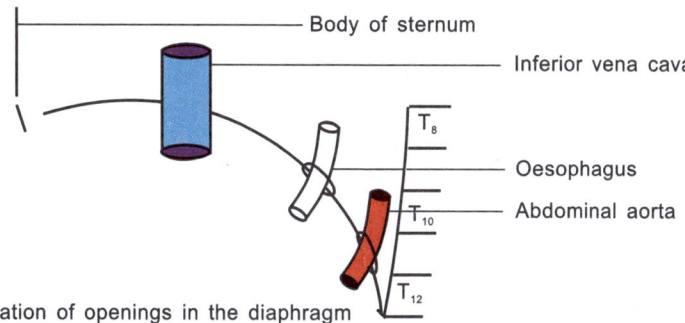 IMP
  a. Arterial supply:
    I. Inferior phrenic artery, first branch of the abdominal aorta.
    II. Musculophrenic, a terminal branch of the internal thoracic artery.
    III. Lower 5 or 6 posterior intercostal, branches of thoracic aorta.
  b. Venous drainage:
    I. Inferior phrenic vein drains into inferior vena cava.
    II. Musculophrenic drains into internal thoracic vein.
    III. Posterior intercostal vein drains into azygos vein.
G. Nerve supply: Sensory and motor.
  a. Sensory: It is divided into
    I. The sensations of the central part are carried by phrenic nerve (C_3, C_4 and C_5).
    II. The sensations from the peripheral part are carried by lower intercostal nerves (T_6 to T_{11}).
  b. Motor: Phrenic nerve ($C_{3,\ 4}$ & $_5$)

2. **Opening in the diaphragm:**
   A. The major opening in the diaphragm

Table 2.14 Showing major openings in the diaphragm

Opening	Level	Situation	Structures passing
a. Caval	Eighth thoracic vertebra	On the right side of central tendon of diaphragm.	I. Inferior vena cava, II. Right phrenic nerve & III. Lymphatics.
b. Oeso-phageal	Tenth thoracic vertebra	The central part of the diaphragm.	I. Oesophagus, II. Vagus nerves & III. Oesophageal branch of left gastric artery & accompanying veins.
c. Aortic	Lower border of twelfth thoracic vertebra	Just to the left of the midline, between the median arcuate ligaments.	Relation from left to right I. Descending thoracic aorta, II. Thoracic duct & III. Azygos vein.

Body of sternum

Inferior vena cava

T_8

Oesophagus

T_{10} — Abdominal aorta

T_{12}

Fig. 2.76 Situation of openings in the diaphragm

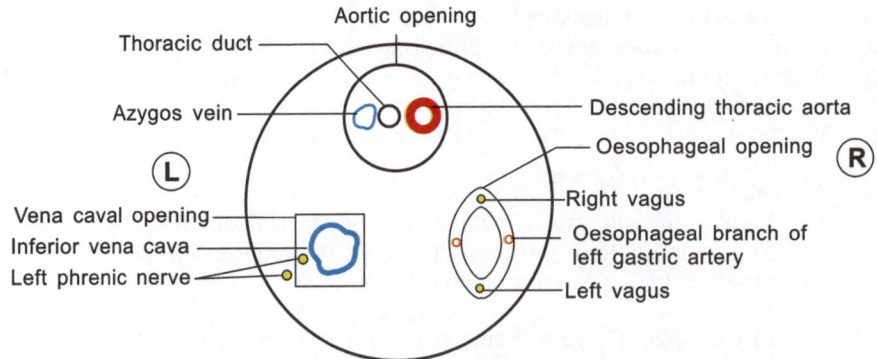

Fig. 2.77 Openings in the diaphragm

B. The minor opening in the diaphragm are as follows:
a. The superior epigastric vessels (and some lymphatics) pass between the xiphoid and costal (7th costal cartilage) origins of the diaphragm. This gap is known as Larry's space or foramen of Morgagni.
b. The musculophrenic vessels pierce the diaphragm at the 8th or 9th costal cartilage.
c. Several small veins pass through minute apertures in the central tendon.

3. **Development:**
A. Germ layer: It develops from the mesoderm.
B. Site: Lateral plate mesoderm.
C. Sources:
a. Septum transversum forms the principal components of the definitive diaphragm. It forms
   I. Central tendon,
   II. Anteromedian part,
   III. Vena caval opening &
   IV. Oesophageal opening.
b. Pleuro peritoneal membranes: It also forms a major contribution to the development of diaphragm. It gives rise to circumferential part in the ventrolateral region.

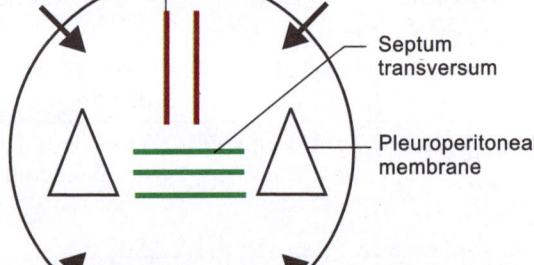

Fig. 2.78 Development of the diaphragm

c. Dorsal mesentery of the oesophagus forms
   I. The posterior part of diaphragm between the oesophageal the aortic openings.
   II. Crura of the diaphragm.
d. Left and right body wall. They form tissue on the periphery of the diaphragm.
D. Anomalies:
a. Diaphragmatic hernias: It is one of the more common anomalies of the diaphragm. The incidence is 1/2000 new born. The diaphragmatic hernia may be of following type depending upon the situation.
   I. Posterolateral,
   II. Posterior,
   III. Retrosternal &
   IV. Central.

b. Accessory diaphragm.
c. Congenital eventration of the diaphragm.

4. Applied anatomy:
A. Hiatus hernia is relatively common (1%) accounting for 98% of the all diaphragmatic hernia. It is manifested by
   a. **H**iccough
   b. **A**naemia  **HARD**
   c. **R**egurgitation
   d. **D**ysphagia
B. *The lesion of the phrenic nerve results into the paralysis of the dome of the diaphragm and the affected dome is pushed upwards.*
C. Irritation of the diaphragm may cause referred pain in the shoulder because of phrenic and supraclavicular nerves have same root value.

LAQ-19 Describe the abdominal aorta under
1. Gross anatomy,   2. Histology,
3. Development and   4. Applied anatomy.

1. Gross anatomy:
A. Introduction:
   a. Origin: It is the continuation of thoracic aorta below the diaphragmatic opening behind the median arcuate ligament.
   b. Termination: It terminates at the lower border of vertebra L_4 by dividing into two common iliac arteries.
   c. Extent: It extends from the lower border of T_{12} to lower border of L_4.
   d. Course: It descends in front of the bodies of L_1 to L_4 vertebrae. It lies slightly to the left of midline.
B. Relation:
   a. Anterior:
      I. Coeliac artery with coeliac plexus.
      II. Superior mesenteric artery.
      III. Left renal vein.
      IV. Body of pancreas with splenic vein.
      V. Gonadal arteries.
      VI. Parietal peritoneum.
      VII. Root of mesentery.
   b. Posterior:
      I. Left border of L_1 to L_4 vertebra with intervertebral disc and anterior longitudinal ligament.
      II. Beginning of the lumbar arteries.
      III. Third and fourth lumbar veins.
      IV. Left psoas major.
   c. Right:
      I. Cisterna chyli.
      II. Lumbar azygos.
      III. Right crus of the diaphragm.

IV. Right coeliac ganglion.

V. Inferior vena cava.

    d. Left:

        I. Left crus of the diaphragm.

        II. Left coeliac ganglion.

        III. Fourth part of duodenum.

        IV. Duodeno jejunal flexure.

        V. Left sympathetic trunk.

        VI. Inferior mesenteric vessels.

C. Branches:

    a. Paired:

        I. Inferior phrenic artery.

        II. Middle suprarenal artery.

        III. Renal artery.

        IV. Gonadal artery.

        V. Common iliac artery.

    b. Unpaired:

        I. Coeliac trunk.

        II. Superior mesenteric artery.

        III. Inferior mesenteric artery.

        IV. Median sacral artery.

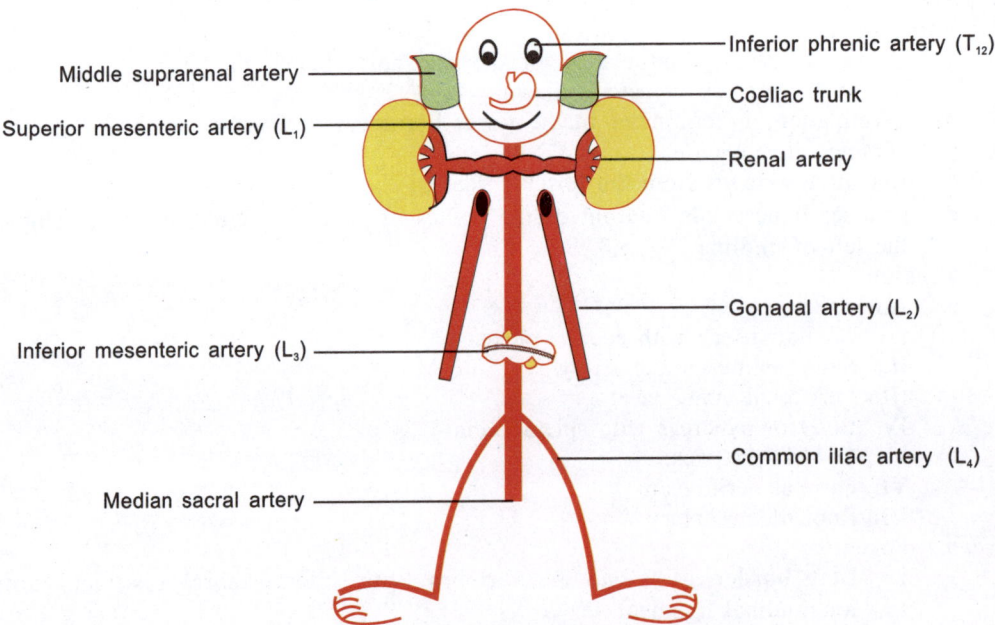

Fig. 2.79 Branches of abdominal aorta

2. **Histology:** The histology of abdominal aorta is same as elastic artery. It consists of three coats

A. Tunica intima consist of

    a. Endothelium lined by simple squamous epithelium.

    b. Subendothelial connective tissue is usually prominent.

B. Tunica media is thickest coat consist of
   a. Elastic fibers.
   b. Internal elastic lamina which is fenestrated and is formed by elastic fibers. It is indistinguishable from the media.
C. Tunica adventitia, a thin walled outercoat.

3. **Development:**
   A. Chronological age: The vascular system appear in the middle of third week.
   B. Germ layer: Mesoderm.
   C. Source: The aorta is developed from the fusion of two primitive dorsal aortae, the fusion extends from the fourth thoracic to fourth lumbar segments.

4. **Applied anatomy:**
   A. In thin individuals the abdominal aorta can be palpated and auscultated.
   B. Aneurysmal dilatation of abdominal aorta is not uncommon. It is usually present at the proximal site where the branches are given.
   C. Coarctation (stenosis of the abdominal aorta), if prerenal, it is more likely to be fatal because of the less blood flow through the kidneys.

LAQ-20	**Describe inferior vena cava under**
	1. Gross anatomy, 2. Development and 3. Applied anatomy.

1. **Gross anatomy:**
   A. Introduction:
      a. Formation: It is formed by the union of
         I. Right common iliac vein.
         II. Left common iliac vein.
      b. Level of formation: It is formed on the right side of body of fifth lumbar vertebra.
      c. Termination: It opens into the lower and posterior part of right atrium and guarded by valves.
      d. Dimensions:
         I. Breadth: 1″
         II. Length: 9″
   B. **Relations:**
      a. Anterior: From above downward it is related to
         I. Posterior surface of liver.
         II. Epiploic foramen.
         III. First part of duodenum.
         IV. Portal vein.
         V. Head of pancreas.
         VI. Third part of duodenum.
         VII. Right gonadal artery.
         VIII. Parietal peritoneum.
         IX. Root of mesentery.
         X. Right common iliac arteries.

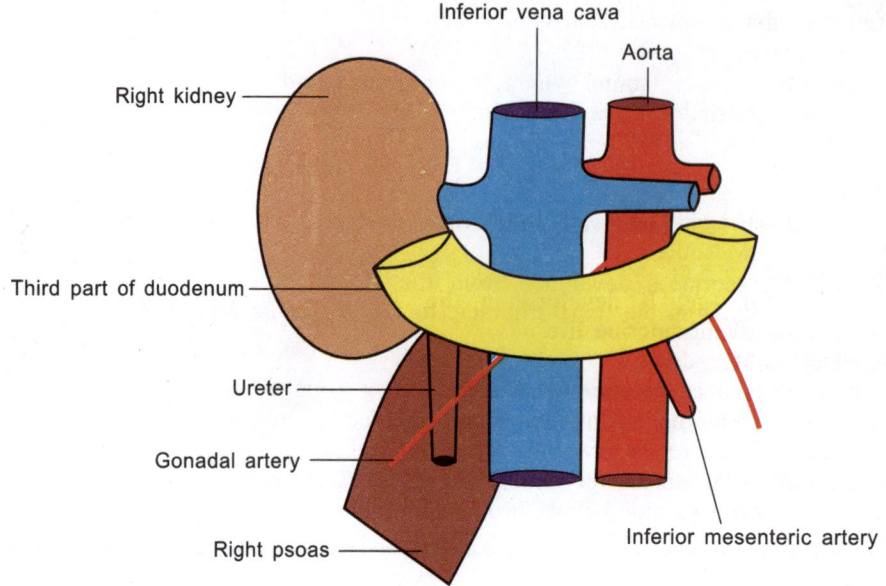

Fig. 2.80 Relations of inferior vena cava

  b. Posterior:
    I. Lower part:
      i. Bodies of lumbar vertebrae.
      ii. Anterior longitudinal ligament.
      iii. Right psoas major muscle.
      iv. Right sympathetic trunk.
      v. Third and fourth lumbar arteries.
    II. Upper part:
      i. Right crus of the diaphragm.
      ii. Right coeliac ganglion.
      iii. Part of suprarenal gland.
      iv. Right renal artery.
      v. Middle suprarenal artery.
      vi. Inferior phrenic artery.
  c. Right side:
    I. Right ureter,
    II. Second part of duodenum and medial border of right kidney,
    III. Hepato-renal pouch of Morison and
    IV. The bare area of the liver.
  d. Left side:
    I. Abdominal aorta,
    II. Right crus of the diaphragm with cisterna chyli and thoracic duct,
    III. Omental bursa and
    IV. Caudate lobe of liver.
C. Tributaries: The tributaries of vena cava are not identical with the branches of the abdominal aorta. Particularly there is no corresponding to the three ventral branches to the gut. Following are the tributaries of the inferior vena cava.
  a. Pair of common iliac veins.

b. Lumbar veins.
   I. Third and fourth pair of lumbar veins drain directly into the inferior vena cava.
   II. First and second drain into ascending lumbar vein.
   III. A pair of renal vein.
   IV. A pair of phrenic vein.
   V. Right gonadal vein.
   VI. Right suprarenal vein and hepatic veins.

2. **Development:**
   A. Chronological age: It develops in the eighth week of intrauterine life.
   B. Germ layer: Mesoderm.
   C. Sources: It is a composite vessel and is developed from the following sources from below upwards

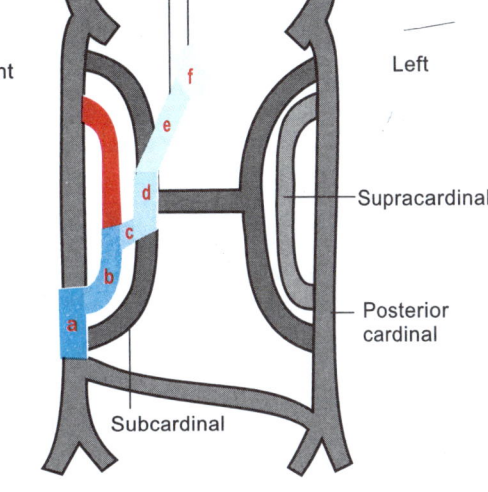

Fig. 2.81 Development of inferior vena cava

   a. From the persistent caudal part of right posterior cardinal vein.
   b. From the right supra-cardinal vein: This part receives third and fourth pairs of lumbar veins.
   c. From the anastomosis between right supra-cardinal and right sub-cardinal veins: This part receives right gonadal vein.
   d. From the upper part of right sub-cardinal vein: This part receives right supra-renal & both renal veins.
   e. From a new vessel: It develops behind the liver and communicates right sub- cardinal vein with commonhepatic vein also called hepatocardiac channel.
   f. From the common hepatic vein: It is developed from supra-hepatic part of right vitelline vein.
      The post-renal segment of the vena cava lies on a more posterior plane than the pre-renal segment. This explain why right testicular artery crosses in front of the vena cava, whereas right renal, middle suprarenal and inferior phrenic arteries pass behind the vein.
   D. Anomalies:
      a. Double inferior vena cavae below the renal veins.
      b. Retro-caval ureter.

3. **Applied anatomy:**
   A. In obstruction of inferior vena cava, a collateral circulation may me established between the tributaries of superior and inferior vena cava by a number of superficial and deep sets of vein.
   B. Thrombosis in the inferior vena cava causes oedema of legs and back.

SN-15   Cisterna chyli

1. **Gross anatomy:**
   A. It is an elongated lymphatic sac.
   B. Length: 5 to 7 cm.
   C. Situation: Infront of first and second lumbar vertebra, immediately to the right of the abdominal aorta.

2. **Tributaries:** Right and left intestinal lymph trunks.

3. **Termination:** Its upper end continues as thoracic duct.

4. **Draining areas:** Intestinal trunk brings lymph from
   A. The stomach to intestine.
   B. Pancreas.
   C. Spleen.
   D. Anteroinferior part of the liver.
   E. All structures below diaphragm (lower half of the body).

5. **Applied anatomy:**
   A. Thoracic duct when obstructed due to filarial infection or growth will give rise to chylothorax, chyluria etc.
   B. Thoracic duct when damaged during operation in the neck the lymph usually follows other channel but if it fails then chylous fistula may result.

SN-16   Perineal body (Central perineal tendon)

1. **Introduction:** It is a pyramidal fibro- muscular mass situated in the midline of perineum.

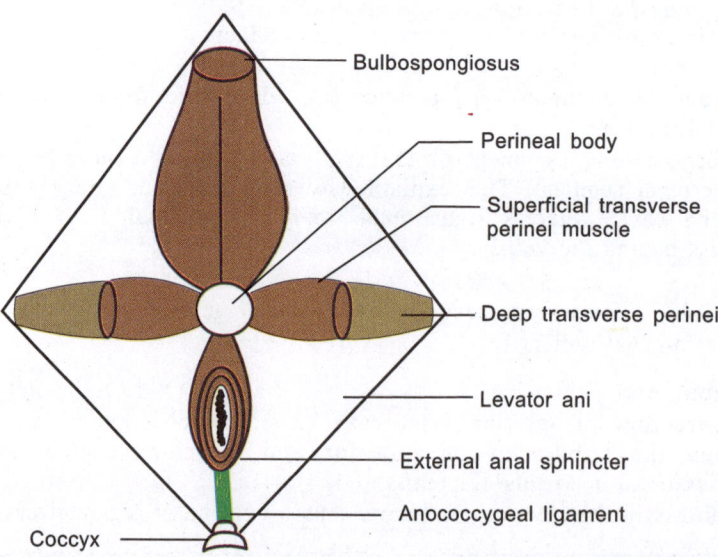

Fig. 2.82 Perineal body

2. **Location:**
   A. Male: It is located close to the bulb of penis.
   B. Female: It is present between anal canal and pudendal cleft.

3. **Formation:** It is formed by 10 muscles, 4 paired and 2 unpaired.
   A. Paired:
      a. <u>B</u>ulbo spongiosus.
      b. <u>S</u>uperficial transverse perinei.
      c. Deep transverse peri<u>n</u>ei.
      d. <u>L</u>evator ani.
   B. Unpaired:
      a. External anal sphincter.
      b. External urethral sphincter.

4. **Development:** It develops from the tip of the urorectal septum.

5. **Applied anatomy:**
   A. In female, it supports the pelvic organs which is a very important support.
   B. Injury to the peroneal body may weaken the pelvic floor and lead to prolapse of the vagina and uterus.
   C. Episiotomy (incision of vulva) is given to facilitate the labor and prevents the rupture of the perineal body in primiparous commonly.
   D. The torn perineal body during parturition, if not properly repaired, leads to wider hiatus urogenatalis.

SN-17	**External anal sphincter**

1. **Formation:** It is formed by the skeletal muscles.

2. **Control:** It is under voluntary control.

3. **Extent:** It surrounds the whole anal canal.

4. **Function:** It keeps the anus and anal canal closed.

5. **Parts:** It is divided into three parts
   A. Subcutaneous part:
      a. It is formed by flat bands.
      b. It is 15 mm in breadth.
      c. It surrounds the lower part of the anal canal.
      d. It is situated deep to the skin & is separated by perianal fascia.
   B. Intermediate or superficial part:
      a. It extends from perineal body to the tip of coccyx.
      b. It is separated from subcutaneous part by perianal fascia.
      c. It is separated from internal anal sphincter by conjoint fibers of levator ani and longitudinal muscle of the rectum and anal canal.
   C. Deep part: It encircles the upper part of the anal canal.

6. **Nerve supply:** It is supplied by pudendal nerve (somatic nerve).

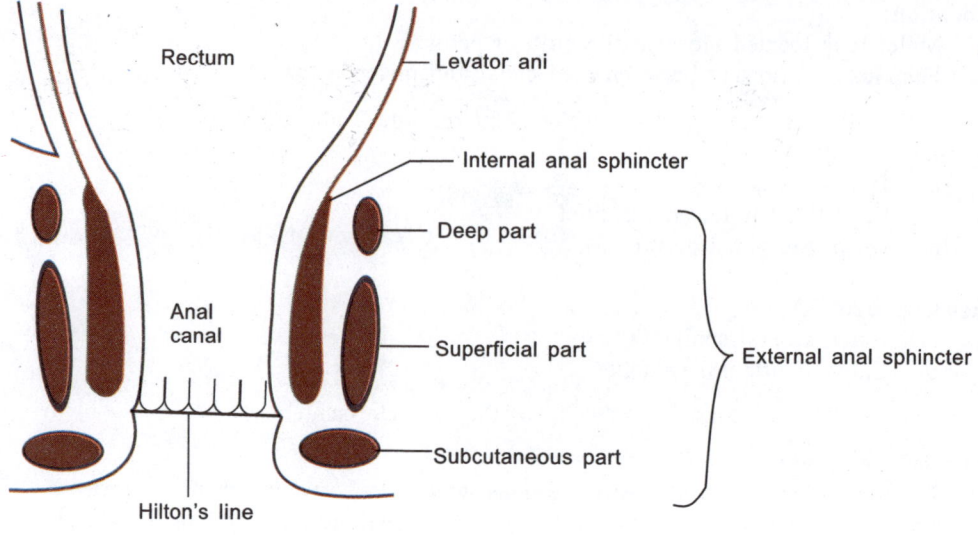

Fig. 2.83 External anal sphincter

| LAQ-21 | **Describe ischiorectal fossa under** |

Describe ischiorectal fossa under
1. Gross anatomy, 2. Boundaries, 3. Contents,
4. Recesses, 5. Spaces, 6. Canals,
7. Applied anatomy.

1. **Gross anatomy:**
   A. Introduction: It is also called ischio anal fossa. It is the wedge shaped space present in the lateral part of anal triangle.
   B. Location: It is present one on either side of anal canal and below the pelvic diaphragm.
   C. Dimension: Length x width x depth 2″ x 1″ x 2″

2. **Boundaries:**
   A. Apex: It is formed by the junction of the obturator and anal fascia (inferior fascia of the pelvic diaphragm).
   B. Base: It is formed by the skin.
   C. Anterior: Posterior border of the perineal membrane.
   D. Posterior:
      a. Lower border of the gluteus maximus.
      b. Sacrotuberous ligament.
   E. Lateral wall:
      a. Obturator internus.
      b. Obturator fascia.
      c. Medial surface of ischial tuberosity.
   F. Medial wall:
      a. In the lower part: External anal sphincter.
      b. In the upper part: Levator ani.

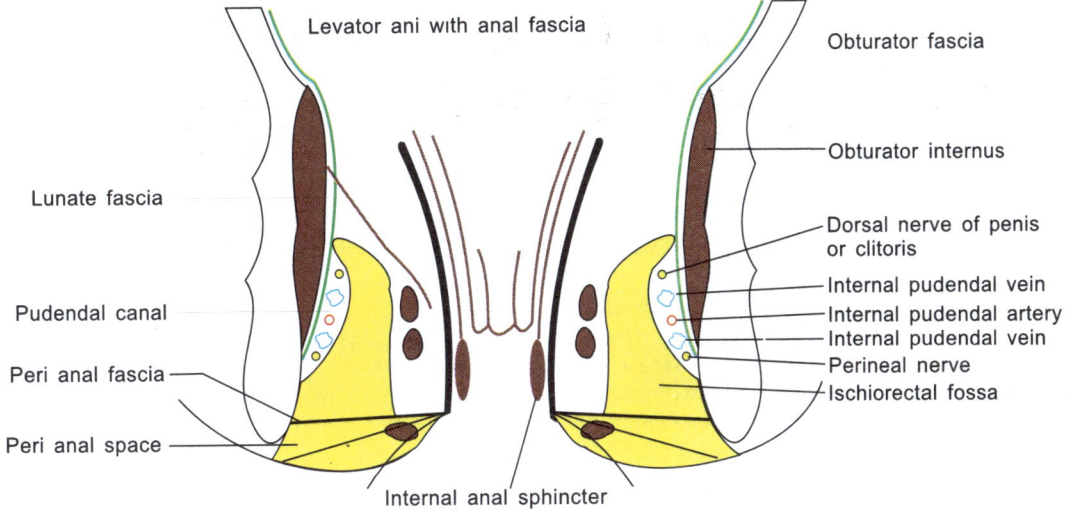

Fig. 2.84 Ischiorectal fossa

3. **Contents:**
   A. Pudendal canal with its content.
      a. Pudendal nerve (ventral division of ventral ramus of S_2, $_3$ and $_4$).
      b. Internal pudendal vessels (anterior division of internal iliac artery).
   B. Posterior scrotal nerve & vessels.
   C. Perforating cutaneous branch of S_2, S_3.
   D. Inferior rectal nerve and vessels.
   E. Pad of fat.
   F. Perineal branch of S_4 nerve. It supplies anterior part of external anal sphincter.

4. **Recesses:** These are narrow extensions of ischiorectal fossae.
   A. Anterior recess: It extends from the urogenital diaphragm and reaches upto the posterior surface of the body of pubis.
   B. Posterior recess: It is smaller than anterior. It is present deep to the sacrotuberous ligament.
   C. Horseshoe recess: It connects 2 ischiorectal fossae behind the anal canal.

5. **Spaces**
   A. Perianal space:
      a. Perianal fascia is a septum which separates the perianal space from the ischiorectal space.
      b. It extends from the white line of Hilton medially to the pudendal canal laterally.
      c. The fat is arranged tightly in the small loculi.
      d. The inflections of this space are, therefore, very painful due to the tension caused by swelling.
   B. Ischiorectal space:
      a. It is deep to the perianal space.
      b. The fat is arranged loosely due to incomplete septi.
      c. The infections of this space is less painful since there is no tension in the swelling.

    d.   Lunate fascia arches over ischiorectal fat and divides it into
        I.   Suprategmental space.
        II.   Tegmental space

6. Canals (Fascial canal, Alcock's Canal): It is the connective tissue sheath in the lower lateral wall of the ischiorectal fossa.

7. Applied anatomy:
    A.   It allows distension of anal canal during passage of faeces. It also allows dilatation of the vagina during parturition when passage of the foetal head literally obliterates the space.
    B.   The loss of the fat results into prolapse of rectum.
    C.   The perineal and ischiorectal spaces are common sites for abscesses. Through the horseshoe recess unilateral abscess may become bilateral.
    D.   Presence of Hiatus of Schwalbe: It is a gap at the apex of the fossa due to defective origin of levator ani from obturator fascia. It is occasionally present. Very rarely pelvic organ may herniate through it into the ischiorectal fossa.
    E.   Psoas abscess may enter the iliac fossa and may travel the ishciorectal fossa along the pudendal vessels.
    F.   An abscess in the ishchiorectal space may burst in the anal canal and produces fistula in ano.

SN-18   Pudendal canal (Fascial canal, Alcock's canal)

1. Introduction: It is the connective tissue sheath in the lower lateral wall of the ischiorectal fossa.
    A.   Location: 2.5 cm above the ischial tuberosity.
    B.   Formation:
        a.   Laterally: Obturator fascia.
        b.   Above: Lunate fascia.
        c.   Below: Falciform process of sacrotuberous ligament.
        d.   Medially: Perianal fascia.
        e.   Extent: From lesser sciatic foramen to deep perineal pouch.

2. Content:
    A.   Pudendal nerve (S_2 - S_4 ventral division of ventral rami) and
    B.   Internal pudendal vessels.
    C.   The arrangement of the structures within the canal are as follows from above downwards:
        a.   Dorsal nerve of penis or clitoris.
        b.   Internal pudendal vein.
        c.   Internal pudendal artery.
        d.   Perineal nerve.

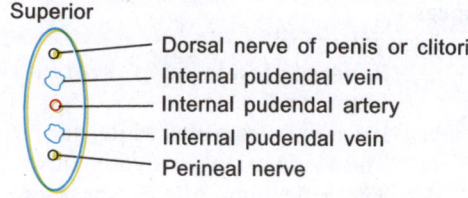

Superior

- Dorsal nerve of penis or clitoris
- Internal pudendal vein
- Internal pudendal artery
- Internal pudendal vein
- Perineal nerve

Inferior

Fig. 2.85 Arrangement of pudendal canal

3. Applied anatomy:
Pudendal nerve is blocked to anaesthetize the perineum, this is called pudendal block. It is given by following methods.
    A.   Transvaginal procedure: A long needle is passed through the vaginal wall and guided by a finger to the ischial spine, which can be palpated per vaginum.

B. Perineal procedure: The ischial tuberosity is palpated subcutaneously through the buttock, and the needle is inserted into the pudendal canal along the medial side of the tuberosity. The canal lies about 1 inch (2.5 cm) deep to ischial tuberosity.

SN-19   **Perineal membrane (Inferior fascia of urogenital diaphragm)**

1. **Introduction:** It is an unyielding sheath of fibrous tissue which separates superficial and deep perineal pouch. It forms the inferior boundary of deep perineal pouch and superior boundary of superficial perineal pouch.

2. **Gross:**
   A. Dimension: AP dimension 3.5 cm.
   B. Disposition: Horizontal in erect posture.
   C. Attachments:
      a. Anteriorly and on either side: Ischiopubic rami.
      b. Posteriorly and on either side: Anterior part of ischial tuberosity.
      c. Anterior border forms the transverse perineal ligament.
      d. Posterior border fuses to perineal body and superiorly to superior layer of urogenital diaphragm. It fuses inferiorly with Colle's fascia.

3. **Structures piercing:**

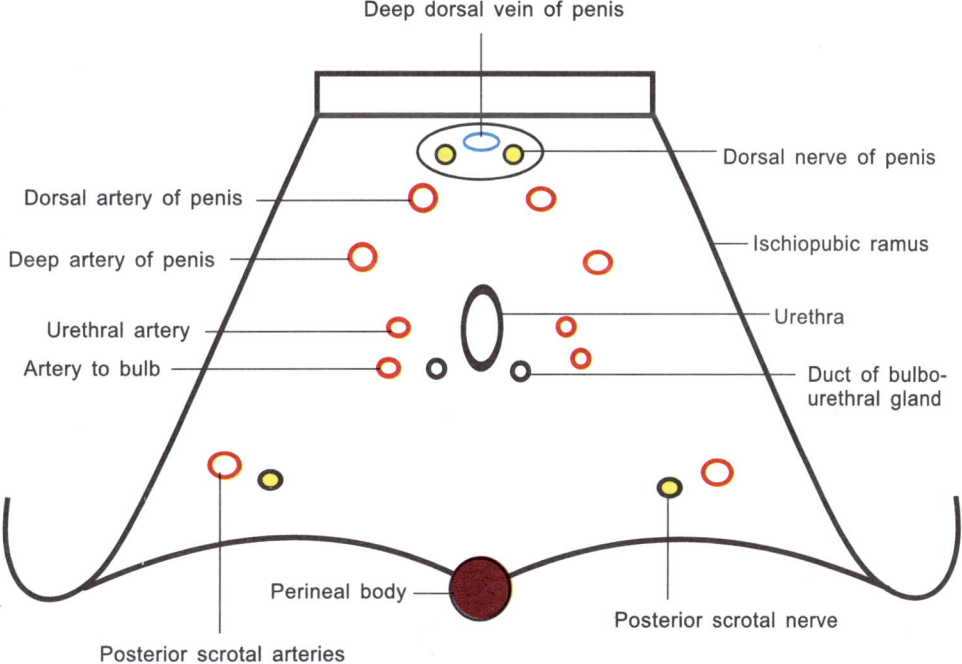

Fig. 2.86 Openings in the perineal membrane in male

A. In male:
   a. Urethra in the midline,
   b. Ducts of bulbourethral gland,
   c. Arteries:
       I. Artery to the bulb,
       II. Urethral artery,
       III. Deep artery of penis &
       IV. Dorsal artery of penis.
       } a branch of artery of penis (a branch of perineal artery).
       V. Posterior scrotal artery, a branch of perineal artery (a branch of internal pudendal artery).
   d. Nerves:
       I. Nerve to the bulb, a branch of nerve to bulbospongiosus (a branch of perineal nerve).
       II. Posterior scrotal nerve.
       III. Branches of perineal nerve to the superficial perineal muscle.
B. In female:
   a. Urethra,
   b. Vagina,
   c. Arteries:
       I. Artery to the bulb of the vestibule,
       II. Deep artery of clitoris,
       III. Dorsal artery of clitoris &
       IV. Posterior labial arteries.
   d. Nerves:
       I. Nerve to bulb of vestibule,
       II. Posterior labial nerve &
       III. Muscular branches of perineal nerve supplying superficial perineal muscles.

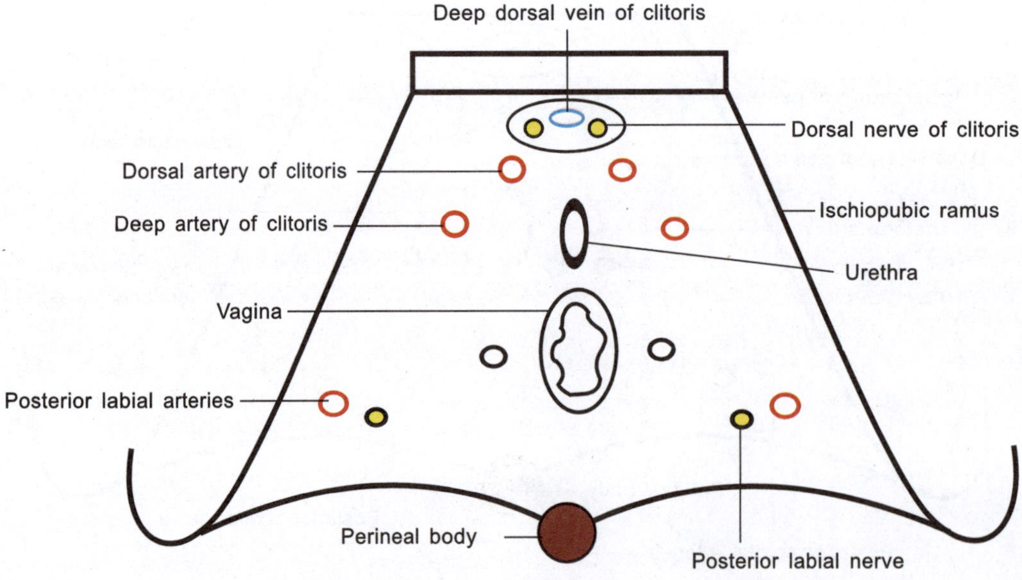

Fig. 2.87 Openings in the perineal membrane in female

4. **Applied anatomy:** Urethra passing through the perineal membrane is called membranous urethra. It is shortest and least dilatable part of urethra and does not contain any glands.

Urogenital diaphragm

1. **Introduction:** It is a musculo-fascial partition across the pubic arch and separates the pelvic cavity from the anterior part of the pelvic outlet.

2. **Formation:**
    A. Sphincter urethrae: It encircles the membranous urethra and consists of superficial and deep fibers.
    B. Deep transversus perinei.

3. **Nerve supply:** Both muscles are supplied by muscular branches of the perineal nerve, branch of pudendal nerve.

4. **Structure piercing:**
    A. In male: Urethra.
    B. In female: Vagina & urethra.

5. **Relations:**
    A. Below: Contents of superficial perineal pouch.
    B. Above:
        a. Apex of prostate (in male) or neck of the urinary bladder (in female).
        b. Anterior fibers of both levator ani muscles.
        c. Anterior recesses of ischiorectal fossae.

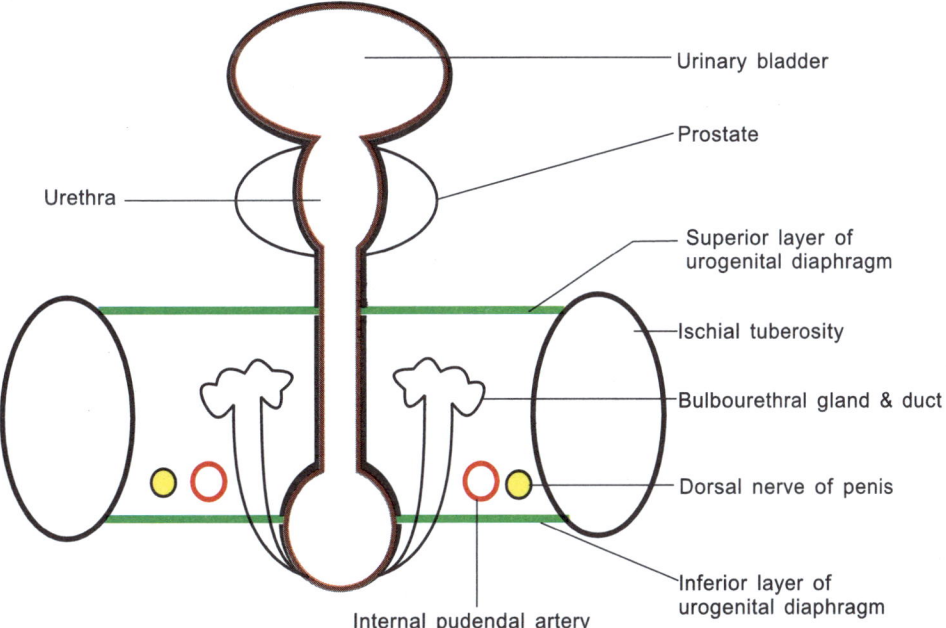

Fig. 2.88 Urogenital diaphragm

C. In front: A triangular gap between arcuate pubic ligament and transverse perineal ligament. It transmits the deep dorsal vein of penis or clitoris.
D. Behind: Ischiorectal fossae and their contents.

6. **Actions:**
   A. It supports the prostate or the bladder.
   B. In female, it constricts the vagina.
   C. It fixes the perineal body.
   D. Sphincter urethrae exerts voluntary control of micturition, and expels the last drops of semen and urine.

7. **Applied anatomy:** Rupture of the urethra is common beneath the pubis by fall on the sharp object. This causes extravasation of the urine.
   A. Rupture of urethra, superficial to the perineal membrane results in extravasation of the urine in the superficial perineal pouch & accumulates in the scrotum - penis - anterior abdominal wall, deep to fascia of Scarpa and extends upto axilla.
   B. Rupture of the urethra, deep to the perineal membrane produces extravasation of the urine in the extraperitoneal space of the pelvis & then accumulates in the anterior abdominal wall.

LAQ-22 — Describe superficial perineal pouch under
1. Introduction, 2. Boundaries, 3. Contents and 4. Applied anatomy.

1. **Introduction:** It is the space between the Colle's fascia and the perineal membrane (inferior layer of urogenital diaphragm)

2. **Boundaries:**
   A. Superficially or floor by Colles' fascia.
   B. Deep or roof by the perineal membrane.
   C. On each side by the ischiopubic rami.
   D. Posteriorly the space is closed by fusion of the perineal membrane with Colle's fascia.
   E. Anteriorly it is opened and is continuous with the spaces of the scrotum, the penis and the anterior abdominal wall.

3. **Contents:**

Table 2.15 Showing contents of superficial perineal pouch

Particulars	Male	Female
A. Structure	a. Crus of penis b. Bulb of the penis and urethra c. Root of the penis	a. Crus of clitoris b. Bulb of the vestibule c. Urethra and vagina
B. Glands	Ducts of bulbourethral gland	Greater vestibular gland

C. Nerves	a. Long perineal nerve from the posterior cutaneous nerve of the thigh.
	b. Three sets of branches from the perineal nerve which are branches of internal pudendal nerve
	  I. Muscular branches
	  II. Nerve to the bulb
	  III.Posterior scrotal nerves in male and labial nerves in female.	

Particulars	Male	Female
D. Muscles	a. **S**uperficial transverse perinei. b. **B**ulbospongiosus. c. **I**schiocavernosus. <u>SBI</u>	

E. Vessels	a. Branches of perineal artery
	   I. In male posterior scrotal artery and in female labial artery
	   II. Transverse perineal artery	

	b. Branches of the artery of penis I. Artery of the bulb	I. Artery of the bulb: Supplying erectile tissue of the vestibular bulb and vagina.

	II. Urethral artery
	   III.Deep artery of penis
	   IV.Dorsal artery of penis
		II. Urethral artery
		III.Deep artery of the clitoris
		IV.Dorsal artery of the clitoris.

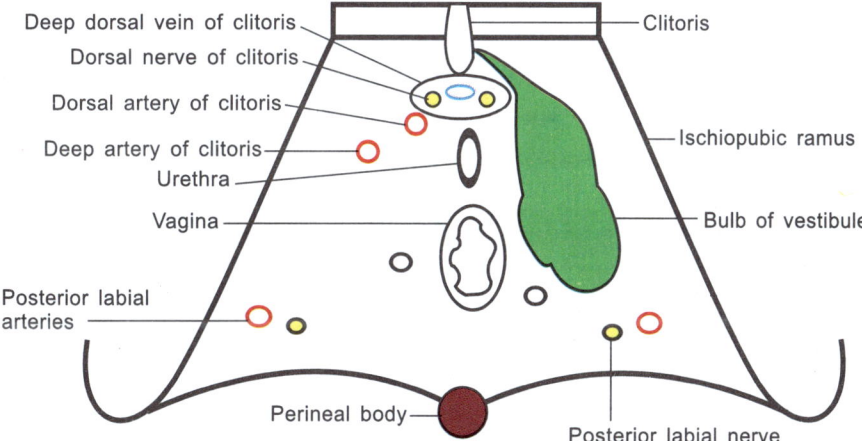

Fig. 2.89 Contents of the superficial perineal pouch in female

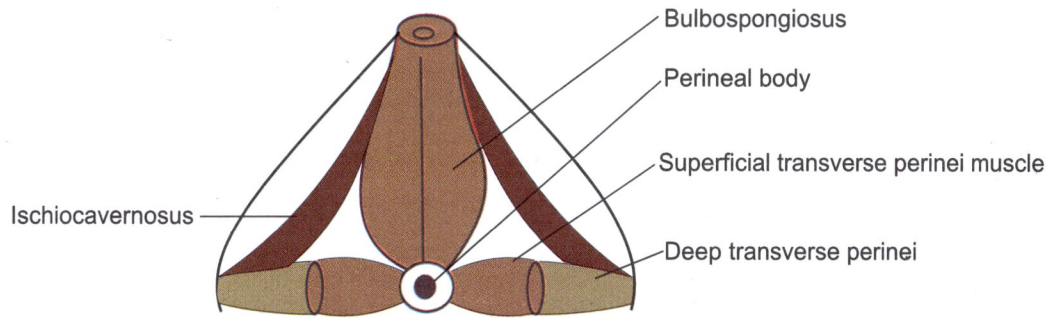

Fig. 2.90 Muscles in the superficial perineal pouch

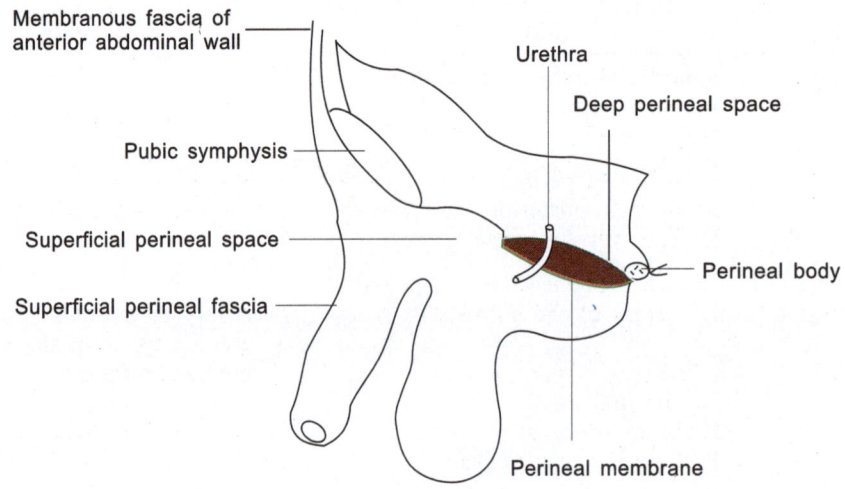

Fig. 2.91 Superficial and deep perineal pouch

4. **Applied anatomy:** Rupture of urethra superficial to the perineal membrane results in extravasation of the urine in the superficial perineal pouch and accumulates in the scrotum - penis - anterior abdominal wall, deep to Scarpa's of fascia and may extend upto axilla.

LAQ-23	**Describe deep perineal pouch under**

   1. **Introduction,**   2. **Boundaries,**
   3. **Contents and**   4. **Applied anatomy.**

1. **Introduction:** It is the space between superior and inferior fascia of urogenital diaphragm.

2. **Boundaries:**
    A. Inferior or superficial layer is by perineal membrane (inferior layer of urogenital diaphragm).
    B. Superior or deep by the superior layer of urogenital diaphragm.
    C. On each side by the ischiopubic rami.
    D. Posteriorly the space is closed by the union of the perineal membrane with the superior fascia of the urogenital diaphragm (fusion of superior and inferior layer of urogenital diaphragm).
    E. Anteriorly it is closed by the union of perineal membrane with the superior fascia of urogenital diaphragm at the transverse perineal ligament.

3. **Contents:**
    A. These can be described in male and female.
        a. In male
            I.   Membranous urethra and
            II. Bulbourethral gland.
        b. In female
            I.   Urethra and
            II. Vagina.

B. Muscles
   a. Sphincter urethrae.
   b. Deep transversus perinei.
C. Nerves
   a. In male dorsal nerve of the penis (pudendal nerve) and in female dorsal nerve of clitoris.
   b. Muscular branches from the perineal nerve.
D. Vessels: Artery of penis, a branch of internal pudendal artery.

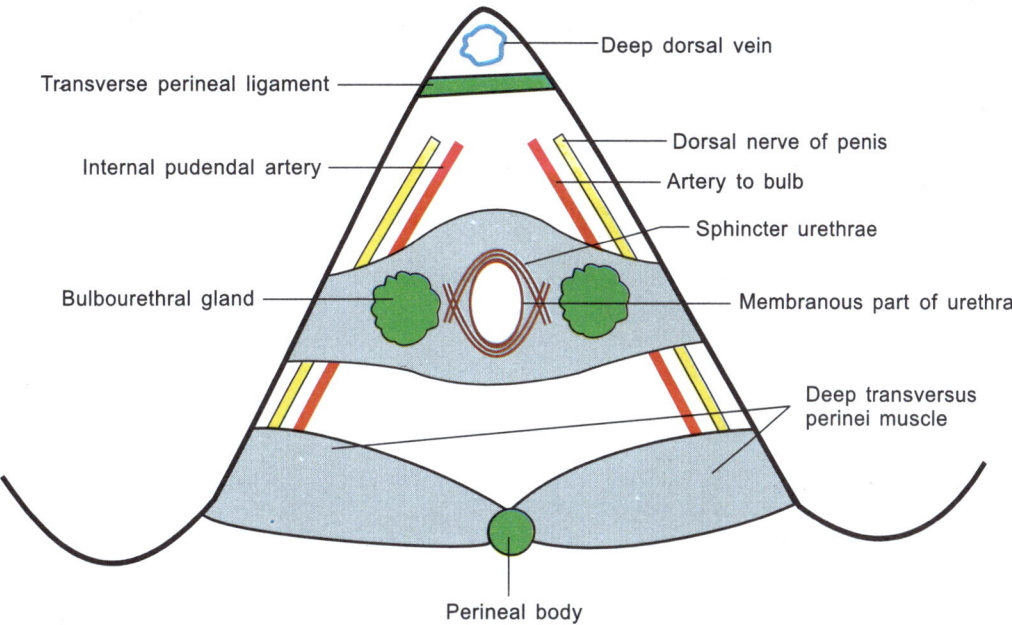

Fig. 2.92 Structures in the deep perineal pouch

4. **Applied anatomy:** Rupture of the urethra (deep to the perineal membrane) produces extravasation of the urine in the extraperitoneal space of the pelvis & then accumulates in the anterior abdominal wall.

LAQ-24 **Describe urinary bladder under**
   1.   **Gross anatomy,**   2.   **Histology,**
   3.   **Development and**   4.   **Applied anatomy.**

1. **Gross anatomy:**
   A. Introduction:
      a. Location: It is present behind the pubic symphysis, in the anterior part of pelvic cavity.
      b. Capacity: **2, 4, 8, 16, 32**
         I. At birth it is **2** ounce (60 ml).
         II. When the capacity of the bladder reaches **4** ounces (120 ml), one gets sense of filling the bladder.

III. When the bladder is filled beyond **8** ounce (240 ml), onegets desire to micturate.

IV. When the capacity of the bladder reaches **16** ounce (480 ml), it become painful.

V. The anatomical capacity of bladder is **32** ounce (960 ml).

B. External features:

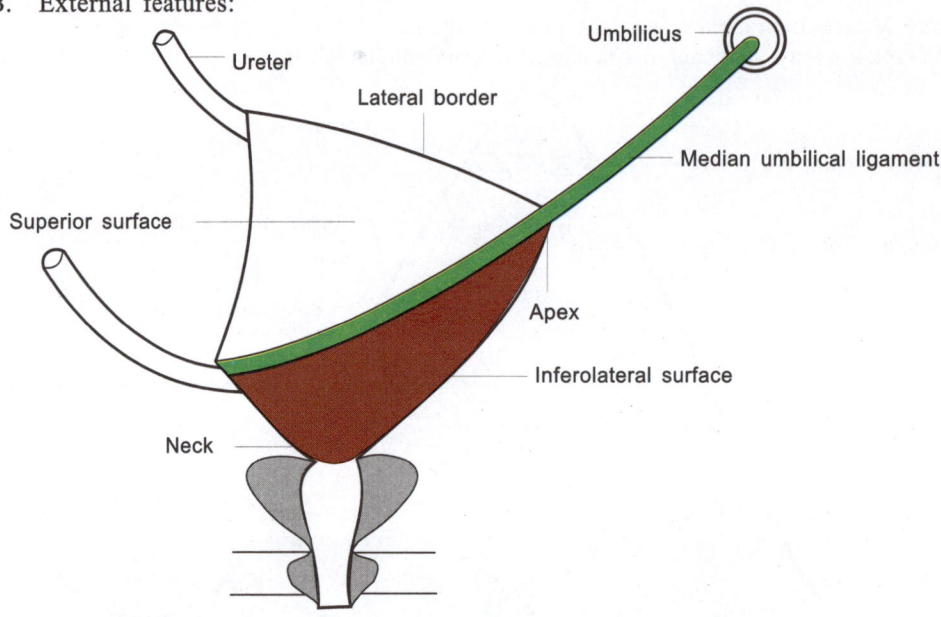

Fig. 2.93 Features of bladder.

a. Shape:
 I. In empty, it is tetrahedral.
 II. In distended, it is ovoid.

b. Apex:
 I. In empty it is directed forward.
 II. In full it is directed towards the umbilicus.

c. Base is directed backwards.

d. Neck is lowest and most fixed part of the bladder.

e. Surfaces:
 I. In empty
  i. One superior and
  ii. Two inferolateral surfaces.
 II. In full
  i. One anterior and
  ii. One posterior.

f. Borders: 4
 I. Left lateral,
 II. Right lateral,
 III. Posterior and
 IV. Anteroinferior.

C. Relations: **Table 2.16** Showing relations of urinary bladder

Particulars	Female	Male
a. Apex	Connected to umbilicus by median umbilical ligament	

b. Base	I. Cervix of uterus
	II. Vagina
		Separated from rectum
		i. In upper part - by
		  - Rectovesical pouch
		  -. Coils of intestine
		ii. In lower part by
		  - Seminal vesicle
		  - Vas deferens

c. Neck - lower and fixed part	Pelvic fascia which surrounds upper part of urethra	Base of prostate

d. Superior surface is covered by peritoneum	Greater part is covered by peritoneum and is related to vesicouterine pouch and contains
	  I. Sigmoid colon
	  II. Terminal part of ileum
		Completely covered by peritoneum & is in contact with
		i. Sigmoid colon
		ii. Terminal part of ileum

e. Inferolateral surfaces are devoid of peritoneum	It is related to
	  I. Pubis
	  II. Pubovesical ligament
	  III.Retropubic fat
	  IV.Levator ani
	  V. Obturator internus
		i. Pubis
		ii. Puboprostatic ligament
		iii.Retropubic fat
		iv. Levator ani
		v. Obturator internus

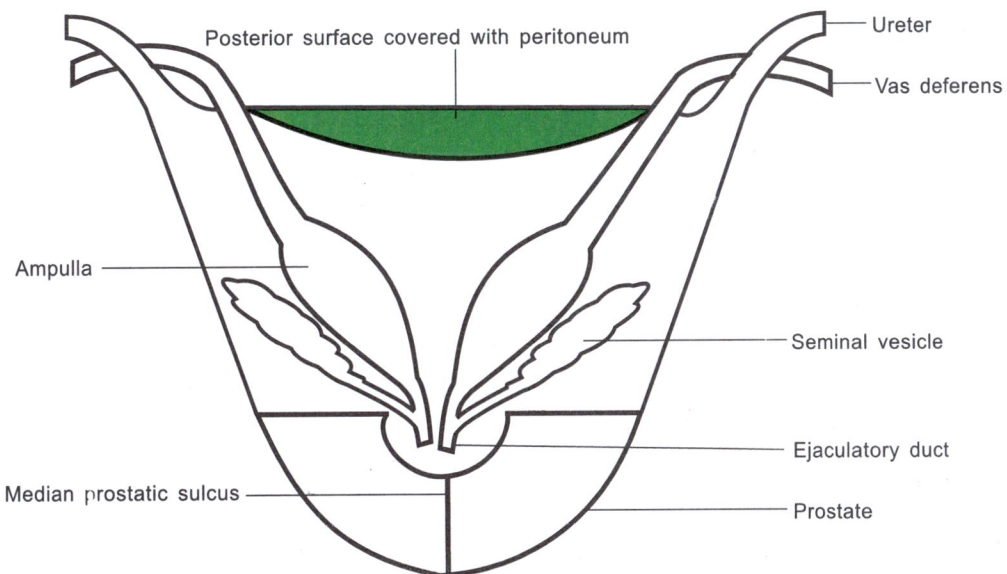

Fig. 2.94 Posterior surface of the bladder

D. Blood supply:
  a. Arterial supply:
    I. Major blood supply to the bladder is by
      i. Superior vesical artery, a branch of internal division of internal iliac artery.
      ii. Inferior vesical artery, a branch of internal division of internal iliac artery.
    II. Minor blood supply to the lower part of the bladder is from
      i. Obturator artery,
      ii. Inferior gluteal artery,
      iii. Uterine artery and   } Branches of internal iliac artery
      iv. Vaginal artery.
  b. Venous drainage: Veins of the bladder do not follow the arteries. They vary in male and female.
    I. In male: Veins form a vesico prostatic plexus between bladder and prostate, which drains backwards to the internal iliac vein.
    II. In female: Veins form a plexus in the base of the broad ligament. And drains backward to the internal iliac vein.

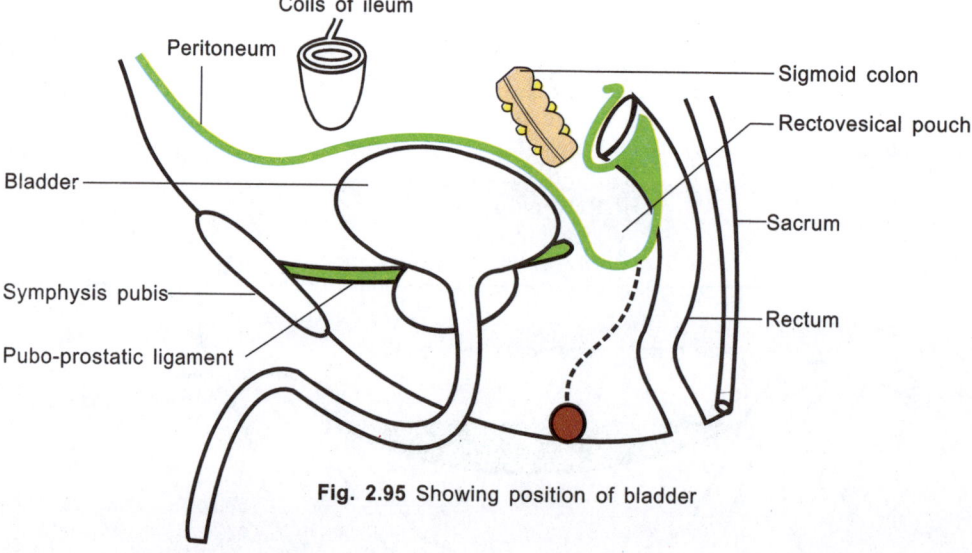

Fig. 2.95 Showing position of bladder

E. Nerve supply: It is mainly by
  a. Parasympathetic fibers, which provide main motor innervation of the bladder. It reaches via pelvic splanchnic nerve (Nervi erigentes $S_{2, 3, 4}$). The <u>emptying of the bladder</u> is done by parasympathetic fibers.
    I. Contraction of the detrusor muscle,
    II. Relaxation of the internal urethral sphincter.
  b. Sympathetic fibers are derived from L_1 and L_2 segments of the spinal cord. For most of the bladder the sympathetic fibers are vasomotor and
    I. Inhibitory to the detrusor and
    II. Motor to the sphincter vesicae.
    This nerve is for the filling of the bladder.
  c. Somatic pudendal nerve: It supplies the external urethral sphincter (sphincter urethrae) which is voluntary.

d. Sensory nerves: It is carried mainly by parasympathetic nerves and partly by sympathetic nerves.
  I. Pain sensation is carried by the lateral spinothalamic tract.
  II. Distension of bladder is carried by the posterior column.
F. Lymphatic drainage: The lymphatics of the bladder follow the course of the arteries and drain into internal and external iliac nodes.

2. **Histology:** The wall of the bladder presents following coats from outside inward.
  A. Serous coat: It is lined by simple squamous epithelium only on the superior surface. In other places it is formed by adventitial coat.
  B. Muscular coat: It possesses three ill defined layers of smooth muscle.
    a. Outer longitudinal,
    b. Middle circular and
    c. Inner longitudinal.
  C. Mucosa: It consists of
    a. Transitional epithelium, which consists of
      I. Deep layer is formed by columnar cells.

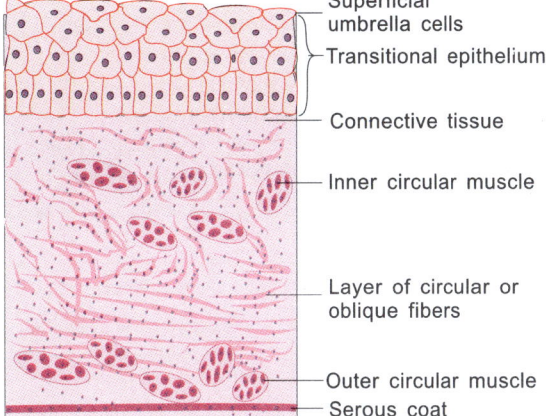

Fig. 2.96 Histology of urinary bladder

      II. Middle layer is formed by polyhedral cells.
      III. Superficial layer is formed by umbrella cells in empty bladder. In distended bladder the cells are squamous type.
    b. Lamina propria: Muscularis mucosa is absent.

3. **Development:**
  A. Chronological age: It develops in the fourth to seventh week of intrauterine life.
  B. Germ layer: The epithelium develops from endoderm and mesoderm and muscles from the mesoderm.
  C. Site: Cloaca.
  D. Source:
    a. Epithelium of the urinary bladder:
      I. Except trigone develops from cranial part of vesicourethral canal (endoderm).
      II. Epithelium of trigone develops from absorbed part of mesonephric duct (mesoderm).
    b. The muscles and the connective tissue develop from intra embryonic splanchnopleuric mesoderm.
  E. Anomalies:
    a. **A**bsence of the urinary bladder. 🗝 **A B C D E F**
    b. **B**ladder may be divided into upper & lower compartment by septum (hour glass bladder).
    c. There may be **c**ommunication with the rectum - vesicorectal fistula.
    d. **D**iverticulum of the urinary bladder. It is usually at the junction of trigone and rest of the bladder.
    e. **E**ctopic vesicae: The lower part of the anterior abdominal wall is absent, the bladder is exposed on the surface of the body.
    f. **F**istula: Allantosis may remain patent entirely & urine passes through umbilicus.

4. **Applied anatomy:**
   A. Lesion of the parasympathetic nerve causes
      a. Loss of control of the micturition,
      b. Retention of urine due to overactivity of sympathetic nerve.
   B. Lesion of the sympathetic nerve fibers causes: Paralysis of the sphincter vesicae and results into dribbling in continence.
   C. Results of both pyramidal tracts lesion (upper motor neuron lesion) results into loss of voluntary initiation of micturition.
   D. Bilateral anterolateral cordotomy results into abolition of pain sensation without awareness of bladder and desire to micturate. This is present in advance stage of cancer of the bladder.
   E. The posterior column lesion (tabes dorsalis - i.e. wasting of the dorsal column), the bladder is atonic and large quantity of urine is collected without any reflex contraction.

LAQ-25	Describe male urethra under

Describe male urethra under
1. **Gross anatomy,**   2. **Histology,**
3. **Development and**   4. **Applied anatomy.**

1. **Gross anatomy:**
   A. Introduction:
      a. Length: 18 to 20 cm
      b. Curvatures: There are 2 curvatures.
      c. Extent: It extends from internal urethral orifice to the external urethral orifice at the tip of the penis.
   B. Divisions:
      a. Prostatic part of the urethra.
         I. Introduction:
            i. Situation: It is present in the prostate gland.
            ii. Peculiarity: *It is widest and most dilated part of the male urethra and is narrowest at the junction with the membranous urethra.*
         II. Internal features: Posterior wall of the prostatic urethra shows following features.
            i. The urethral crest, a median longitudinal ridge of mucous membrane.
            ii. The colliculus seminalis, an elevation on the middle of the urethral crest.
            iii. The prostatic utricle, a blind sac about 6 mm long, which lies within the prostate.
            iv. There is an orifice on the elevation through which prostatic utricle opens into the urethra.
            v. On each side of this orifice there are openings of the ejaculatory ducts.
            vi. There are two vertical grooves called as prostatic sinuses situated one on each side of urethral crest.
            vii. Each sinus presents the openings of 20 to 30 prostatic glands.
      b. Membranous part of urethra:
         I. Introduction: It passes through the deep perineal space and pierces the perineal membrane. About 2.5 cm below and behind the pubic symphysis.
            i. It is the second narrowest and least dilatable part of the male urethra.
            ii. It is surrounded by sphincter urethrae (external urethral sphincter).

iii. The bulbo urethral glands are placed one on each side of the membranous urethra and their ducts open into the spongy part of urethra.

II. Internal features: There are many urethral glands which also open into the membranous urethra.

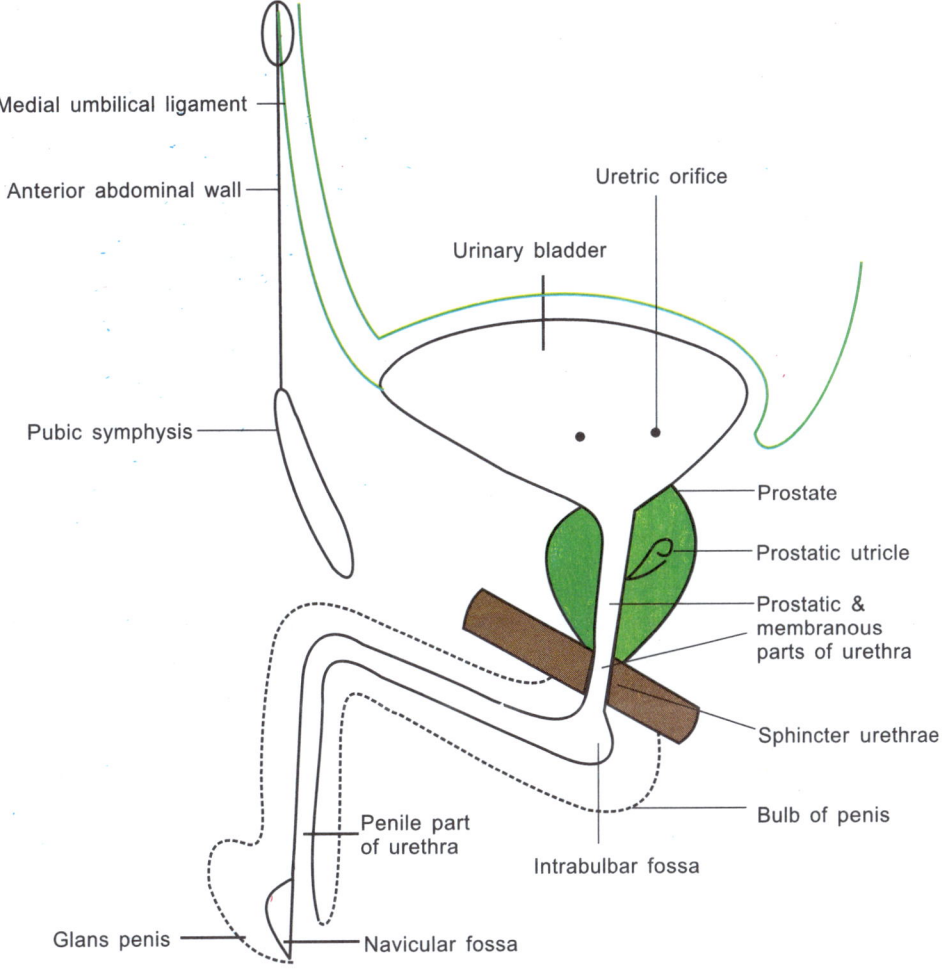

Medial umbilical ligament

Anterior abdominal wall

Uretric orifice

Urinary bladder

Pubic symphysis

Prostate

Prostatic utricle

Prostatic & membranous parts of urethra

Sphincter urethrae

Penile part of urethra

Bulb of penis

Intrabulbar fossa

Glans penis

Navicular fossa

Fig. 2.97 Internal features of male urethra

c. Spongy part or penile part of the urethra:
   I. Introduction: It is so called because it lies in the corpus spongiosum of penis.
   II. Situation: It lies in the corpus spongiosum and hence partly in the superficial perineal pouch and partly in the body of penis and also in the glans penis.
   III. Extent:
      i. Begins: From the membranous urethra or from perineal membrane.
      ii. Ends: It opens to the exterior by an orifice called the external urethral orifice. It is a vertical slit of 6 mm long. It is the narrowest part of the urethra. It is guarded by two lips called labia.

    IV. Dimension:
        i.   Length: 15 cm.
        ii.   Diameter: 6 mm in the body of penis.
    V. Course: It first ascends upwards and forwards in the superficial pouch up to the symphysis pubis and then descends down in the flaccid condition of the penis.
    VI. Dilatations:
        i.   Intrabulbar fossa: It lies in bulb of the penis. It bulgis into the floor and to each side. Hence looks like a trapezium in cross section.
        ii.   Fossa terminalis: It is also called fossa navicularis which lies within the glans penis.

C. Blood supply:
    a. Arterial supply: There is no single artery to the urethra. The blood supply is from any adjacent vessels as it passes through the prostate, sphincter urethrae and corpus spongiosum. These are
        I.   Inferior vesical,
        II.   Middle rectal,   } Supply pelvic part of urethra.
        III. Internal pudendal &
        IV. Urethral branch of the artery to the bulb of   } Supply supraperineal and penile part of urethra.
            penis (a branch of internal pudendal artery).
    b. Venous drainage: Veins correspond to the arteries and drain into internal iliac veins.
D. Nerve supply: Most of the urethra is supplied by autonomic nerves, and terminal part by somatic nerves.
    a. Sympathetic fibers are derived from the superior hypogastric plexus; the preganglionic fibers come form L_1 and L_2 segments.
    b. Parasympathetic fibers are derived from pelvic splanchnic nerves, carrying preganglionic fibers from S_2, S_3 and S_4 segments.
    c. Somatic fibers are derived from the urethral branches of the pudendal nerves.
E. Lymphatic:
    a. The lymphatics from prostatic and membranous parts drain into internal and external iliac lymph nodes.
    b. The lymphatics from spongy part drains into deep inguinal and sometimes into external iliac lymph nodes.

2. Histology: It presents 3 coats from outside inward.
A. Muscular coat: The prostatic urethra shows mainly longitudinal muscle.
    Rest of the urethra demonstrates inner longitudinal and outer circular layers of the smooth muscle.
B. Submucous coat consists of erectile vascular tissue.
C. Mucous membrane presents regional variation.
    a. Above the colliculus: It is lined by transitional epithelium.
    b. Between the colliculus and the terminal fossa: It is lined by stratified columnar epithelium.
    c. Distal to terminal fossa: It is lined by stratified squamous nonkeratinized epithelium.

3. Development:
A. Chronological age: It develops at the end of third month of intrauterine life.
B. Germ layer: Endoderm, ectoderm and mesoderm.

C. Sources:
  a. Prostatic part
    I. Above the opening of ejaculatory duct.
      i. Anterior and lateral wall develops from caudal part of vesicourethral canal, which is of endodermal in origin.
      ii. Posterior wall develops from absorbed part of mesonephric duct (mesoderm), which is mesodermal in origin.
    II. Below the opening of ejaculatory duct develops from pelvic part of definitive urogenital sinus, which develops from endoderm.
  b. Membranous part develop from pelvic part of definitive urogenital sinus, which is endodermal in origin.
  c. Penile part develops from phalic part of definitive urogenital sinus, which is endodermal in origin.
  d. Terminal part develops from ectoderm.

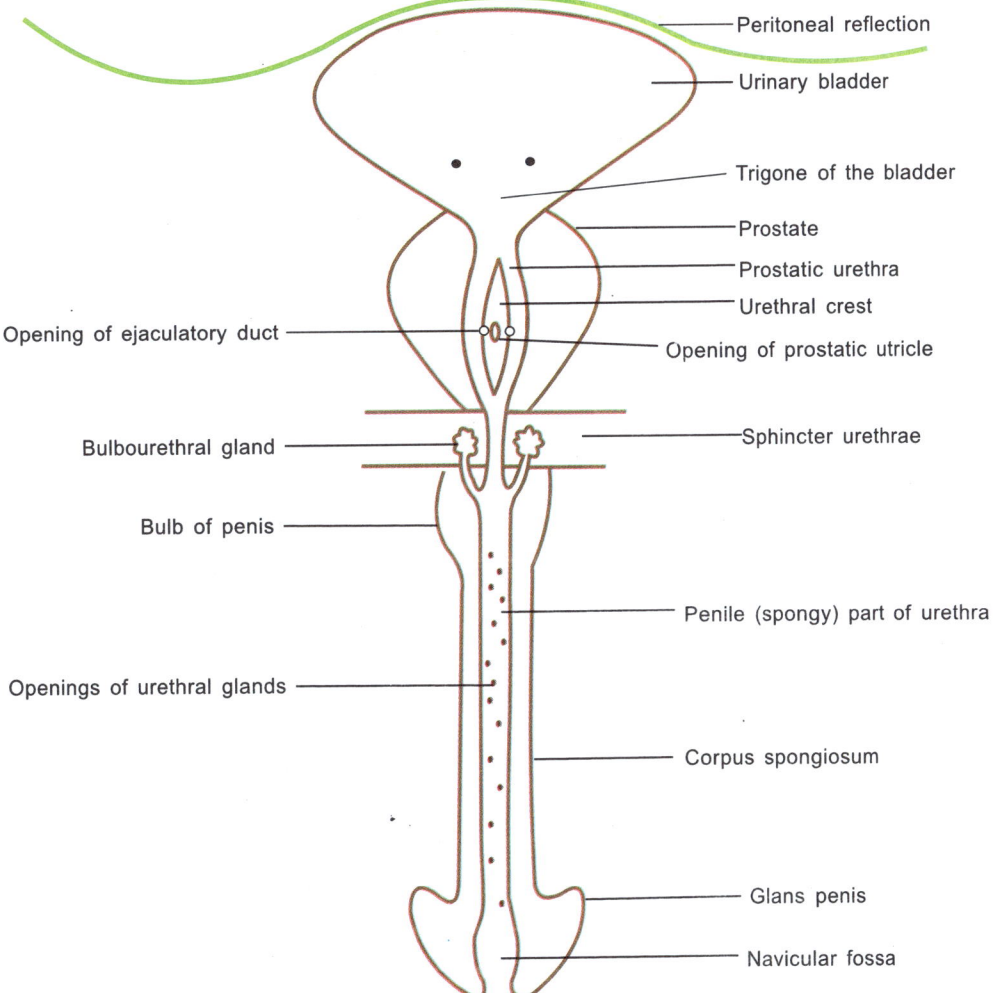

Fig. 2.98 Male urethra

D. Anomalies:
   I.   Hypospadiasis: The urethra opens anywhere on the undersurface of the penis.
   II. Epispadiasis: The urethra opens on dorsal surface of penis close to anterior abdominal wall.
   III. Ectopia vesicae: The deficient infra umbilical part of anterior abdominal wall.

3. Applied anatomy:
   A. In retention of urine, a rubber or metal tube is passed into the bladder through the urethral meatus is called catheterization. While catheterization, the normal curvatures of the urethra should be kept in mind. The forceful insertion of metallic instruments may create false passage in the urethra.
   B. Rupture of the urethra is common beneath the pubis by fall on sharp object. This causes extravasation of urine.
      I. Rupture of urethra superficial to perineal membrane results in extravasation of urine in superficial perineal pouch & urine accumulates in scrotum - penis - anterior abdominal wall deep to fascia of scarpa - extends upto axilla.
      II. Rupture of urethra (Deep to perineal membrane) produces extravasation of urine in the pelvic extraperitoneal space and urine accumulates in the anterior abdominal wall.
   C. Urethritis is an inflammation of urethra.

LAQ-26 — Describe the ovary under
1. **Gross anatomy,**   2. **Histology,**
3. **Development and**   4. **Applied anatomy.**

1. Gross anatomy:
   A. Introduction:
      a. General introduction: It is a female gonad which forms the ova.
      b. Situation: It is located in ovarian fossa.
      c. Dimension: 3 x 1.5 x 1 cm (length x breadth x thickness).
   B. External features:
      a. Surface:
         I. Medial &
         II. Lateral.
      b. Borders:
         I. Anterior or meso-ovarian border.
         II. Posterior border is free border.
      c. Pole:
         I.   Upper broader
         II. Lower narrower
         III. Axis ·
            i. Multiparous: Horizontal.
            ii. Nulliparous: Vertical.
   C. Relations:
      a. Peritoneal:
         I. Ovary is entirely covered with peritoneum except along the meso-ovarian border i.e. Anterior border where peritoneum is continuous with the posterior layer of broad ligament.

      II.   Suspensory ligament of the ovary extends from upper pole of ovary to external iliac vessels. It contains ovarian vessels.

  b. Visceral:
      I.   Upper pole is related to uterine tube and external iliac veins.
      II. Lower pole is related to pelvic floor.
      III. Anterior border: Uterine tube & obliterated umbilical artery.
      IV. Posterior border:
         i.   Uterine tube.
         ii. Ureter.
      V.   Lateral surface: Ovarian fossa, & related to obturator vessels and obturator nerve separated by peritoneum, which is lined by parietal peritoneum.
      VI. Medial surface: Covered by uterine tubes.

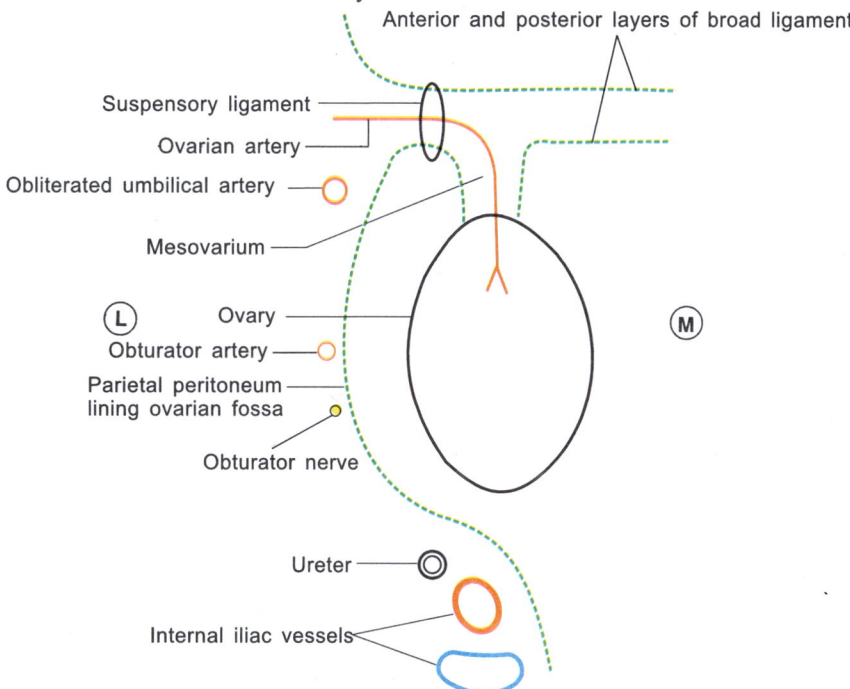

Fig. 2.99 Relations of the ovary

D. Blood supply:
  a. Arterial supply: The ovary is supplied by the ovarian artery, a branch of the abdominal aorta from just below the renal artery. The vessel runs down behind the peritoneum. It crosses the ureter obliquely and crosses the brim of the pelvis. It enters the suspensory ligament. It gives a branch to the uterine tube which runs between the layers of the broad ligament and anastomosis with the uterine artery.
  b. Venous Drainage: The ovarian veins form a plexus in the mesovarium and the suspensory ligament which is called pampiniform plexus. The plexus drains into a pair of ovarian veins which accompany the ovarian artery. They usually combine as a single trunk before their termination.

      Right ovarian vein opens into the inferior vena cava and left ovarian vein opens into left renal vein.

E. Nerve supply: It is formed by ovarian plexus. The fibers of the plexus are formed by
  a. Sympathetic (vaso constrictor) fibers reach the ovary from the aortic plexus along its blood vessels. The pre-ganglionic fibers arises from T_{10} to T_{11} segments of the spinal cord.
  b. Parasympathetic fibers may reach the ovary from the inferior hypogastric plexus via uterine artery.
  c. Sensory fibers accompany the sympathetic nerves so that the ovarian pain may be referred along the umbilicus.
F. Lymphatic drainage: The lymphatics of the ovary drain to para-aortic nodes along side the origin of ovarian artery.

2. **Histology:** It shows following layers from inside out
A. Simple cuboidal epithelium.
B. Tunica albuginea, a thin layer of connective tissue.
C. Cortex shows various stages of ovarian follicle.

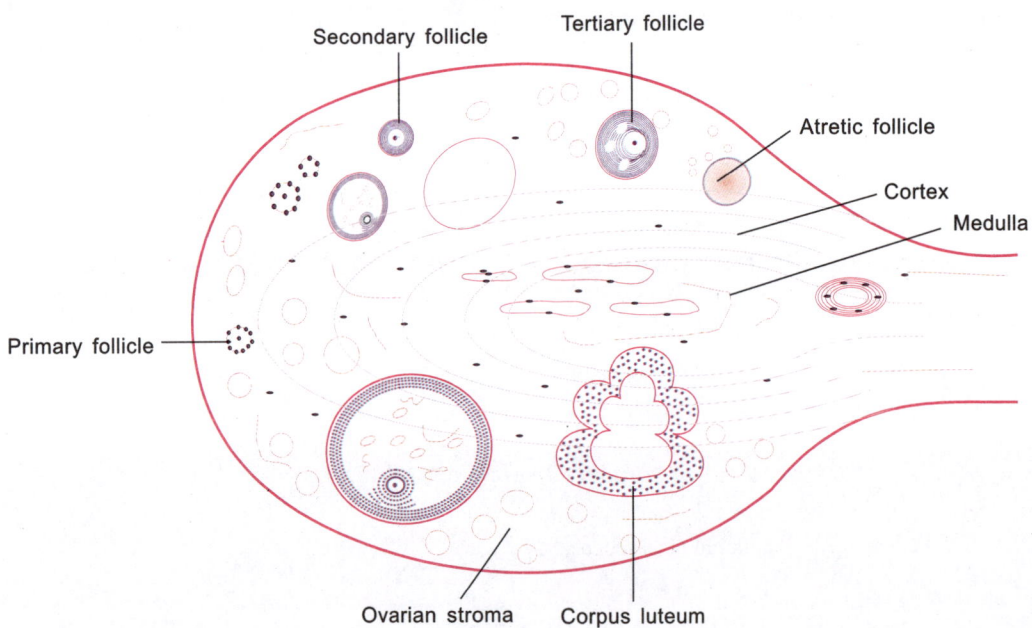

Fig. 2.100 Histology of ovary

3. **Development:**
A. Chronological age: It develops in the seventh week of intrauterine life.
B. Germ layer: Endoderm.
C. Site: Wall of the yolk sac close to the allantois.
D. Sources:
  a. Ovary develops from the coelomic epithelium lining the medial side of the nephrogenic cord.
  b. The surface epithelium of the female gonad forms cortical cords. In the fourth month these cords form primitive germ cell.
  c. Descend of the gonads is considerably less in the female than male and the ovary is finally settle just below the rim of the true pelvis.

4. **Applied anatomy:**
   A. Prolapse of ovaries: It is frequently displaced in the pouch of Douglas, it can be palpated by per vaginal examination.
   B. The carcinoma of ovary is common, and accounts for 15% of all cancers and 20 % of gynaecological cancers.
   C. Krukenberg's tumor: It is transcoelomic migration of cancer cells from mammary gland to ovary and forms a tumor called Krukenberg's tumor.
   D. Oophoritis: It is the inflammation of ovary. It may produce localized peritonitis of the ovarian fossa and eventual irritation of the obturator nerve. This results into pain on the medial side of thigh.

SAQ-10 — Ovarian fossa

1. **Introduction:** It is a fossa present in the pelvis which contains ovary, the female gonad.

2. **Boundaries:** It is bounded
   A. Anteriorly by obliterated umbilical artery.
   B. Posteriorly by
       a. Ureter and
       b. Internal iliac artery.

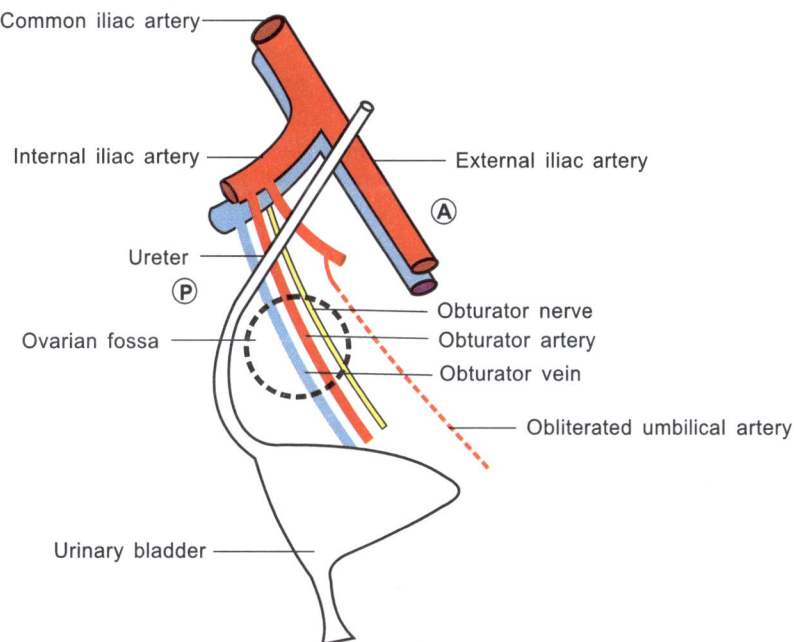

Fig. 2.101 Boundaris of the ovarian fossa

3. **Applied anatomy:** The inflammation of the ovary produces localized peritonitis of the ovarian fossa and eventual irritation of the obturator nerve. This results into pain on the medial side of thigh.

LAQ-27   Describe uterine tube under
1.   Gross anatomy,   2.   Histology,
3.   Development and   4.   Applied anatomy.

1.   Gross anatomy:
- A.   Introduction:
  - a.   General introduction: These are the tortuous ducts which convey the ova from the ovary to the uterus. The spermatozoa introduced into the vagina pass into the uterus and then into the uterine tubes. The fertilization usually takes place in the ampullary part of the fallopian tube.
  - b.   Length: About 10cm (4 inches)
- B.   External features: Parts of uterine tube are as follows
  - a.   Infundibulum: It is a funnel shaped lateral end of uterine tube. It bears finger like processes called fimbriae and is therefore called fimbriated end. One of the fimbriae is longer than the others and is attached to be tubal pole of the ovary. It is known as ovarian fimbriae. At the lateral end the uterine tube opens into the peritoneal cavity through its abdominal ostium. It is about 3 mm in diameter.
  - b.   Ampulla: It is thin walled, dilated and tortuous and forms approximately lateral $2/3^{rd}$ of the tube. It is about 4 mm in diameter.
  - c.   Isthmus: It is narrow, rounded and cord like.
  - d.   The interstitial part of the uterine tube is about 1 cm long and lies within the wall of the uterus.

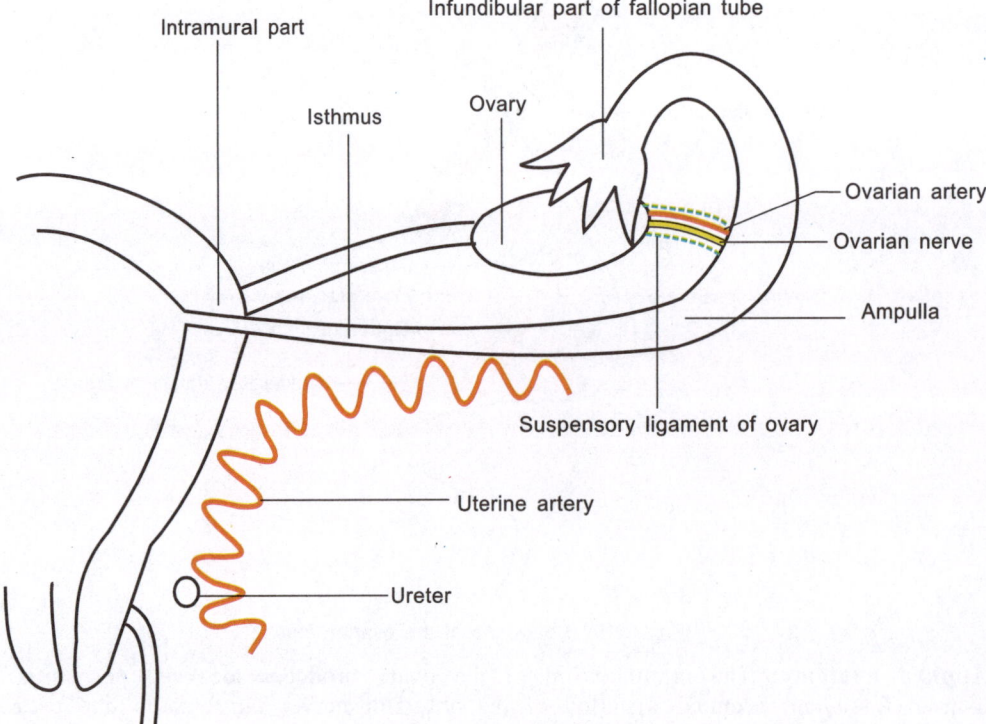

Fig. 2.102 The parts, relations and blood supply of the uterine tube

C. Course and relations:
  a. The ampulla arches over the ovary and is related to the anterior & posterior border of the ovary. It is also related to upper pole and medial surface of the ovary.
  b. The uterine tube lies in the upper free margin of the broad ligament of uterus. The part of the broad ligament between the attachment of the mesovarium and the uterine tube is known as mesosalpinx.
D. Blood supply:
  a. Arterial supply: The uterine tube is supplied by tubal branch of ovarian artery. The tubal artery runs below the tube between the layers of the broad ligament. It anastomoses with the tubal branches of uterine artery in the broad ligament.
  b. Venous drainage: The veins run parallel with the arteries. The veins of the tube join the pampiniform plexus and drain into the uterine veins.
E. Nerve supply: The uterine tubes are supplied by both the sympathetic and parasympathetic nerves.
  a. The sympathetic fibers are derived from the hypogastric plexuses. They are vaso motor in function.
  b. Parasympathetic fibers are derived from S_2, S_3, S_4. They inhibit peristalsis and produce vasodilatation.
F. Lymphatic drainage:
  a. The lymphatics of the fallopian tube join the lymphatics of the ovary and drain into lateral aortic and para aortic nodes.
  b. The lymphatics from the isthmus accompany the round ligament of the uterus and drain into the superficial inguinal nodes.

2. **Histology:** It consists of
  A. Muscular coat: It consists of inner circular and outer longitudinal layer of the smooth muscle.
  B. The mucous membrane shows numerous branching fold which fill the lumen of the tube
  C. Mucosa: It is lined by ciliated columnar epithelium.

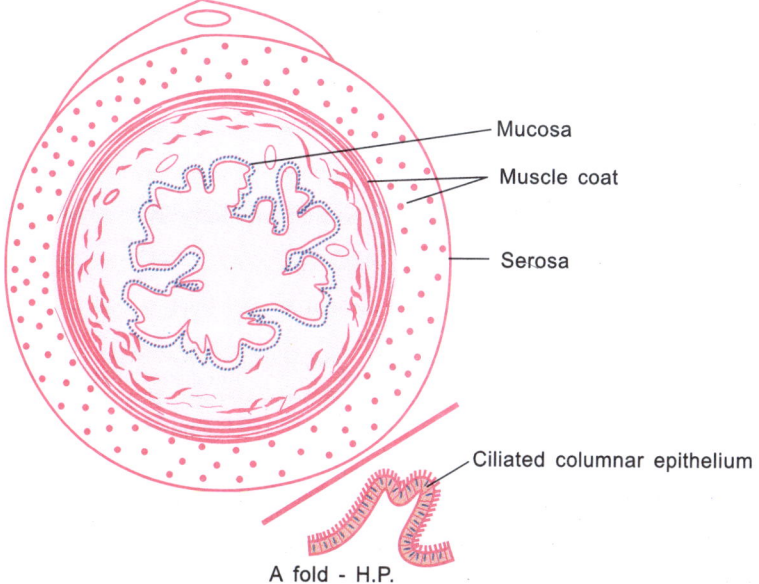

A fold - H.P.

Fig. 2.103 Histology of uterine tube

3. **Development:**
   A. Chronological age: It develops in the eighth week of intrauterine life.
   B. Germ layer: Mesoderm.
   C. Site: Intermediate mesoderm.
   D. Sources:
      a. Proximal unfused vertical part of the paramesonephric duct forms the fallopian tube.
      b. Fimbria are formed from the invagination of the paramesonephric duct into the coelomic epithelium.
   E. Anomalies:
      a. Absence of the uterine tubes on one or both the sides.
      b. The tubes may be partially or completely duplicated on one or both the sides.
      c. There may be atresia of the tubes.
      d. Hydatid (of Morgagni): The cranial end of the paramesonephric duct does not contribute to the infundibulum of the uterine tube and may persist as a vesicular appendage called as hydatid of Morgagni.

4. **Applied anatomy:**
   A. Salpingitis: Inflamation of the uterine tube is called salpingitis.
   B. Sterility: Inability to conceive is called sterility. The most common cause of sterility in the female is blockage of the fallopian tube. It may be congenital or may be caused by tuberculosis infection. The patency of the tube is investigated by
      a. Insufflation test (Rubin's test): Normally, air pushed into the uterus passes through the tubes and leaks into the peritoneal cavity. This leakage produces a hissing or bubbling sound which can be auscultated over the iliac fossae.
      b. Hysterosalpingography is a radiological technique by which the cavity of the uterus and the lumina of the tubes can be visualized, after injecting a radiopaque oily dye into the uterus.

LAQ-28 **Describe uterus under**
   1. **Gross anatomy,**   2. **Histology,**
   3. **Development and**   4. **Applied anatomy.**

1. **Gross anatomy:**
   A. Introduction: It is a child bearing organ present in the pelvic cavity.
   B. External features:
      a. Axis of uterus
         I. Anteversion (*ante* prior to or infront of, *version* relation of uterus with the vagina around transverse axis through external os of cervix): The forward lipping or tilting of an organ, displacement in which the organ is tipped forward but is not bend at an angle as occurs in anteflexion.
            However it is defined as forward angle between the axis of cervix and that of vagina, measuring 90°.

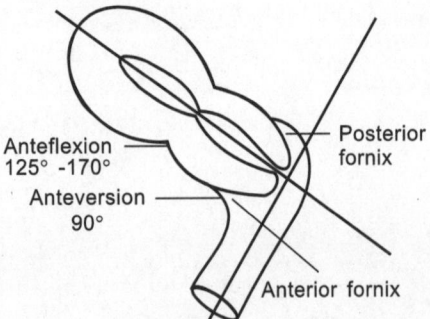

Fig. 2.104 Anteflexion and anteversion of the uterus.

II. Anteflexion: Forward angle between the body and the cervix, at the isthmus measuring 135°, provided bladder and rectum are empty.

b. Supports of uterus: The most fixed part of the uterus is cervix. The urinary bladder, vagina attached to the uterus, maintain the position of the uterus.

e.g. Distention of the bladder.

Gravity during recumbency.

I. Axis: The maintenance of the anteversion axis is an important pre-requisite for the support of uterus.

II. Perineal body:
   i. It is a pyramidal shaped fibromuscular node and is formed by paired and unpaired muscles.
   ii. Functions: It maintains the integrity of the pelvic floor.

III. Muscles:
   i. Levator ani which is formed by
      - Pubovaginalis and
      - Puborectal sling.
   ii. Functions of levator ani:
      - It constricts the vagina from the side and maintains the anorectal flexure.
      - It prevents the prolapse of the uterus.
      - In damaged puborectal sling, the anorectal angulation becomes straight and this results into prolapse of the rectum.

IV. Ligaments:

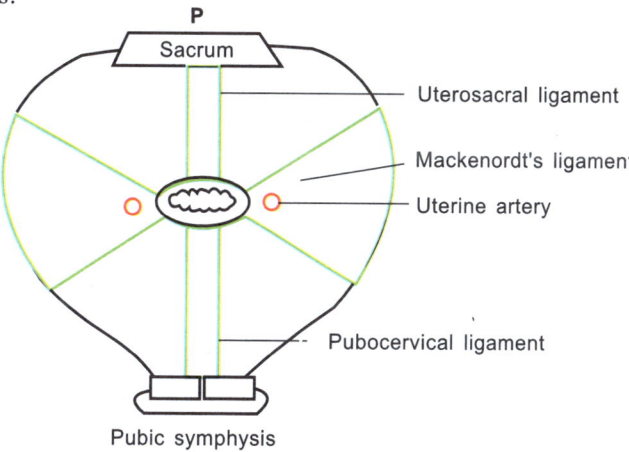

Fig. 2.105 Ligaments of the uterus

   i. Mackenrodt's ligament: It keeps the cervix in the midline. It prevents the downward displacement of uterus through vagina.
   ii. Uterosacral ligament: It is condensation of pelvic fascia that extends from cervix, embraces, the rectouterine pouch and attach to fascia over piriformis. They are best palpated in rectal examination. They keep the cervix braced backward against the forward pool of the round ligaments on the fundus and so maintain the body of uterus in anteversion.
   iii. Pubo cervical ligament: It prevents excessive traction of cervix by counter acting uterosacral ligament. It keeps the cervix in position.

  iv. Round ligament of uterus.

  V. Tone of the muscles of the abdominal wall maintains intra-abdominal pressure. In weakness of the muscle tone, sigmoid colon and small intestine exert pressure upon the uterus.

C. Blood supply:

  a. Arterial supply: It is chiefly by uterine arteries, which are branches of internal iliac artery. It passes medially across the pelvic floor, in the base of the broad ligament, above the ureter. It reaches the uterus at the supravaginal part of the cervix. It gives a branch to the cervix and anastomosis with the branch of ovarian artery. It gives branches which penetrate the walls of the uterus. The artery is tortuous for the expansion of the uterus during pregnancy.

  b. Venous drainage: The veins of the uterus form a plexus along the lateral border of the uterus. The plexus drains through the uterine, ovarian and vaginal veins into the internal iliac veins.

D. Nerve supply: The uterus is richly supplied by both sympathetic and parasympathetic nerves, through the inferior hypogastric and ovarian plexuses.

  a. Sympathetic nerves (T_{12}, L_1) produce uterine contraction and vasoconstriction.

  b. The parasympathetic nerves ($S_{2, 3, 4}$) produce uterine inhibition and vasodilatation. However, these effects are complicated by the pronounced effects of hormones on the genital tract.

Pain sensations from the body of the uterus pass along the sympathetic nerves, and from the cervix, along the parasympathetic nerves.

E. Lymphatic: The lymphatics pass with each veins to the internal iliac group of lymph node. The lymphatics of the uterus forms three intercommunicating networks. Endometrial, myometrial and sub-peritoneal. These plexuses drain into lymphatics on the side of uterus. The lymphatics of the uterus are divided into three area.

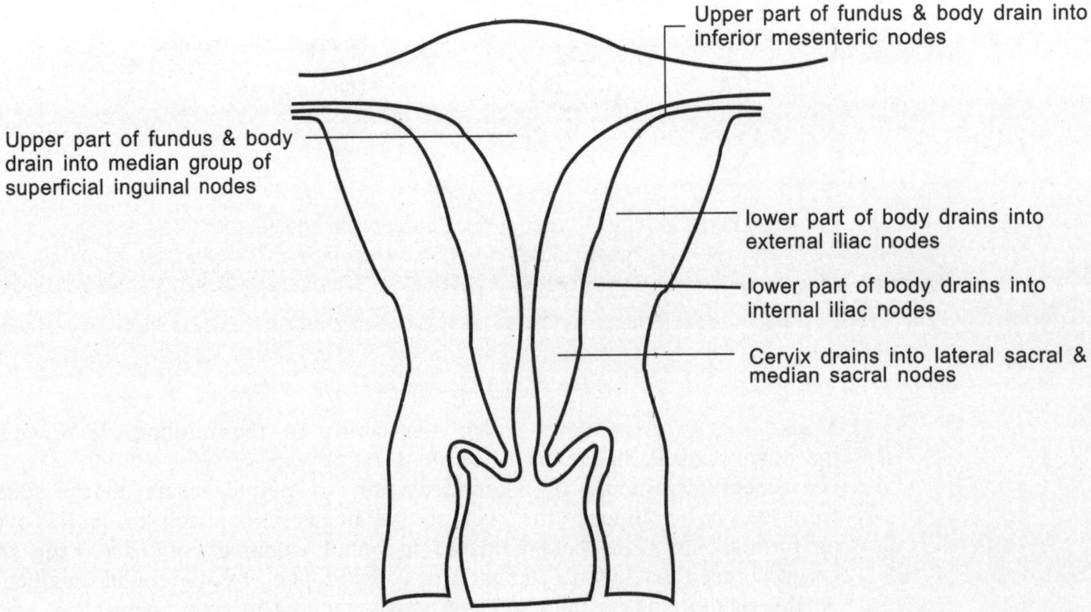

Upper part of fundus & body drain into inferior mesenteric nodes

Upper part of fundus & body drain into median group of superficial inguinal nodes

lower part of body drains into external iliac nodes

lower part of body drains into internal iliac nodes

Cervix drains into lateral sacral & median sacral nodes

Fig. 2.106 Lymphatic drainage of the uterus

a. The lymphatics from the fundus and upper part of the body drain mainly to aortic lymph node and partly to the superficial inguinal lymph nodes along the round ligament of uterus.

b. The lymphatics from the lower part of the body pass to the external iliac lymph nodes.

c. The lymphatics from the cervix pass to the external iliac, internal iliac and sacral lymph nodes.

2. **Histology:** The uterus consists of

A. The mucous membrane called endometrium. It is lined by the simple columnar epithelium. It rests on the connective tissue. It shows numerous tubular glands which are dipped into the stroma. The appearance of the endometrium varies depending upon the phase of the menstrual cycle.

a. In the proliferative phase, the endometrium is relatively thin and the glands are straight

b. In the secretory phase the endometrium is much thick. The uterine glands are long, dilated and tortuous. They have saw toothed margin in the section. The blood vessels are more conspicuous. The stroma is divisible into three part

 I. The superficial layer is called stratum compactum in which the cells are closely packed.

 II. Middle stratum spongiosum, which is relatively loose.

 III. Stratum basale in which the cells are densely packed.

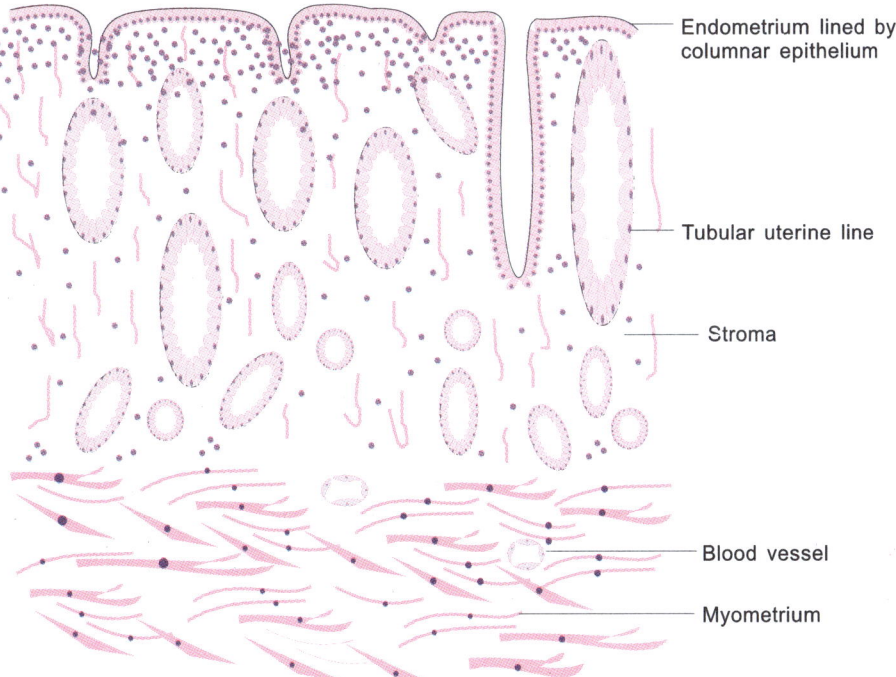

Fig. 2.107 Histology of the uterus

B. Thick layer of muscle called myometrium. It consists of various layers. But these are difficult to make out as a fibers running various direction.

3. **Development:**
   A. Chronological age: It develops in the eighth week of intrauterine life.
   B. Germ layer: Mesoderm.
   C. Site: Intermediate mesoderm.
   D. Sources:
      a. Epithelium of the uterus develops from the fused paramesonephric ducts.
      b. The myometrium is derived from the surrounding mesoderm.
      c. The caudal unfused part partially gets embedded within the substance and forms fundus of the uterus.
   E. Anomalies:
      a. One of the relatively common anomalies is the uterus bicornis in which the uterus has two horn entering a common vagina.
      b. The less common anomalies are
         I. The lumen may be partially, or completely, subdivided by a septum.
         II. The entire uterus may be absent.
         III. One half of the uterus may be absent (unicornuate uterus).
         IV. The uterus may remain rudimentary.
         V. There may be atresia of the lumen either in the body or in the cervix.
         VI. The cervix may be absent.

4. **Applied anatomy:**
   A. Sometimes the uterus passes downwards into the vagina which is called prolapse of the uterus. It is caused by the weakness of the various supports of uterus.
   B. Hysterectomy is the operation for the removal of the uterus.
   C. Insertion of a foreign body into the uterus can prevent implantation of a fertilized ovum. This is the basic principle underlying the use of various intrauterine contraceptive devices for preventing pregnancy.
   D. Caesarean section: The delivery of the child is done by opening the abdomen and uterus. It is commonly done for the cephalopelvic disproportion.

LAQ-29 — Describe prostate under
1. Gross anatomy, 2. Histology, 3. Age changes & 4. Applied anatomy.

1. **Gross anatomy:**
   A. Introduction:
      a. General introduction: It is an accessory gland of male reproductive system. It adds 30% of bulk to the seminal fluid. There is no counter part in the female.
      b. Situation: It is situated in the lesser pelvis.
      c. Dimension: Breadth is more than the length.
         I. The anteroposterior: 2 cm.
         II. Vertical: 3 cm.
         III. Transverse: 4 cm.
      d. Shape:It resembles inverted cone.
   B. External features:
      a. Surfaces: It has a base, apex and three surfaces
         I. Anterior surface
         II. Posterior surface and

III. Inferolateral surface

b. Base is fused with the neck of bladder and perforated by urethra. Apex is blunt and prostatic urethra emerges from the front of the apex to become membranous urethra.

c. Consistency: It is firm in consistency and is formed by fibromuscular stroma.

d. Lobes: It has five lobes
   I. Anterior lobe: It is present in front of prostatic urethra. There is no glandular tissue.
   II. Posterior lobe: It is the part of the prostate present behind the prostatic urethra and connects two lateral lobes. It is a common site of beginning of primary carcinoma.
   III. Median or middle lobe: It lies behind the upper part of urethra and is present in front of the ejaculatory duct. It produces an elevation in the lower part of trigone of the bladder, known as the uvula vesicae.
   IV. Lateral lobes lie one on each side of urethra.

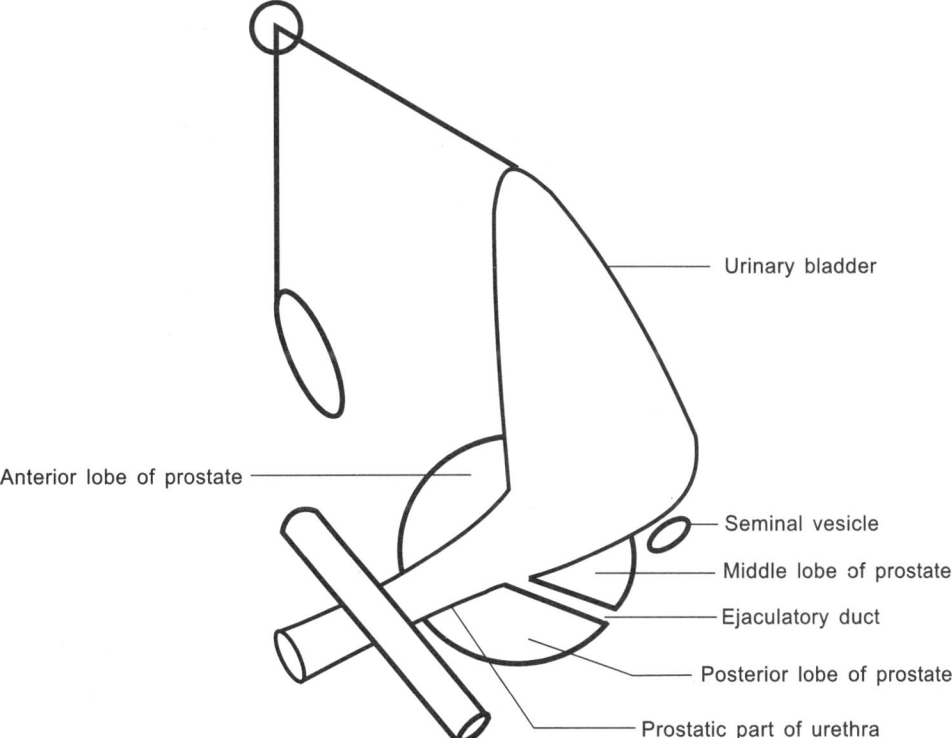

Fig. 2.108 Sagittal section of bladder & prostate showing lobes of prostate

e. Capsules: It has two capsules
   I. True capsule: It is formed by condensation of the fibrous connective tissue around the peripheral part of the gland. It contains no venous plexus.
   II. False capsule: It lies out side the true capsule and is derived from the pelvic fascia. The prostatic venous plexus is embedded in it. Posteriorly it is avascular and is formed by the recto vesical fascia of Denonvilliers.

f. Structures within prostate
    I. The prostatic urethra is present at the junction of anterior 1/3rd and posterior 2/3rd of prostate.
    II. The prostatic utricle is a blind sac, one end of which opens into the urethra.
    III. The ejaculatory ducts open into the prostatic urethra on each side of the opening of the prostatic utricles.

C. Relations: Visceral relations:
    a. Anteriorly:
        I. Retropubic space and
        II. Pubic symphysis.
    b. Superiorly: Neck of urinary bladder.
    c. Posteriorly: Rectum.
    d. Inferiorly: Urogenital diaphragm and pelvic diaphragm.
    e. Laterally: It is clasped by levator prostatae.

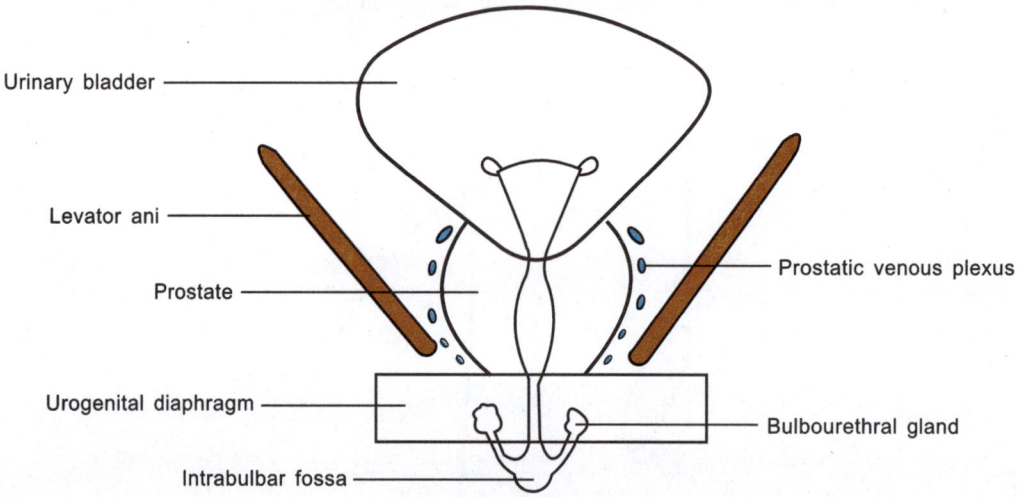

Urinary bladder

Levator ani

Prostate

Urogenital diaphragm

Intrabulbar fossa

Prostatic venous plexus

Bulbourethral gland

Fig. 2.109 Relations of the prostate

D. Blood supply:
    a. Arterial supply: The prostate is supplied by
        I. Prostatic branch of inferior vesical artery which is the main artery of the prostate.
        II. Small branches of middle rectal artery.
        III. Small branches of internal pudendal arteries.
        Branches of these arteries form a large outer or sub-capsular plexus and small inner or periurethral plexus. The greater part of the gland is supplied by the sub-capsular plexus.
    b. Venous drainage: The veins form a plexus and lie between true and false capsule. The veins form a rich plexus around the sides and the base of the gland. The plexus receives the deep dorsal vein of the penis. It communicates with the vesical plexus and forms vesicoprostatic plexus, situated between the bladder and prostate. There are no valves in these veins and hence there is a free communication between the prostatic and vertebral venous plexuses through which the malignant cells of the prostate spreads to vertebral column, skull and central nervous system.

E. Nerve supply:
   a. Sympathetic nerve is derived from inferior hypogastric plexus.
   b. Parasympathetic nerve is derived from pelvic splanchnic nerve. It contains thick nerves and numerous large ganglia. The plexus contains sympathetic and parasympathetic nerves. The secretions of the prostate are produced by sympathetic and discharged by parasympathetic nerve (pelvic splanchnic nerve).

F. Lymphatic drainage: The lymphatic of the prostate pass across the pelvic floor to the nodes on the side wall of the pelvic. It passes along the internal iliac vessels. It mainly drains into
   a. Internal iliac lymph node and
   b. Sacral group of lymph node.

2. **Histology:** It is a fibromusculo glandular tissue. It contains
   A. fibrous stroma,
   B. Smooth muscle and
   C. The acini of varying shapes and sizes.
      It contains large cavities which are lined by columnar epithelium. There is infolding of the epithelium which is a distinguishing feature. It is divided into
      a. Outer larger zone: It contains large branched glands with ducts which curve backwards and opens into prostatic utricle.
      b. Inner smaller zone: It contains
         I. Submucous glands opening in prostatic sinuses.
         II. Simple mucosal glands thrown into folds.
   D. Small rounded masses of uniform or laminated structures are found within the lumen of the follicles. They are called amyloid bodies or corpora amylacea. These are more abundant in older individuals. This consists of condensed glycoprotein. They are often calcified.
   E. The fibromuscular tissue forms a conspicuous feature of the section of the prostate.

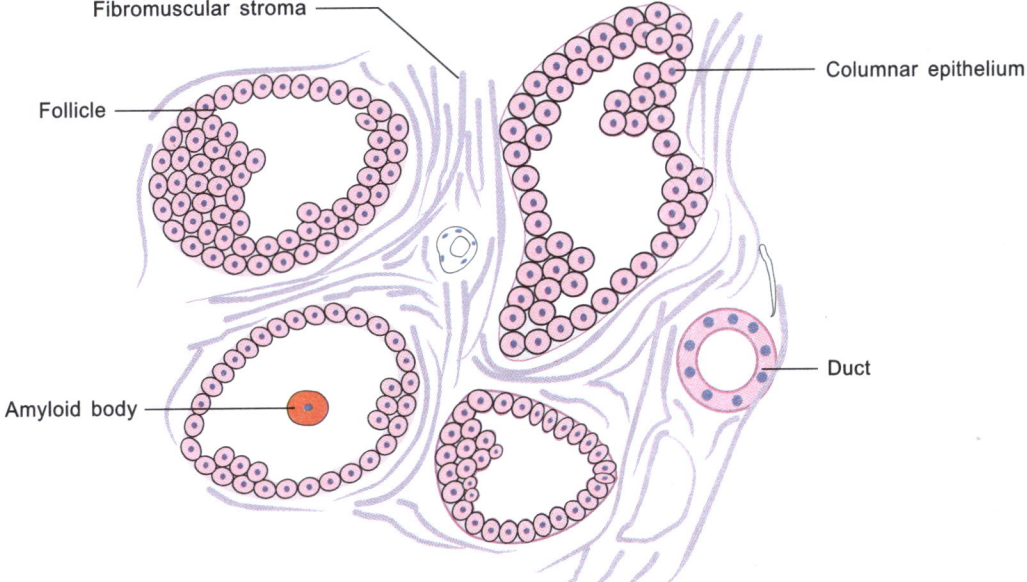

Fig. 2.110 Histology of prostate

3. **Age changes in prostate:**
   A. At birth prostate is made up mainly of stroma which consists of simple ducts.
   B. During first six weeks the epithelium of the duct and of the prostatic utricle undergoes hyperplasia and squamous metaplasia.
   C. Between 9 to 14 years there is a proliferation of duct system and the glands slowly increase in size.
   D. At puberty: It becomes double in size. The stroma in condensed and markedly reduced.
   E. From 20 to 30 years there is a proliferation of glandular elements and the infolding of the glandular epithelium.
   F. From 30 to 45 the size remains constant.
   G. After 45 to 50 years the prostate is either enlarge or reduced in size.

4. **Applied anatomy:**
   A. Benign hypertrophy of prostate occurs in the middle lobe. It is a local proliferation of the internal zone or central region, the region of mucosal or periurethral gland.
   B. Primary carcinoma occurs in the peripheral zone.
   C. In prostatectomy: Capsule is left behind along with venous plexus.
   D. The prostate is a common site of carcinoma. It can spread to vertebral column & skull because of communication of prostatic & vertebral venous plexuses.
   E. The enlargement of the prostate in old age is benign growth and is called BPH.
   F. Prostatitis: It is an inflamation of the prostate gland.
   G. The prostatic adenoma is removed by transurethral route. The resectoscope is passed along the urethra to a point proximal to the seminal colliculus so that the external urethral sphincter is not damaged during resection.
   H. An abdominal suprapubic incision into the retropubic space gives a wide exposure to the organ.

LAQ-30 Describe rectum under
1. Gross anatomy, 2. Development and 3. Applied anatomy.

1. **Gross anatomy:**
   A. Introduction:
      a. General introduction: It is the distal part of the large gut.
      b. Situation: It is situated in the posterior part of lessor pelvic in front of lower three pieces of sacrum and the coccyx. It begins as a continuation of the sigmoid colon at the level of vertebra S_3. It ends by becoming continuous with the anal canal.
      c. Length: 12 cm.
   B. External features:
      Course and direction: The rectum lies in the median plane at the beginning and at the end but it shows two types of curvature in its course.
      a. Two anteroposterior curves
         I. The sacral flexure of the rectum follows the concavity of the sacrum and coccyx.
         II. The perineal flexure of the rectum is the backward bend at the anorectal junction.

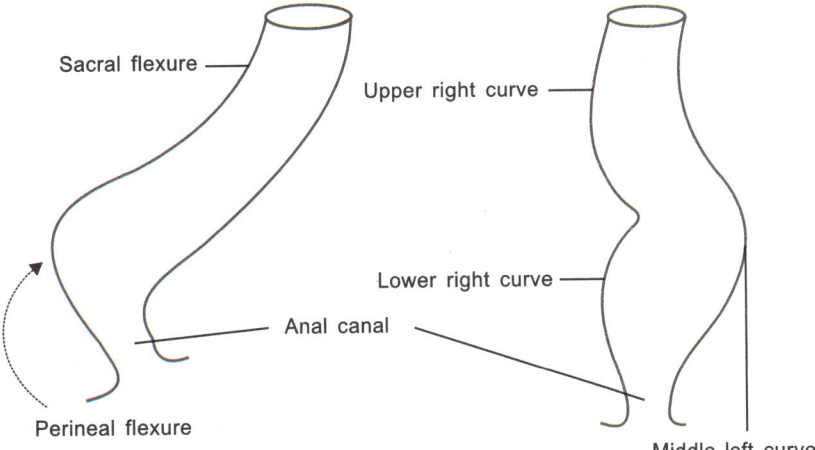

Fig. 2.111 Curvatures of rectum

 b. 3 lateral curves.
  I. Upper lateral curve is convex to the right.
  II. Middle lateral curve is convex to the left and is most prominent.
  III. Lower lateral curve is convex to the right.
C. Relations:
 a. Peritoneal relation:
  I. In upper one-third the peritoneum covers the anterior and lateral part of the rectum.
  II. In the middle one-third the peritoneum covers only anterior part.
  III. In the lower one-third there is no peritoneum.

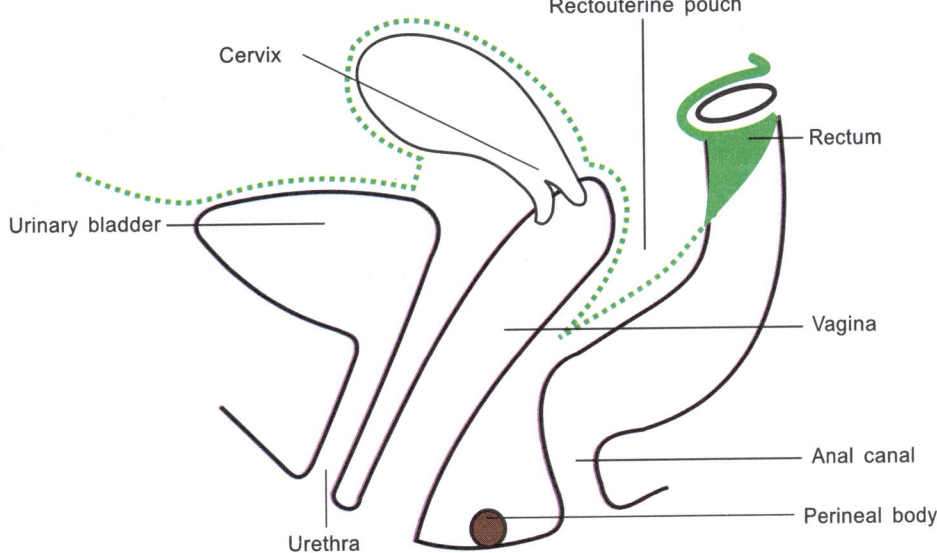

Fig. 2.112 Relations and peritoneal reflections of rectum

b. Visceral relations:
  I. Anteriorly:
    i. Male:
      - Upper 2/3rd:
        * Coils of intestine and ⎫ In rectovesical pouch
        * Sigmoid colon. ⎭
      - Lower 1/3rd:
        * Urinary bladder,
        * Terminal part of the ureters,
        * Seminal vesicles,
        * Deferent ducts and
        * Prostate.
    ii. Female:
      - Upper 2/3rd: Recto uterine pouch containing coils of small intestine.
      - Lower 1/3rd: Lower part of the vagina.
  II. Posteriorly: They are same in male and female.
    i. Lower 3 pieces of the sacrum, the coccyx and the anococcygeal ligament.
    ii. Piriformis, the coccygeus and the levator ani.
    iii. The median sacral, the superior rectal and the lower lateral sacral vessels.
    iv. The sympathetic chain with the ganglion impar, the anterior primary rami of $S_{3, 4, 5}$ and first coccygeal nerve, and the pelvic splanchnic nerves, lymph nodes lymphatics and fat.

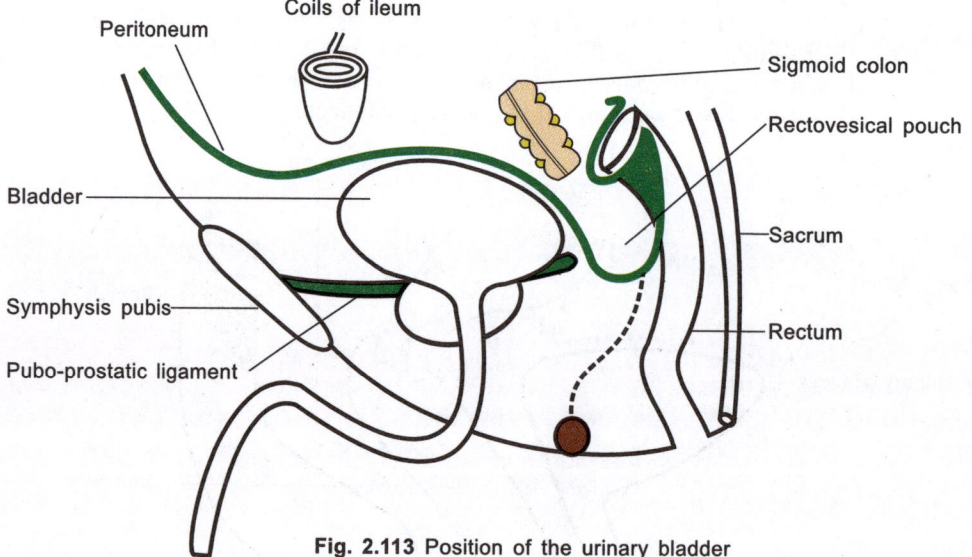

Fig. 2.113 Position of the urinary bladder

D. Blood supply:
  a. Arterial supply:
    I. The main blood supply of rectum is by superior rectal artery. It is the continuation of inferior mesenteric artery.
    II. The muscle wall of the rectum receives from the middle rectal artery which is branch of internal iliac artery.
    III. Small branches from the median sacral artery supply the back of the rectum.

b. Venous drainage: There is very free anastomosis between the tributaries of the venous system.
   I. Superior rectal vein: The tributaries of this vein begin in the anal canal. They pass upward in the rectal sub-mucosa, pierce the muscular coat and unite to form superior rectal vein which continues upward as inferior mesenteric vein.
   II. Middle rectal vein: It drains mainly the muscular wall of rectal ampulla and open into internal iliac vein.

E. Nerve supply: It is supplied through superior rectal and inferior hypogastric plexuses.
   a. The sympathetic fibers are derived from L_1 and L_2. These are vaso-constrictor and inhibitory to the rectal musculature and motor to the internal sphincter.
   b. Parasympathetic fibers are derived from S_2, $_3$, $_4$. These are motor to the musculature of rectum and inhibitory to the internal sphincter. The sensations of the distension of the rectum are also carried by parasympathetic nerve. Pain sensations are carried by both parasympathetic and sympathetic.

F. Lymphatic drainage: The lymphatics of the rectum run along the arteries. The lymph vessels in the mucous membrane provide the first filter. The lymphatic vessels pierce the wall of the rectum and travel to lymph nodes.
   a. The lymphatics from more than upper half of the rectum pass along the superior rectal vessels to the inferior mesenteric nodes after passing through the pararectal and sigmoid nodes.
   b. The lymphatics from the lower half of the rectum pass along the middle rectal vessels to the internal iliac nodes.

2. **Development:**
   A. Chronological age: It develops in the fourth week of intrauterine life.
   B. Germ layer: Endoderm and mesoderm.
   C. Site: Caudal part of hindgut.
   D. Source:
      a. The epithelium of the upper part of rectum is derived from the epithelium of the hindgut.
      b. The epithelium of the lower part of rectum is derived from dorsal part of endodermal cloaca.
      c. The smooth muscles and the connective tissues are derived from splanchnic mesoderm, surrounding the cloaca.
   E. Anomalies:
      a. Imperforate anus: The commonest cause of imperforate anus is persistence of the anal membrane.
      b. Congenital rectovesical or rectourethral fistula.
      c. Congenital rectovaginal fistula.
      d. Ectopic anus.

3. **Applied anatomy:**
   A. Per rectal examination: The following structures can be palpated by a finger passed per rectum.
      a. In male the posterior surface of prostate, seminal vesical and vasa differentia is palpated.
      b. In females the perineal body, cervix is palpated.
   B. Proctoscopy and sigmoidoscopy: The interior of the rectum and anal canal can be examined under direct vision with special instruments, like a proctoscope or a sigmoidoscope.

C. Prolapse of rectum: It may be
   a. Incomplete or mucosal prolapse of the rectum.
   b. Complete prolapse or procidentia is the condition in which the whole thickness of the rectal wall protrudes through the anas.

LAQ-31   Describe anal canal under
1. Gross anatomy,   2. Development and
3. Applied anatomy.

1. **Gross anatomy:**
  A. Introduction:
    a. General introduction: The terminal part of large intestine is called anal canal. It is devoid of
      I. Sacculations,
      II. Taenia coli,
      III. Appendices epiploicae,
      IV. Mesentery and
      V. Peritoneum.
    B. Situation: It is situated in the anal triangle between two ischiorectal fossae.
    c. Length: It is 4 cm long, & situated about 4 cm in front of the tip of the coccyx.
    d. Direction: Downwards, & backwards.
  B. External features:
    Extent: It extends from anorectal flexure (½" below & 1" in front of tip of the coccyx) to the vertical slit between two buttocks.
  C. Relations:
    a. Anterior relations are the structure at the base of urogenital triangle.
      I. Perineal body
      II. In male
        i. Bulb of penis
        ii. Bulbospongiosus muscle
      III. In female: Lower part of vagina.
    b. Posterior: Anococcygeal ligament.
    c. Laterally:
      I. In the upper part: Levator ani.
      II. In the lower part: External anal sphincter.
  D. Interior of the anal canal: It is divided by pectinate and Hilton's white line into three parts
    a. Upper part (above the pectinate line):
      I. Length is 15 mm.
      II. It is lined by mucous membrane which shows 6 - 10 vertical folds, these folds are called anal column of Morgagni. They are prominent in children but often not in adults.
      III. The lower end of the anal columns are united to each other by short transverse fold of mucous membrane. These folds are called anal valves.
      IV. Above each valve there is a depression which is called anal sinus. There are about ten mucous secreting anal glands which open into the anal sinuses.
      V. The anal valve together form a transverse line called as pectinate line.

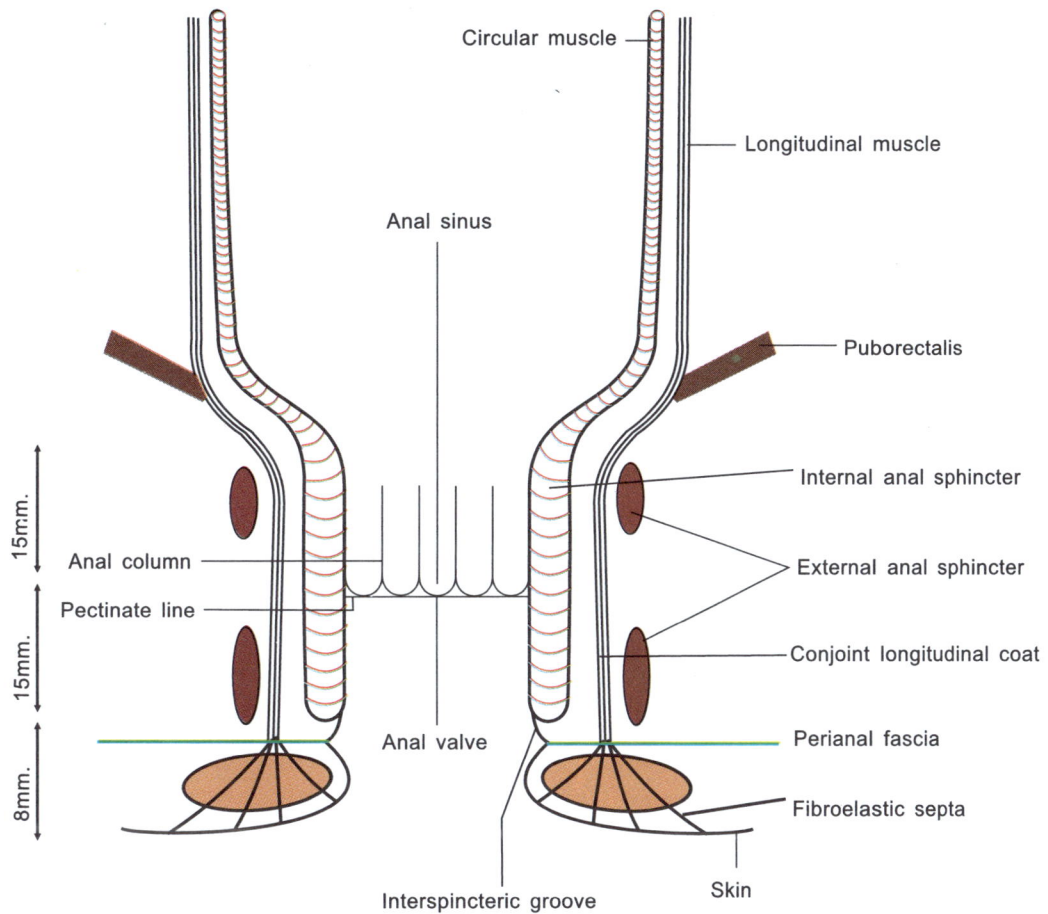

Fig. 2.114 Interior of anal canal

b. Middle part:
(between pectinate and Hilton's line)
I. This region is called pecten or transitional zone. There is no abrupt change as in oesophagus to stomach.
II. The lower limit of the pecten has a whitish appearance, hence it is called as white line of Hilton.
III. It is about 15 mm in length.
IV. It is lined by mucous membrane, which is bluish in appearance. It contains dense venous plexus which lies between mucosa and muscle coat.
V. Mucous is less mobile as compared the mucosa of the upper part. <u>Anal fissures are present in this zone.</u>

c. Lower part (cutaneous) (below Hilton's line):
I. It is about 8 mm long.
II. It is lined by true skin containing sweat glands, sebaceous glands and hair follicle. The lining epithelium is stratified squamous keratinised.

Table 2.17 Showing blood supply, nerve supply and lymphatic of anal canal

Particulars	Above the pectinate line	Below the pectinate line
E. Blood Supply a. Arterial	Superior rectal artery, a continuation of the inferior mesenteric artery. (The artery of the hind gut)	Inferior rectal artery, a branch of the internal pudendal artery is the main artery.
b. Venous	Upper part is drained into portal system via superior rectal vein.	Lower part is drained into systemic vein via inferior rectal vein.
F. Nerve Supply a. Sympathetic	Superior hypogastric plexus (L_1, L_2) and autonomic nerve. (S_2, S_3, S_4)	Lower area is supplied by pudendal nerve (somatic nerve) via inferior rectal nerves. This area possesses all modalities of cutaneous sensation.
b. Parasympathetic	Pelvic splanchnic (S_2, S_3, S_4) This area is insensitive to modalities of cutaneous sensation.	------
G. Lymphatic	Lymphatics are drained into internal iliac nodes.	Lower area is drained into horizontal set of superficial inguinal lymph nodes.

2. **Development:**
   A. Chronological age: It develops in the seventh week of intrauterine life.
   B. Germ layer: Endoderm and ectoderm.
   C. Site: Terminal part of the hind gut.
   D. Sources:
      a. Superior two-third of the anal canal develops from terminal part of the hind gut.
      b. Inferior one-third develops from the proctodeum.
   E. Anomalies:
      a. Imperforate anus occurs about one in every 5000 infants. It is more common in males. It results from abnormal development of urorectal septum.
      b. Anal agenesis: The anal canal may and blindly.
      c. Anal stenosis.

3. **Applied anatomy:**
   A. Anal fissure: The lower end of anal columns are connected by small folds called anal valves. In chronic constipated persons the anal valves may be torn due to faecal mass catching on fold of mucous membrane. The elongated ulcer is called anal fissure, which is very painful.
   B. Perianal abscess is due to the trauma to anal mucosa caused by faecal matter.
   C. Anal fistulae are due to the spread of inadequately treated anal abscess. If the abscess opens only on one surface it is called sinus.
   D. Incontinence associated with rectal prolapse is due to trauma and spinal cord injury.
   E. Haemorrhoides are saccular dilatations of the internal rectal venous plexus. They occur above the pectinate line and are therefore painless.

They bleed profusely during straining at stool.
a. Predisposing conditions
   I.   Portal hypertension in cirrhosis
   II. Pregnancy
   III. Cancerous tumor.
   IV. Chronic constipation
b. Causes
   I.   Familial tendency associated with leg vein varicosities.
   II. Most dependant part of portal circulation
   III. Supported loosely by connective tissue
   IV. Valveless
   V.   Venous return decreases during defecation.
c. The details of the piles is described in the following table.

Table 2.18 Showing details of the piles

Particulars	Internal	External
I. Site	Upper half of anal canal	Lower half of anal canal
II. Constitution	i. Superior rectal artery ii. Superior rectal vein iii. Mucosa iv. Submucosa	i. Inferior rectal vein ii. Mucous membrane ii. Skin
III. Position	3, 7, 11'O Clock. This is a primary site.	Position may be anywhere
IV. Degree	1^0 - Within anal canal 2^0 - Extruded on defecation 3^0 - Prolapse on defecation and remains outside	--
V. Nerve supply	Autonomic	Inferior rectal nerve
VI. Clinical feature	Painless, sensitive to stretch.	Painful to touch, pain and pressure.

SN-21 Internal iliac artery

1. **Introduction:** This is artery supplying the external genitalia, structures in the lateral pelvic wall, pelvic organs and gluteal region.

2. **Origin:** It arises as one of the terminal branch of common iliac artery.

3. **Termination:** It terminates by dividing into anterior and posterior division.

4. **Distribution:** It supplies
   A. Pelvic organs
   B. Perineal
   C. Gluteal region
   D. Iliac fossa

5. **Course:**
   A. It begins in front of the sacroiliac joint at the level of intervertebral disc between L_5 and sacrum. It lies medial to psoas major muscle.

B.　It runs downwards and backwards and ends near the upper margin of greater sciatic notch by dividing into anterior and posterior division.

6.　**Relations:** The artery is related
A.　Anteriorly:
　　a.　Ureter
　　b.　In females to the ovary and lateral end of uterine tube.
B.　Posteriorly:
　　a.　Internal iliac vein,
　　b.　Lumbosacral trunk &
　　c.　Sacroiliac joint.
C.　Laterally:
　　a.　External iliac vein and
　　b.　Obturator nerve.
D.　Medially:
　　a.　Peritoneum and
　　b.　Tributaries of internal iliac vein.

7.　**Branches:**
A.　Anterior division:
　　a.　In the male
　　　　I.　Superior vesical artery,
　　　　II.　Obturator artery,
　　　　III.　Middle rectal artery,
　　　　IV.　Inferior vesical artery,
　　　　V.　Inferior gluteal artery and
　　　　VI.　Internal pudendal artery.
　　　　The last two are the terminal branches.
　　b.　In female: It gives off seven branches. The inferior vesical artery is replaced by the vaginal artery. The uterine artery is the seventh branch.
B.　Posterior division:
　　a.　Iliolumbar,
　　b.　Lateral sacral and
　　c.　Superior gluteal arteries.

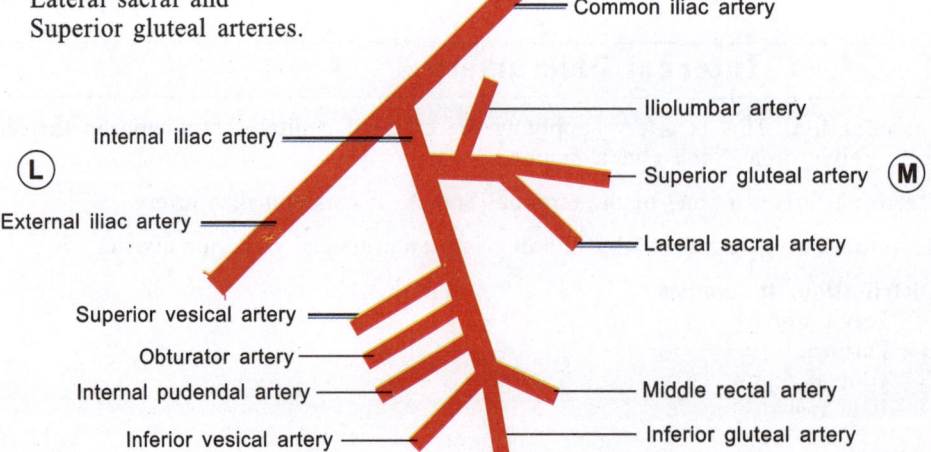

Fig. 2.115 Branches of the right internal iliac artery

GENERAL HISTOLOGY

SECTION THREE

SAQ-1	Simple squamous epithelium	193
SN-1	Columnar epithelium	193
SN-2	Pseudostratified epithelium	194
SN-3	Stratified squamous epithelium	194
SN-4	Transitional epithelium	195
SAQ-2	Loose areolar tissue	196
SN-5	Hyaline cartilage	197
SN-6	Articular cartilage	198
SN-7	Fibrocartilage	198
SN-8	Elastic cartilage	199
SN-9	Compact bone	199
SAQ-3	Sarcomere	201
SN-10	Cardiac muscle	201
SN-11	Elastic artery	202
SN-12	Muscular artery	203

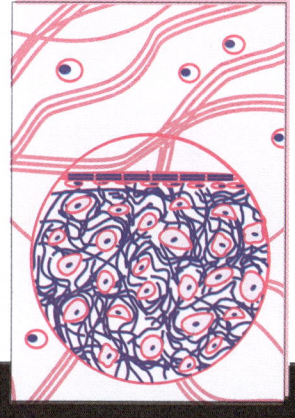

SAQ-1   Simple squamous epithelium

1. **Introduction:** The cells of the simple squamous epithelium are flat and have length, breadth but no thickness.

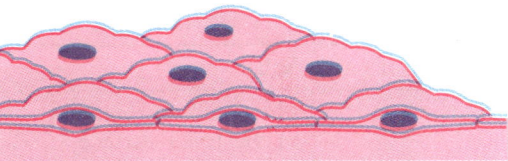

Fig. 3.1 Simple squamous epithelium

2. **Peculiarities:**
   A. Cells are single layer, irregular which are thin and plate like.
   B. The cells on surface view looks polygonal, or mosaic.
   C. Cells lie in contact with basement membrane.
   D. The nucleus is round and centrally situated.
   E. Profile or side view shows bulging of nucleus.
   F. The junction between cells is marked by zonulae occludentes.

3. **Functions:**
   A. The tight junctions between the cells prevent passage of different substances through them.
   B. It helps in transport of material across the cell.
   C. It facilitates movement of viscera in serous cavities.

4. **Sites:**   **SAHEB**
   A. **S**erous membrane.
   B. **A**lveoli of lung.
   C. **H**enles loop.
   D. **E**ndothelium of blood vessel.
   E. **B**owman's capsule.

SN-1   Columnar epithelium

1. **Introduction:** The cells are column like or rectangular (on vertical section).

2. **Peculiarities:**
   A. The cells of the simple columnar epithelium are arranged in single layer.
   B. All the cells touch basal lamina.
   C. The height of the cells is more than width.
   D. The nucleus is elongated.

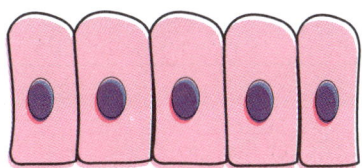
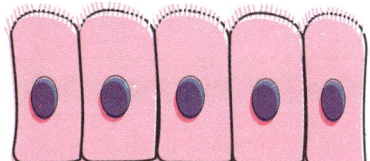
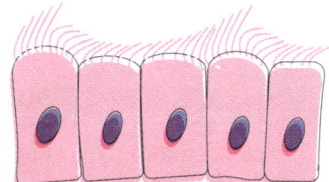

Fig 3.2 Columnar epithelium   **Fig 3.3** Ciliated columnar   **Fig 3.4** Columnar epithelium with microvilli

3. **The characters of different sub-type of columnar epithelium:**

Table 3.1 Showing characters of different sub-type of columnar epithelium

Particulars	Simple	Ciliated	Microvilli
A. Size of cell	Tall	Tall	Tall
B. Nucleus	Elongated and nearer to the basal surface than luminal surface	Elongated	Elongated
C. Peculiarities	--	Cilia present	Microvilli present
D. Functions	a. Absorption b. Secretion	Movements of particles	Movement of particles
E. Situation	I. Gastrointestinal tract (from stomach to rectum) II. Gall bladder	I. Bronchi, bronchioles II. Central canal of spinal cord. III. Efferent ductules IV. Fallopian tube	Jejunum

---

SN-2   Pseudostratified epithelium

(*Pseudo* false)

1. **Introduction:** The simple columnar epithelium giving appearance of stratified (multi layered) epithelium is called pseudostratified epithelium.

2. **Peculiarities:**
   A. The cells are of variable height.
   B. All cells lie on the basement membrane.
   C. All the short cells do not reach lumen.
   D. The nucleus is situated at the base.
   E. It gives the appearance of many layered.

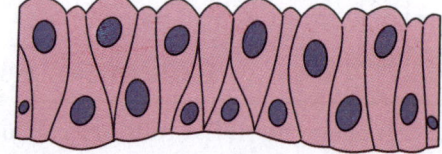

Fig 3.5 Pseudostratified epithelium

3. **Classification:** The pseudostratified epithelium is divided into following types:
   A. Pseudostratified non-ciliated: The luminal surface of the cells do not bear cilia. e.g. male urethra, vas deferens.
   B. Pseudostratified ciliated columnar: The luminal surface of the cells bear cilia. e.g. upper respiratory tract, trachea and larger bronchi.

SN-3   Stratified squamous epithelium

1. **Introduction:** The multilayered epithelium having squamous cells on the top.

2. **Morphology:**
   A. The deepest cells are columnar.
   B. The middle cells are cuboidal or polyhedral.
   C. The superficial cells are flat or squamous.

4. **Classification:** The stratified squamous epithelium is divided into following types depending upon the presence and absence of keratin.

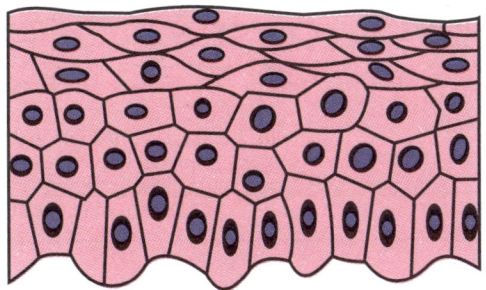

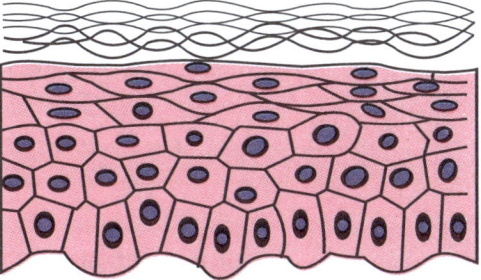

Fig 3.6 Stratified squamous non-keratinized epithelium

Fig 3.7 Stratified squamous keratinized epithelium

Table 3.2 Showing characters of the stratified squamous keratinized and non-keratinized

Particulars	Stratified squamous keratinized	Stratified squamous non keratinized

A. Superficial cells
  a. Viability
  b. Nucleus
  c. Structure
	
	No
	Absent
	Keratin
		
		Viable
		Present
		-

B. Function	To prevent wear and tear	-
C. Site	Dry surface	Wet surface
D. Situation	Skin, vagina, external acoustic meatus.	Oral cavity, tongue, pharynx, oesophagus, lip, cornea

---

SN-4   **Transitional epithelium (urothelium)**

1. **Introduction:** The cells of the transitional epithelium is multilayered, having capacity for distension.

2. **Arrangement of cell:**
    A. The deepest cells are columnar.
    B. The middle cells are pear shaped.
    C. Ths superficial cell are umbrella like.

3. **Peculiarities:**
    A. The deepest cells rest on the basement membrane.
    B. The cells are arranged in 5-6 layers.
    C. The cells are connected by desmosomes.
    D. The cells can be stretched considerably.
    E. The plasma membrane of the surface cell is embedded in lipid which make it resistant to toxins.
    F. It shows mitosis.

4. **Site:**
   A. Pelvis of the kidney,
   B. Ureter &
   C. Urinary bladder.

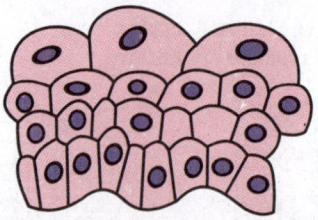

Fig 3.9 Stretched transitional epithelium

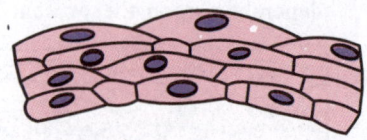

Fig 3.9 Relaxed transitional epithelium

SAQ-2   Loose areolar tissue

1. **Introduction:** It is connective tissue made up of bundles of fibers which encloses large spaces called areola.

2. **Structure:**
   A. Made up of bundle of fibers.

Table 3.3 Showing different types of fibers and their details

Particulars	Collagen	Reticular	Elastic
a. Synonyms	White	Argyrophil	Yellow
b. Gross I. External i. Arrangement of fibers	Runs in bundle	Runs in single	Runs in single
ii. Diameter	7-12 μm	-	-
iii. Nature	Straight, wavy	Thin	Fine, straight,
iv. Branching	bundles branch individual fibres do not branch	Present	Highly refractile, spiraling
v. Anastomosis	Present	Absent	Present
vi. Composition	Tropocollagen	Reticulin	Elastin protein elastin
II. Characters i. Elasticity	No	No	Yes
ii. Toughness	Yes	No	Yes
iii. Flexibility	Yes	Yes	Yes
III. Action on i. Boiling	Forms gelatin	-	
ii. Acid		No	Resistant
c. Stained with	H and E	Silver staining	Orcein
d. Example	Tendons, Ligament, Capsule & Dermis of the skin.	Spleen, Lymph-node & Bone narrow.	Walls of blood vessel, Vocal cords & Ligamentum flava.

B. Cells:
    a. Fibroblast,
    b. Macrophages,
    c. Mast cells,
    d. Lymphocytes,
    e. Fat cells,
    f. Pigment cells and
    g. Plasma cells.

3. **Abundant intercellular space.**

4. **Site:** Superficial fascia, ligamentum flava, basement membrane.

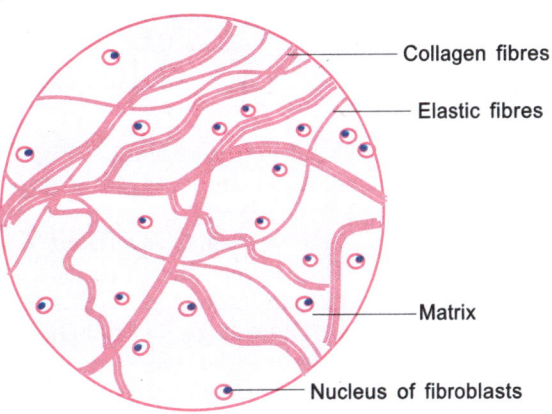

Fig. 3.10 Loose areolar tissue

SN-5   Hyaline cartilage

(*Hyalos* glass, transparent)

1. **Introduction:** The basic tissue which forms skeleton of some organs e.g. larynx.

2. **Peculiarities:**
    A. It is transparent.
    B. It contains homogenous intracellular substance.
    C. It is basophilic i.e. stains blue with Haematoxylin and Eosin stain.
    D. The perichondrium may or may not present.

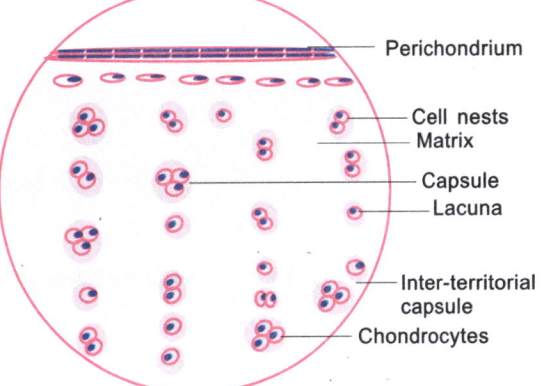

Fig 3.11 Hyaline cartilage

3. **Structures:**
    A. Cells:
        a. The cartilage cells are called chondrocytes.
        b. They are present in cell nests.
        c. They are in groups.
        d. The cells are kept together by dense matrix.
        e. The matrix around the cell nests is stained deeper and is called lacunar capsule.
        f. The matrix in between the cell nests is stained pale and is called interstitial matrix.
    B. Ground substance: It contains collagen fibres.

4. **Functions:**
    A. It resists compressive forces.
    B. It resists tensile forces.

5. **Site:**
    A. Larynx: Thyroid, cricoid, arytenoid cartilage.
    B. Bronchi part of nasal septum lateral wall of nose epiphyseal plate.

SN-6   Articular cartilage

1. **Introduction:** It is a type of hyaline cartilage which covers the articular surfaces of bones.

2. **Features:**
   A. The perichondrium is absent.
   B. The chondrocytes are arranged in three layers.
      a. Superficial layer:
         I. Cells are small and flattened.
         II. They lie parallel to surface.
      b. Intermediate layer:
         I. Cells are large and round.
         II. They may be single or arranged in groups and are obliquely placed..
      c. Deep layer: The cells are placed vertically.
   C. Matrix: Contains numerous collagen fibers.
   D. Calcified matrix:
      a. It is present in deepest layer.
      b. Cartilage cells may get converted into bone.

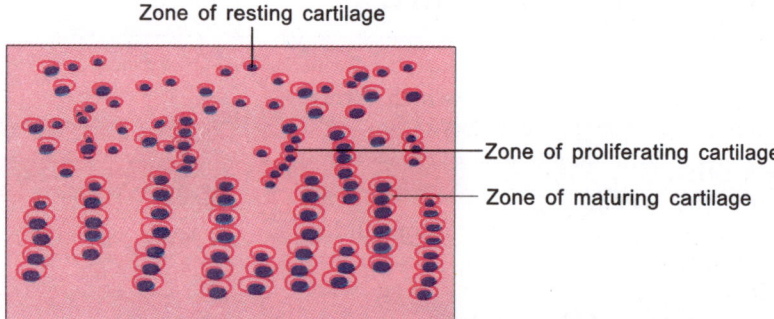

Fig 3.12 Articular cartilage

3. **Nutrition is achieved from surrounding synovial fluid.**

4. **Functions:**
   A. It provides smooth surfaces which prevent friction.
   B. It acts as a shock absorber.

5. **Site:** It lines most of the articular surfaces of synovial joints except temporomandibular joint which is lined by fibrocartilage.

SN-7   Fibrocartilage (White fibrocartilage)

1. **Introduction:** It is a type of cartilage which looks very much like dense fibrous tissue.

2. **Structure:**
   A. The cartilage cells are surrounded by capsule.
   B. The matrix contains plenty of collagen fibers.
   C. The perichondrium is absent.
   D. It contain type I collagen fibers.

E. The fibers merge with surrounding connective tissue.

F. It is less cellular.

3. **Nutrition:** From surrounding fluid by diffusion.

4. **Functions:**

A. It overcomes great tensile strength.

B. It has little elasticity.

5. **Sites:**

A. Glenoidal labrum.

B. Secondary cartilagenous joints.

C. Acetabular labrum.

D. Meniscus.

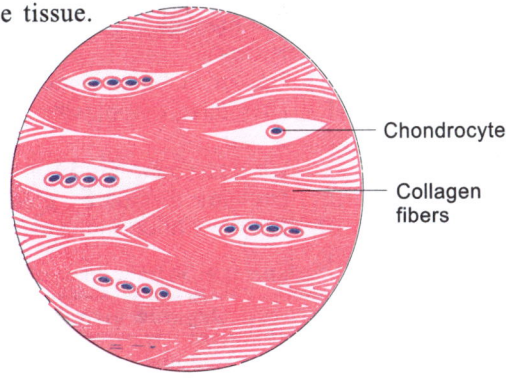

Fig. 3.13 Fibrocartilage

| SN-8 | **Elastic cartilage (Yellow fibrocartilage)** |

1. **Introduction:** It is type of cartilage which is made up of elastic fibers.

2. **Structure:**

A. It contains cartilage cells.

B. It contains elastic fibers, which branches anastomoses.

C. The perichondrium is present.

3. **Peculiarity:** Requires special method for staining.

4. **Site:**

A. **E**piglottis,

B. Pinna of **e**ar.

C. Lateral part of **e**xternal acoustic meatus.

D. Medial part of **E**ustachian tube.

The word elastic cartilage and examples of the elastic cartilage starts with the letter E

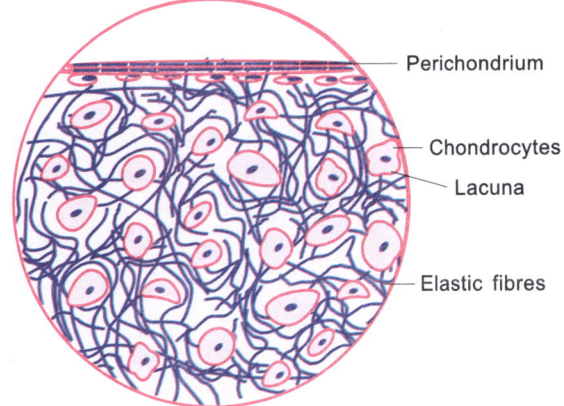

Fig. 3.14 Elastic cartilage

| SN-9 | **Compact bone** |

1. **Introduction:** It is a specialized connective tissue with mineralized matrix.

2. **Structure:**

A. Following cells are present

a. Osteogenic cells

I. They are precursors of osteoblasts.

II. They are present in cellular layer of periosteum.

b. Osteoblasts

I. They are active, large and basophilic cells. They are present during bone formation.

      II. The nucleus is round and eccentric.
  c. Osteocytes
      I. Present in fully formed bone in lacunae.
      II. They have cytoplasmic processes.
  d. Osteoclasts
      I. They are bone modelling cells.
      II. They are formed by giant cells.
      III. They are multinucleated and eosinophilic.

B. Matrix:

Table 3.4 Showing the elements of the compact bone

Organic elements	inorganic elements
a. Dense bundle of collagen fibers. b. Ground substance. I. Hyaluronic acid. II. Protein polysacharides.	Calcium phosphate $Ca_3(PO4)_2$ Calcium carbonate $CaCO_3$ Calcium chloride $CaCl_2$ Magnesium chloride $MgCl$

C. Osteon (Haversian system)
  a. It consists of the central Haversian canal which conduct vessels, lymphatics and nerves.
  b. In is present only in compact bone.
  c. There are 18-50 concentric lamellae.
  d. The spaces between lamellae are called lacunae. They contain osteocytes.
  e. Canaliculi: These are fine channels containing cytoplasmic processes of osteocytes.

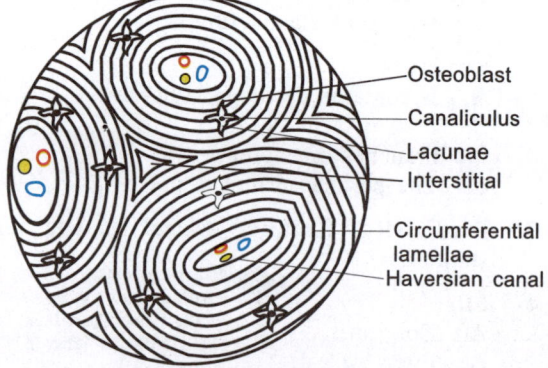

Fig. 3.15 Compact bone

D. Lamellae: There are three types of lamellae.
  a. Concentric lamellae are present around the Haversian canal.
  b. Interstitial lamellae are present between two Haversian system. They do not belong to any Haversian system.
  c. Circumferential lamellae: These are of two types.
      I. Outer circumferential around bone.
      II. Inner circumferential.

E. Periosteum: It has two layers
  a. Outer: Fibrous which contains collagen fibers.
  b. Inner: Cellular layer contains osteocytes.

F. Sharpey's fibres: Enter from periosteum to outer circumferential lamellae.

G. Volkman's canal: It pierces lamellae and connects Haversian system to periosteum. It runs transversely.

H. Site:
  a. Shaft of long bone.
  b. Outer layer all compact bones.

I. Blood supply of compact bone is by nutrient artery. Osteocytes get nutrition from nutrient artery.

SAQ-3   Sarcomere

1. **Introduction:** It is the segment of myofibril between two `Z' disc.

2. **Importance:** It is basic contractile unit of the striated muscle.

3. **Each myofibril:**
   A. Diameter: 1-2 μ
   B. Length: As long as muscle fibre.
   C. Character: Light and dark zone under light microscope, causes difference in the refractive index
   D. Filaments:
      a. Actin &
      b. Myosin.

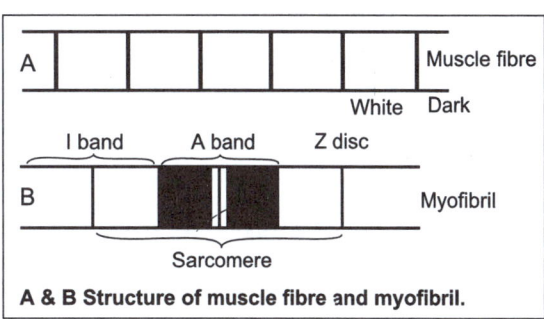

A & B Structure of muscle fibre and myofibril.

Fig 3.16 Sarcomere

4. **Dark zone:** Anisotropic (A band)
   H band is clear area in A band.
   M line is thickened central part of H band.

5. **Light zone:** Isotropic (I band)
   The centre of the light zone is called Z disc (Krause's membrane).

6. **Sarcomere:** Half of I + A + half of I

7. **During contraction:** Actin filament slide between myosin filament towards the centre of sarcomere. Z discs are brought closer shortening of contractile unit. A band remains same.

SN-10   Cardiac muscle

It is a striated and involuntary muscle.

1. **Fibers:** Each fiber of the muscle is called myocyte. It branches and anastomoses to form syncitium.

2. **Nucleus:** Each myocyte contains one nucleus which is placed centrally.

3. **Length of myocyte:** 50 μm.

4. **Width of myocyte:** 18 μm.

5. **Sarcoplasm:** Contains mitochondria.

6. **Striations:** Not very prominent, as few myofibrils are present.

7. **Peculiarity:** It contains large amount of glycogen, myoglobin and is rich in capillary network.

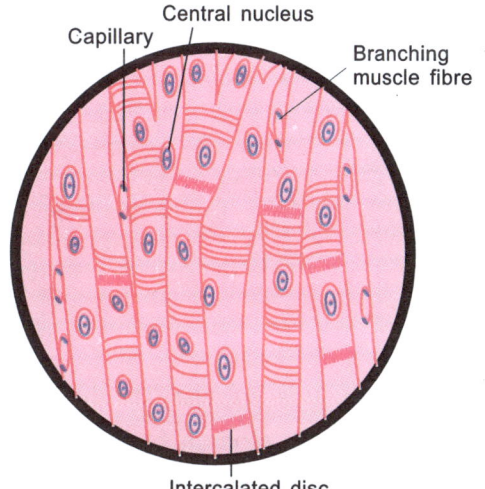

Fig 3.17 Cardiac muscle

8. **Intercalated discs:** Junction between myocyte, appears dark stained transverse lines, lies opposite the `I' band. It has two parts
   A. Transverse portion
   B. Lateral portion
      Due to transverse and lateral portion intercalated disc appears stepwise.

9. **Gap junctions:** Cell membrane and adjacent myocytes are connected by desmosome and is called gap junction.

| SN-11 | **Elastic artery** |

1. **Synonymous:** It is an large size artery　　called elastic artery.

2. **Layers:** It consists of 3 layers
   A. Tunica intima:
      a. It is innermost coat and lined by simple squamous epithelium.
      b. It contains elastic fibers.
      c. The subendothelial layer is prominent and contains elastic fibers
      d. The internal elastic lamina is present but indistinguishable.
   B. Tunica media:
      a. It is a middle and thickest coat.
      b. It consist of concentric layer of fenestrated elastic fibers.
      c. It also contains little amount of smooth muscle and collagen fibers.
   C. Tunica adventitia:
      a. It is thin and contains elastic fibers.
      b. The fibers merge with external elastic lamina.

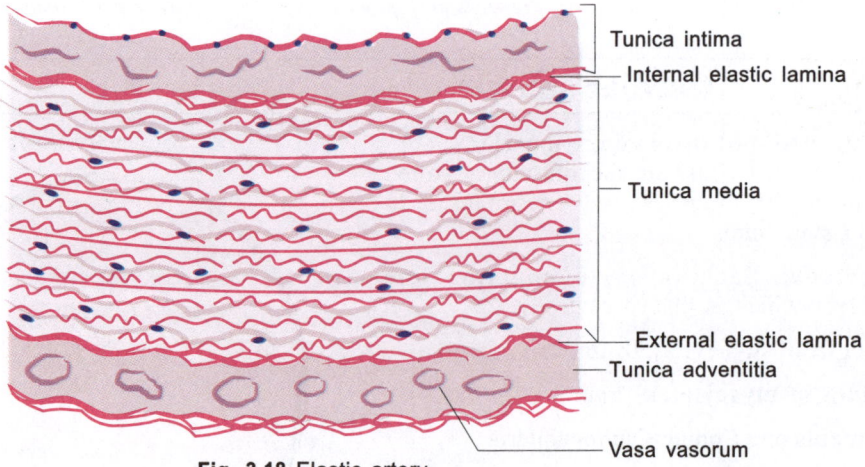

Fig. 3.18 Elastic artery

3. **Lumina:** It is irregular. The diameter of the lumina is more than the thickness of wall.

4. **Functions:** It conducts blood from heart to the different parts of body.

5. **Examples:** Aorta, large arteries of head and neck.

SN-12 Muscular artery

1. **Synonymous:** It is the medium size artery   (distributing artery).

2. **Layers:** It consists of three layers
   A. Tunica intima:
      a. It shows folded appearance
      b. The internal elastic lamina is prominent and wavy.
   B. Tunica media: It shows plenty of smooth muscle cells, arranged concentrically.
   C. Tunica adventitia:
      a. It is as thick as media.
      b. The diameter of the lumina is less than thickness of wall.

3. **Functions:** It regulates the flow of the blood in different regions.

4. **Examples:** Most of the arteries of body distal to the continuation of subclavian artery branches of common carotid, thoracic and abdominal aorta.

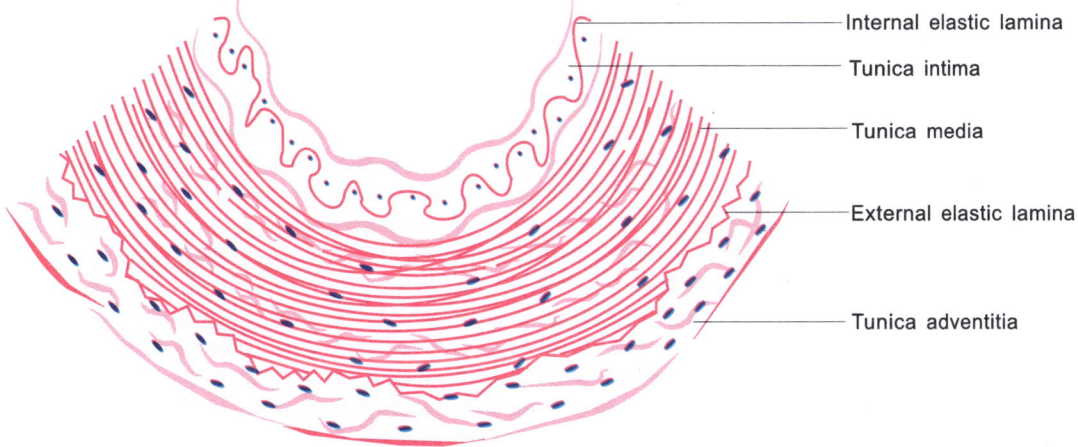

— Internal elastic lamina
— Tunica intima
— Tunica media
— External elastic lamina
— Tunica adventitia

Fig. 3.19 Muscular artery

EMBRYOLOGY

SECTION FOUR

SN-1	Mitosis	207
SN-2	Meiosis	209
SN-3	Spermatogenesis	211
SAQ-1	Spermiogenesis	213
SAQ-2	Sperms	213
SN-4	Capacitation of sperm	214
SN-5	Oogenesis	21
SN-6	Graafian follicle	215
SN-7	Fertilization	216
SN-8	Implantation	218
SN-9	Blastocyst	219
SN-10	Decidua	220
SN-11	Amnion	221
SN-12	Yolk sac	223
SN-13	Primitive streak	224
SN-14	Notochord	226
SN-15	Connecting stalk	227
SN-16	Somites	228
SN-17	Umbilical cord	228
SN-18	Intra embryonic mesoderm	229
SN-19	Allantois	230
SN-20	Trophoblast	231
SN-21	Placenta	232
SN-22	Types of placenta depending upon shape	235
SN-23	Types of placenta depending upon attachment	235
SAQ-3	Placenta praevia	236
SN-24	Chorion	237
SN-25	The maternal-foetal barrier	238
SN-26	Coelomic wall epithelium	239
SAQ-4	Surface ectoderm epithelium	239
SAQ-5	Septum transversum	340
SN-27	Neural crest	240

| SN-1 | **Mitosis** |

Mitos thread, *schisis* cleavage

The type of cell division where threads appear during cleavage of somatic cell, and results in distribution of identical copies of parent cell into two daughter cells.

1. **Interphase:** Cells do not actively divide but elongate. With onset of mitosis chromosomes undergo coiling condensation. Chromosome contains two parallel subunits called chromatids connected by centromere .

    A. Before mitosis: Chromosome number is diploid and DNA is tetraploid.
    B. After mitosis:
        a. Chromosomes remain diploid and
        b. DNA material becomes diploid in amount.

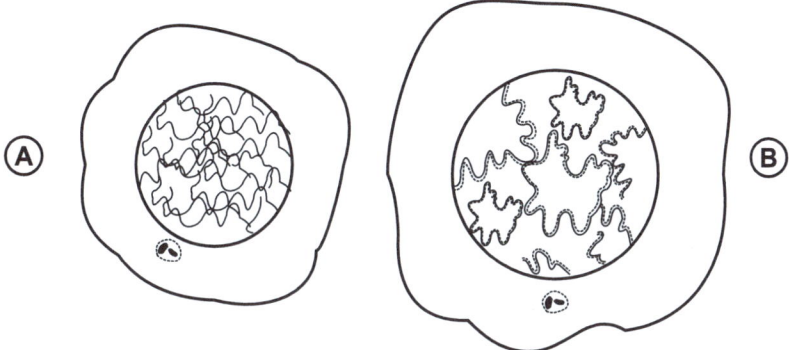

Fig 4.1 Interphase - A) Early interphase: Chromosomes are seen as extended threads.
B) Late interphase: There is duplication of DNA material.

2. **Phases:**

    A. Prophase (*Pro* before): It is the first stage of cell division.
        a. Chromatids are shortened.
        b. Chromosomes are recognised as a structure of chromatids and centromere.
        c. Centrioles separate and start migrating to each pole.
        d. Spindle and asters are formed, together called as diaster.
        e. Nucleolus and nuclear membrane disappear.

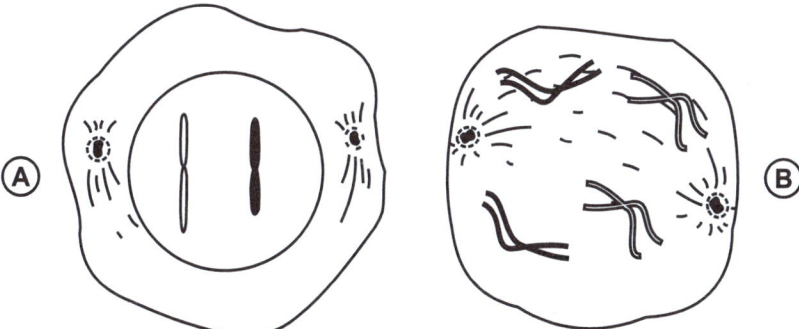

Fig. 4.2 Prophase - A) Early prophase: Chromosomes seen prominently. Centrioles move from each other.
B) Late prophase: The nuclear membrane disappears and spindle is formed

B. Metaphase (*meta* after): It is the cell division after prophase,
   a. Chromosomes migrate towards equators,
   b. Spindle occupies central position and
   c. Centromeres are attached to microtubules.

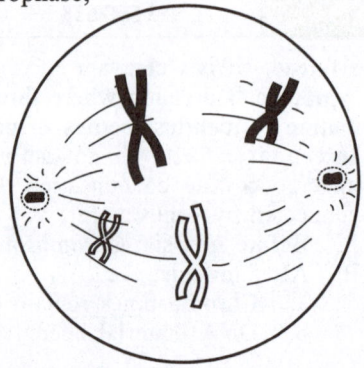

Fig. 4.3 Metaphase - Chromosomes are attached to spindle and are arranged on equator.

C. Anaphase (*Ana* apart): It is the cell division where the chromosomes move apart
   a. Cytoplasmic division starts with appearance of cleavage furrow.
   b. Chromosomes divide but splitting occur at centromere (centromere is double structure).
   c. Such chromosomes start migrating to each end.

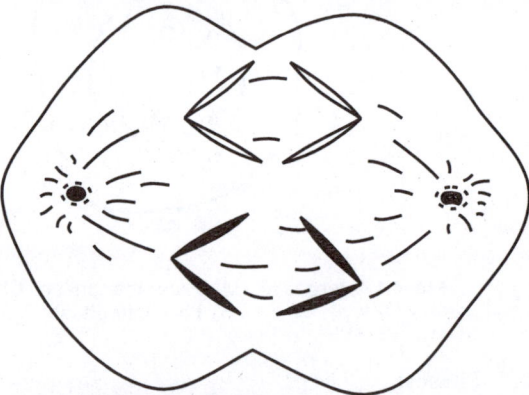

Fig. 4.4 Anaphase - Centromeres split. There are two pairs of chromosome. Each pair moves to one pole.

D. Telophase (*Telo* end): It is the end phase of cell division.
   a. Nuclear membrane reappears.
   b. Nucleoli reappear.
   c. Chromosomes are grouped at each end with diploid number.

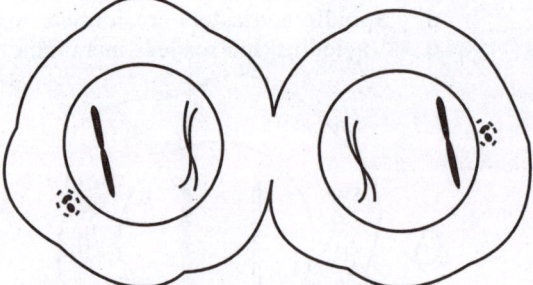

Fig. 4.5 Telophase - Nuclear membranes are formed. Chromosomes become less prominent

3. **Applied anatomy:** Radiation causes change in number of chromosomes and formation of abnormal chromosomes.

SN-2 Meiosis

1. **Meiosis:** It is the cell division occurring only in the germ cells, where exchange of genetic material takes place. The daughter cells are not identical. It occurs just before the formation of the gamete. The number of chromosomes are reduced to half.

2. **Peculiarities:**
   A. Pairing of homologous chromosomes occur only in meiosis and not in mitosis.
   B. After fertility diploid number is restored.
   C. The genetic exchange occurs in homologous chromosomal pairs.
      a. In interphase there is a replication of DNA.
      b. DNA is tetraploid and chromosome is diploid
         I. Meiosis I is a reduction division. At the end a meiosis I each cell contains haploid number of chromosomes.
         II. Meiosis II: The haploid number of chromosomes is maintained. It resembles mitosis but differs in two respects
            i. There is no DNA replication prior to this.
            ii. Second meiotic division follows meiosis I without interphase.

3. **Site:** Meiosis occurs in the germ cells i.e. Spermatogonium in case of male and oogonium in case of female.

4. **Stages:** Meiosis includes first and second meiotic division.
   A. First meiotic division: This consists of
      a. Prophase: It is a long and complex and has various stages.

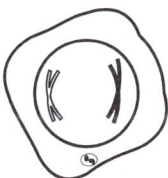

Fig. 4.6 Leptotene

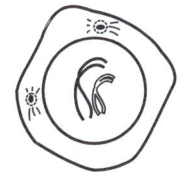

Fig. 4.7 Zygotene

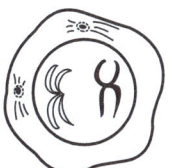

Fig. 4.8 Pachytene

   I. Leptotene (*leptos* slender, *tene* ribbon): The chromosomes appear as individual threads, the one end of which is attached to nuclear membrane. They appear beaded due to the presence of centromere.

   II. Zygotene: The homologous pairing of chromosomes takes place.
      i. Point to point pairing occurs.
      ii. Each pair is a bivalent.
      iii. The limited pairing occurs in X and Y chromosomes.

   III. Pachytene (*pachy* thick):
      i. Coiling condensation takes place.
      ii. Centromere and two chromatids becomes prominent in chromosome.
      iii. Each bivalent pair consists of 4 chromatids and forms tetrad.
      iv. Crossing over: It is an important event. The two central chromatids (one belonging to each chromosome of the bivalent) become coiled over each other so that they cross at a number of points.

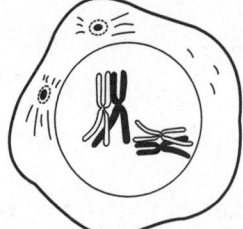

Fig. 4.9 Diplotene

IV. Diplotene (*diplotene* duplication): This stage is characterised by longitudinal separation of members of bivalent, without split in the centromere. Crossing over is complete. *In female the growth of the primary oocyte is arrested in diplotene and prolongs upto ovulation.*

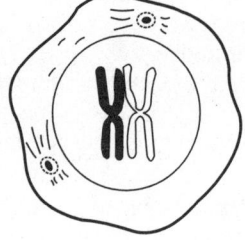

Fig. 4.10 Diakenesis

V. Diakenesis
  i. The chiasmata start resolving.
  ii. The chromosomes further becomes condensed and coiled..
  iii. They start migrating towards equator.
     At the end of prophase I nucleoli and nuclear membrane disappears.

b. Metaphase I
  I. It resembles mitotic metaphase.
  II. Chromosomes are attached by centromere. The spindle is formed.
  III. Homologous pairs lie parallel to equator with one member on each side of equator.

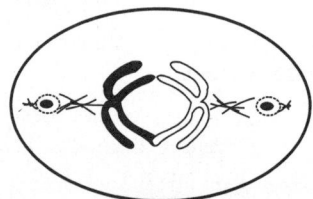

Fig. 4.11 Metaphase

c. Anaphase: The whole chromosomes with two chromatids goes to one pole while other chromosome of homologous pair goes to other side. Such migration of bivalent pairs is at random.

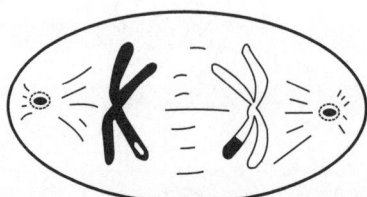

Fig. 4.12 Anaphase

d. Telophase: The chromosome in each cell is reduced to haploid number.

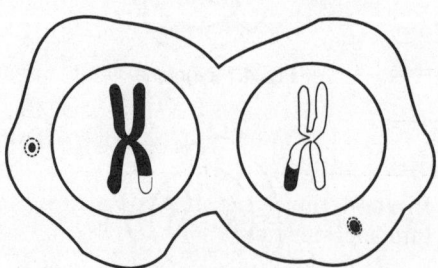

Fig. 4.13 Telophase

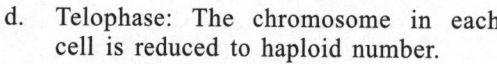

B. The second meiotic division is followed by a short interphase. It differs from usual interphase in that there is no duplication of DNA. It is similar to mitosis. However, the daughter cells are not identical in genetic content.

5. **Significance:**
   A. First meiotic division provides
      a. Genetic variability through the process of crossing over.
      b. Random distribution of homologous chromosomes to daughter cells.
   B. Second meiotic division provides
      a. Germ cells with haploid number of chromosome and
      b. Haploid amount of DNA.
      c. It is similar to mitosis except chromosomes in daughter cell, which are not alike.

6. **Applied anatomy:**
   A. Abnormalities of form
      a. Giant (large): Spermatozoa is too large.
      b. Dwarf (small): Spermatozoa is too small.
      c. Duplication of head, body or tail.
      d. Ovum may have unusually large nucleus.
   B. Chromosomal abnormalities:
      a. Non disjunction is failure of separation of two chromosomes at anaphase.
         I. Trisomy: There are forty seven chromosomes, there being three identical instead of one of the normal pairs e.g.
            i. Mongolism or
            ii. Down's syndrome: Trisomy 21.
         II. Presence of extra X or Y chromosome e.g.
            i. 47, XXX abnormal female.
            ii. 47, XXY: Klinefelter syndrome - abnormal male.
            iii. 47, XYY: Abnormal male.
      b. Abnormal number of chromosomes: There are only forty five chromosomes. Here one pair is represented by single chromosome. 45, X e.g. XO Turner's syndrome. Gamete may have diploid number of chromosomes so that zygote will have 46 + 23 (i.e. 69).
      c. Abnormalities in the shape in the morphological chromosome:
         I. Translocation: Part of a chromosome may get attached to a chromosome of a different pair.
         II. Deletion part of chromosome may be lost.
         III. Duplication of genes.
         IV. Inversion: Chromosome may get inverted before joining the opposite chromosome.

SN-3   Spermatogenesis

1. **Introduction:** It is the complex series of changes by which spermatogonia are transformed into spermatozoa.

2. **Site:**
   A. It takes place in seminiferous tubules.
   B. It is controlled by testosterone.

C. It begins at puberty and continues up to the old age.

3. **Duration:** Sixty four days, are required to complete one cycle of spermatogenesis. These complex series of changes do not take place in all parts of seminiferous tubules simultaneously.

4. **Stages:** The following are the stages
   A. Spermatocytosis: It involves series of mitotic divisions from which spermatogonium A is converted to primary spermatocyte. Primary spermatocyte is comparatively larger cell due to increased nuclear and cytoplasmic material.
   B. Meiosis: Primary spermatocyte (diploid) soon enters into first meiotic division, transforms into secondary spermatocyte (haploid). It is changed into spermatid by second meiotic division. Spermatids have haploid number of chromosomes.
   C. Spermiogenesis: It involves series of changes by which spermatid (non-motile) is converted into an elongated (motile) sperm.

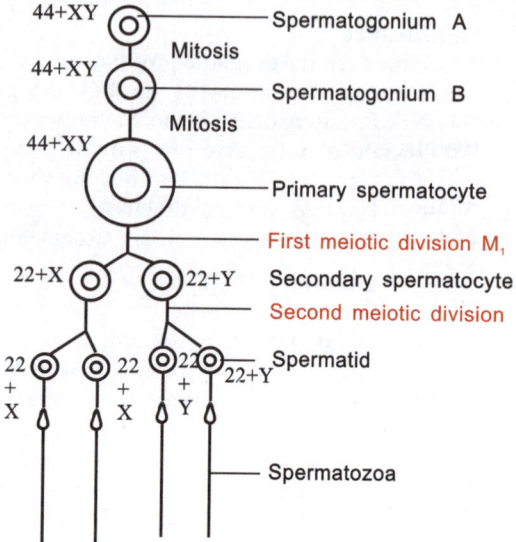

Fig. 4.14 Stages in spermatogenesis

5. **End result of spermatogenesis :** In one cycle 4 motile sperms are formed from one primary spermatocyte which possess haploid number of chromosomes.

6. **Amount of ejaculation** is 2-3 ml.
   A. Each ml contains 100 million sperms.
   B. The life of the sperm is 24 - 48 hours.
   C. Rate of motility is 1.5.to 3 mm/min.
   D. Contents of semen are
      a. Sperm and
      b. Chemicals and enzymes: Citric acid, lactic acid, pyruvic acid, fructose, proteolytic enzymes, prostaglandins, innositol and sorbitol.

7. **Anomalies:** They can be grouped in
   A. Morphological
      a. Double heads
      b. Poorly motile
   B. Numerical
      a. Oligospermia: Less than 10 million per ml.
      b. Azospermia: Zero sperm count.

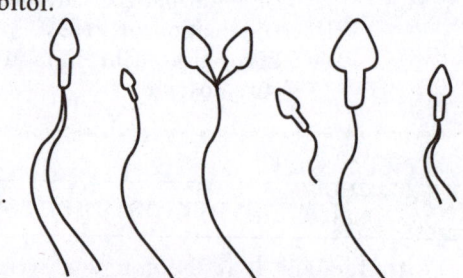

Fig. 4.15 Anomalies of spermatozoa

SAQ-1   Spermiogenesis

Spermiogenesis: It involves series of changes by which spermatid (non-motile) is converted into an elongated (motile) sperm. The cell organelle transform into following structure.

1. Golgi complex forms acrosomal cap on upper two-third of circumference of the head of the sperm. It helps in penetration of the cells of corona radiata and zona pellucida (secondary oocyte). It contains enzymes viz. Namely acrosin, acid phosphatase, proteases and hyaluronidase.
2. The nucleus is converted into head of the sperm. The specific number of chromosome is maintained i.e. haploid number of chromosome.
3. Mitochondria are arranged in helical form around axoneme of the middle piece. It provides energy for motility.
4. Centrioles are of two types:
   A. Proximal centriole is present at the neck.
   B. Distal centriole is present in tail of sperm, which helps in motility.
5. Residual body: The excess of cytoplasm is shed off which is engulfed by cells of Sertoli.

SAQ-2   Sperm

1. **Introduction:** It is a male gamete, smaller than the female gamete i.e. ovum and is about 45-50 mm in length. It is a motile cell.

2. **Parts:** It has following parts.
   A. Head:
      a. Shape: Ovoid / pyriform.
      b. Size: 4 mm.
   B. Tail: Principle piece
      a. Neck: It is constricted part distal to head.
      b. Middle piece: It contains a motor element - axoneme (central doublet with peripheral doublet) which is surrounded by the coarse fibres in middle piece and principle piece. The mitochondria is absent in principle piece.
      c. Proximal piece and
      d. Terminal piece.

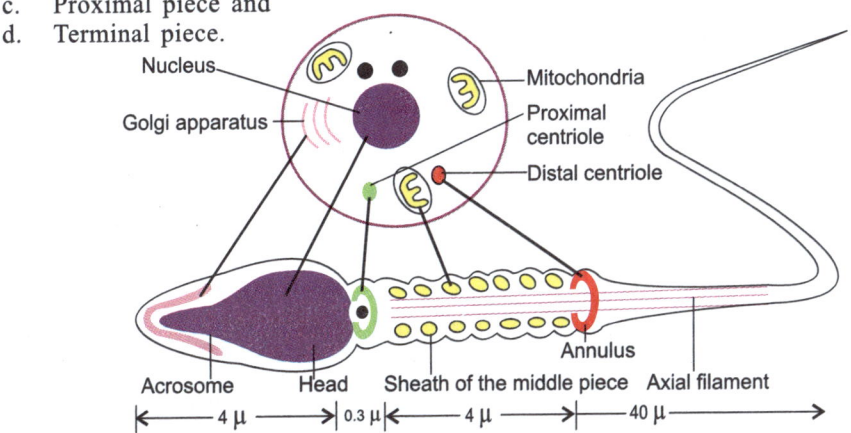

Fig. 4.16 Parts of spermatozoon and their derivation

SN-4 | Capacitation of sperm

It is the final stage of maturation of sperm.

It lasts for period of 7 hours.

It occurs in the female genital tract.

During this time, a glycoprotein coat and seminal plasma proteins are removed from the plasma membrane that overlies the acrosomal region. Capacitated sperm shows no morphological changes except increase of the activity.

The capacitated sperm comes in contact with corona radiata because of following factors.

1. An interaction between the zona pellucida and head of the sperm. It includes release of acrosin which helps in digestion of zona pellucida.

2. Action of tubal mucosal enzyme.

3. Movements of the tail of sperm.

SN-5 | Oogenesis

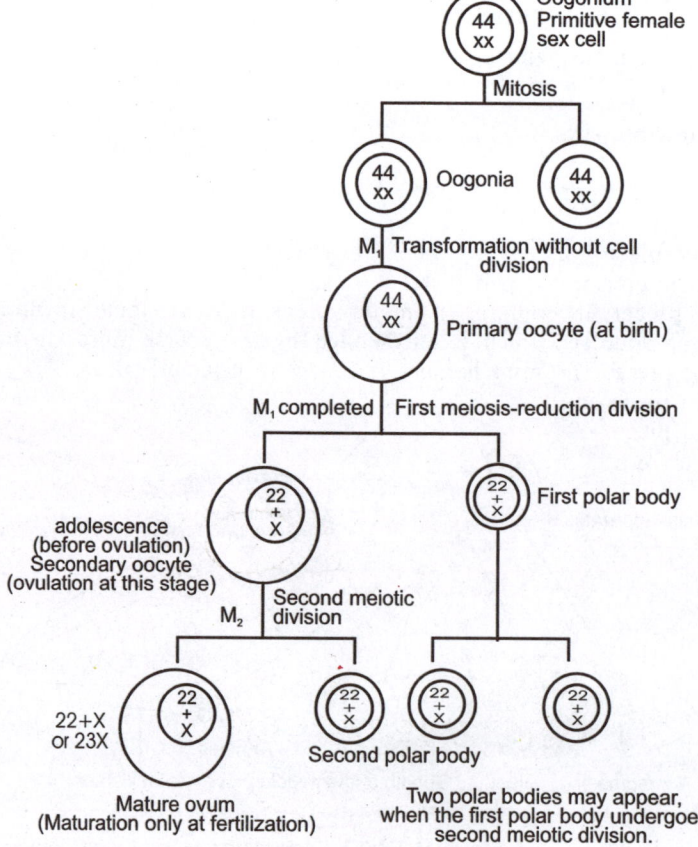

Fig. 4.17 Stages in oogenesis

1. **Introduction:** It is a process involving complex changes by which oogonia are converted into ova, the female gamete.

2. **Site:** It takes place in ovary and fallopian tubes. It begins in the intra uterine life and continues till menopause.

3. **Duration:** It takes 12 - 60 years to complete one cycle of oogenesis. The female gonad is ovary. It has an outer part the cortex and inner part medulla. The cortex contains large cells called oogonia. All oogonia are produced before birth.
   The oogonium enlarges and is called primary oocyte.
   A. Primary oocyte divides by first meiotic division (reduction) into two secondary oocyte. One of two secondary oocyte contains half number of chromosomes and almost all of its cytoplasm. Second of two secondary oocyte contains only half number of chromosomes and no cytoplasma and is called first polar body. The first polar body is therefore formed merely to get rid of unwanted chromosomes.
   B. Secondary oocyte gets arrested into metaphase. It divides into ovum and second polar body by second meiotic division. This occurs only at the time of fertilization.

4. **The number of germ cells at different chronological age:**
   A. In intrauterine life there are 7 million germ cells.
   B. At birth there are 1 million oogonia.
   C. At puberty there are 40,000 oocyte.
   D. The women sheds about 500 secondary oocyte throughout her life.
   E. At each ovulation 1 secondary oocyte is shed.

5. **Ovulation:** Liberation of the secondary oocyte from the ovary is called ovulation.

SN-6   Graafian follicle

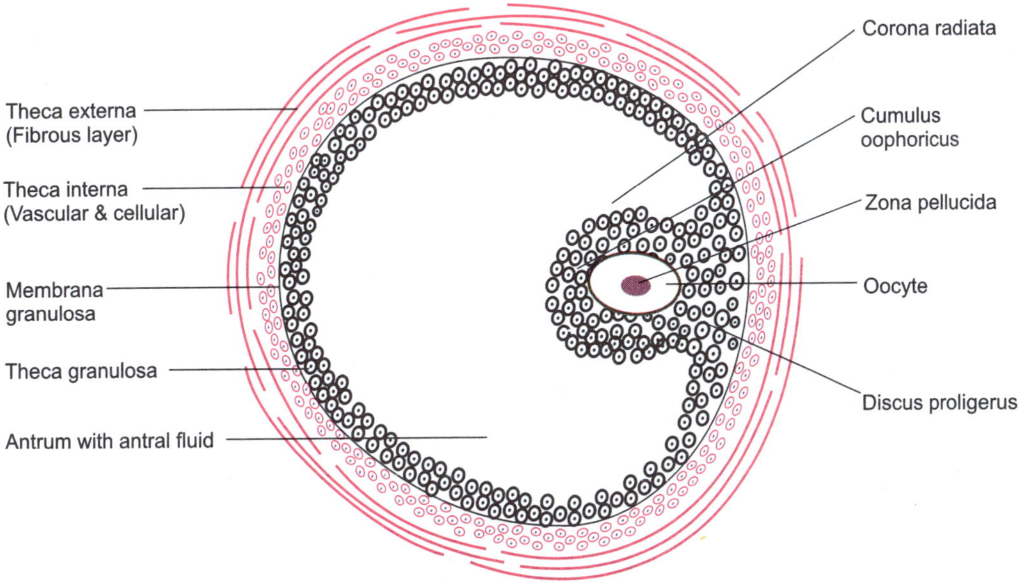

Theca externa (Fibrous layer)

Theca interna (Vascular & cellular)

Membrana granulosa

Theca granulosa

Antrum with antral fluid

Corona radiata

Cumulus oophoricus

Zona pellucida

Oocyte

Discus proligerus

Fig. 4.18 Structures in the Graafian follicle

The ovum develops from oogonia present in the cortex of ovary. These oogonia are surrounded by cells that form stroma. These stromal cells form Graafian follicle. The stages in the formation of Graafian follicle are as follows

1. **Follicular cells:** Some of the cells of stroma becomes flattened and surround oocyte and ultimately give rise to ovarian follicle and hence they are called follicular cells.

2. **Primordial follicle:** The flattened follicular cells become columnar. The follicle upto this stage is called primordial follicle.

3. **Zona pellucida** (*zona* belt, *pellucida* transparent): It is a transparent belt present between follicular cells and oocyte.
   Functions of the zona pellucida:
   A. It protects the oocyte.
   B. It prevents sticking to the endometriun.
   C. It prevents entry of micro molecules into oocyte.
   D. It prevents entry of more than one sperm into oocyte.

4. **Membrana granulosa:** The follicular cells proliferate and contain granules and hence are called granular cells. They form several layers of cells called membrana granulosa.

5. **Antrum (cavity):** The cavity appears within the membrana granulosa. The cavity of the follicle increases rapidly in size. This results into thinness of wall of the follicle. The oocyte now lies eccentrically in the follicle.

6. **Cumulus oophoricus** (*cumulus* accumulation of cells, *ovaricus* surrounding ovum): The follicular cells surrounding oocyte are called cumulus oophoricus.

7. **Discus proligerus** (*discus* flat plate, *proligerus* producing offspring): The cells attached to the wall of follicle are given the name discus proligerus.

8. **Theca interna** (*theca* cover): The cells surrounding the membrana granulosa become condensed and forma theca interna. They secrete hormone called oestrogen and the cells are called thecal gland.

9. **Theca externa:** The fibrous tissue surrounding the follicle gets thickened and are called theca externa.

SN-7	**Fertilization**

1. **Introduction:** It is the fusion of male and female pronuclei (sperm and secondary oocyte). To form the zygote.

2. **Site:** Fertilization occurs in the ampulla of the fallopian tube.

3. **Time:** It occurs within 24 hrs of ovulation.

4. **Pre-requisite** (capacitation): It requires to cross 3 barriers
   A. The cells of the corona radiata,
   B. Zona pellucida and
   C. Vitelline membrane.

5. **Mechanism:**
   A. Cells of corona radiata are disintegrated by the enzyme hyaluronidase.
   B. Zona pellucida is digested by enzyme acrosin and neuraminidase.

C. Many sperms get embedded in zona pellucida but when one sperm reaches vitelline membrane.
   a. Calcium wave spreads in secondary oocyte and second meiosis completes with the formation of ovum.
   b. The cortical granules are released.
D. The cortical granules react with zona pellucida and make it impermeable to other sperms (i.e. acro reaction is inhibited).
E. Only head enters the cytoplasm and gets changed into male pronucleus, DNA replication takes place (chromosome number may be 22X or 22Y).
F. Female pronucleus is also formed.
G. Nuclear membrane disappears and mixing of chromosomes occur.
H. It results into diploid number of chromosome.
I. The zygote is formed.
J. The cleavage starts.

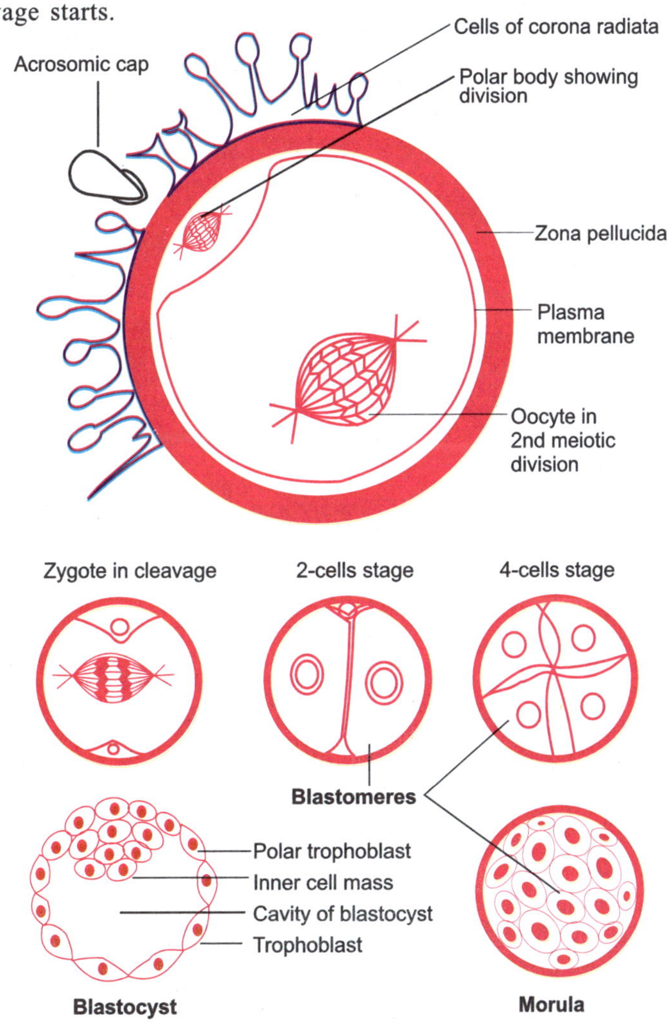

Fig 4.19 Fertilization

6. **Results of fertilization:**
   A. The oogenesis cycle is complete.
   B. The chromosomal number is restored.
   C. The sex is determined.
   D. The cleavage starts.
   E. The genetic combination leads to variations in human species.

7. **Effects:**
   A. On ovary: The corpus luteum changes to corpus luteum of pregnancy.
   B. On uterus: The secretory changes starts in the endometrium.
   C. On zygote: The cleavage starts.
   In vitro fertilization: The pre-ovulatory oocyte is taken out with laproscopy and is fertilized outside.

| SN-8 | **Implantation** |

1. **Introduction:** The process by which blastocyst gets embedded in the endometriun is called implantation.

2. **Time:** On 7th day after fertilization.

3. **Site:** Endometrium of posterior wall of fundus of uterus.

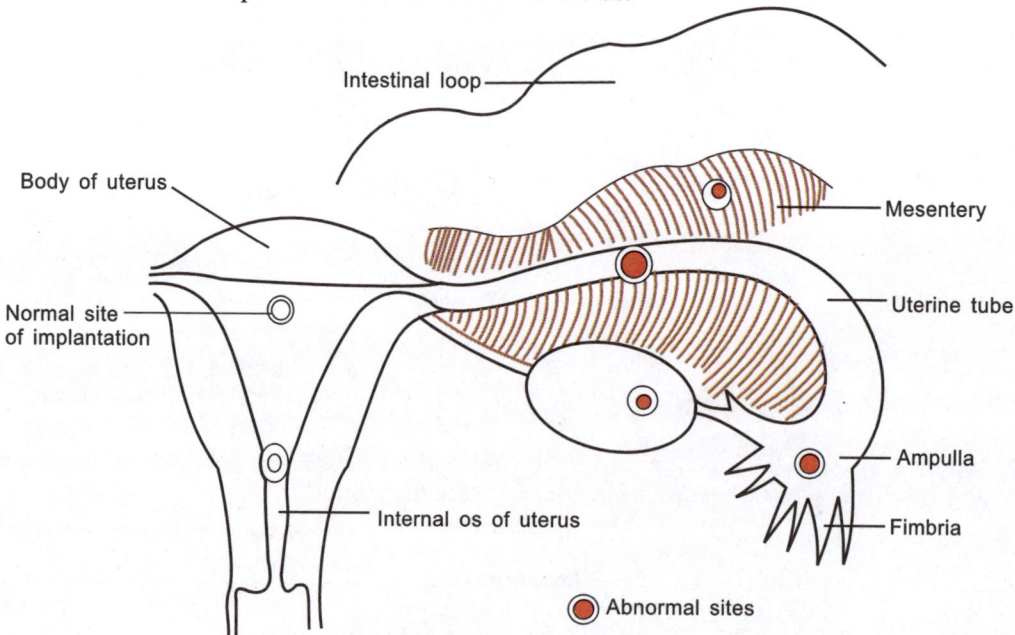

Fig. 4.20 Normal and abnormal sites of implantation

4. **Cells:** The responsible cells are cells of trophoblast. They have the property of adhesion, invasion and erosion.

5. **Types of implantation are:**
   A. **Interstitial:** The blastocyst is embedded into stratum compactum endometrium. e.g. human.
   B. **Central:** The blastocyst is embedded in the cavity of uterus e.g. cow.
   C. **Eccentric:** The blastocyst is embedded in the crypts of uterus e.g. Rat.

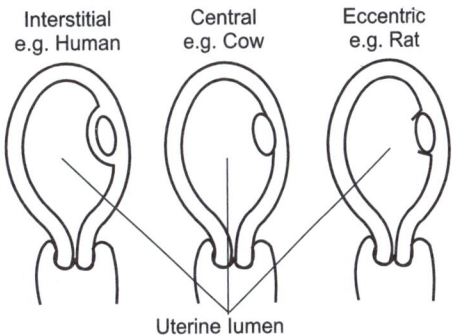

Fig 4.21 Types of implantation

6. **Pre requisite:**
   A. Dissolution of zona pellucida.
   B. Preparation of the endometrium. It is facilitated by progesterone, which is secreted by corpus luteum. This is called decidual reaction.

7. **Actual process:**
   A. The zona pellucida disappears.
   B. The trophoblast adheres to endometrium.
   C. The trophoblast penetrates endometrium by proteolytic action.
   D. The cells of the trophoblast proliferate.

8. **Results of implantation:**
   A. Trophoblast differentiates into two layers:
      a. Cytotrophoblast &
      b. Syncytiotrophoblast.
   B. Inner cell mass differentiates into epiblast cells, hypoblast cells with amniotic cavity and yolk sac cavity.

9. **Abnormal sites of implantation of the ovum:**
   A. Implantation within the uterus
      Placenta praevia (*prae* infront): The placenta is attached to lower uterine segment completely or partially. It is characterized by painless haemorrhage in last trimester particularly in the eighth month of pregnancy.
   B. Implantation outside the uterus
      a. Tubal,
      b. Cervical,
      c. Peritoneal and
      d. Ovarian.

10. **Applied anatomy:** Excessive or deeper implantation results into post partum haemorrhage. E.g. Placenta accreta, placenta increta and placenta percreta.

SN-9   Blastocyst

1. **Introduction:** A blastula having a fluid filled cavity is called blastocyst.

2. **Chronological age:** *It is formed between __fourth to fifth day__ of fertilization*

3. **Parts:**
   A. Blastocoele and
   B. Inner cell mass (embryoblast).
   C. Trophoblast.

4. **Formation:** Cells of morula are of two types.
   A. Cells forming the embryoblast which give rise to embryo proper.
   B. Trophoblast cells which are subdivided into
      a. Polar: Polar cells gives rise to chorion frondosum.
      b. Mural: Mural cell gives chorion levae. The cavity of the blastocyst is called blastocoele.

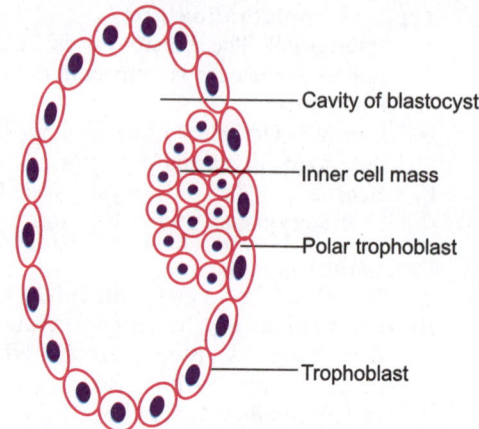

Fig. 4.22 Blastocyst

SN-10   Decidua

(*Decidua* falling off)

1. **Introduction:** The uterine endometrium after implantation is called decidua.

2. **Decidual reaction:** After implantation the endometrial glands accumulate glycogen and lipid secretion and this is called decidual reaction.

3. **Following changes occur**
   A. Nuclei becomes rounded.
   B. The number of cytoplasmic organellae increase.
   C. The volume of the cytoplasm increases.
   D. The vascularity of the cell increases.

4. **Hormones responsible for the changes are**
   A. Progesterone.
   B. HCG (Human chorionic gonadotropin).

5. **Functions:**

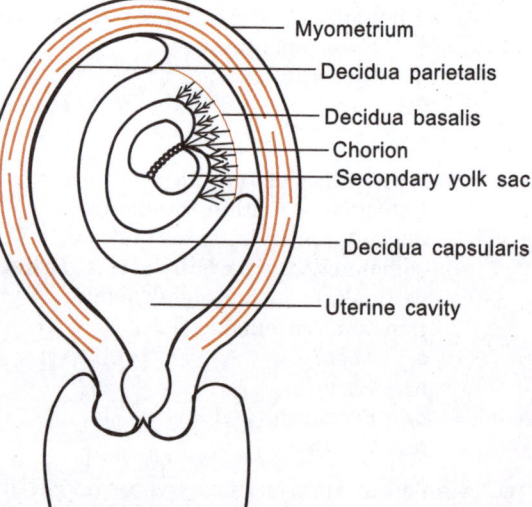

Fig. 4.23 Decidua

   A. It gives mechanical support to the fertilized ovum and forms a suitable site for implantation.
   B. It provides nutrition to blastocyst.
   C. The decidua basalis forms maternal part of placenta and takes temporary function of placenta.

6. **Part of decidua:**
   A. Decidua basalis: The endometrium towards embryonic pole / base of embryo.
   B. Decidua capsularis: The endometrium towards abembryonic pole (towards uterine cavity).

C. Decidua parietalis: The endometrium of remaining part.

7. **Fate:**
  A. The decidua basalis undergoes marked development and forms the maternal surface of placenta.
  B. The decidua capsularis and parietalis are stretched and fuse and undergo atrophy. With the increase in size of amniotic cavity following changes occur.
    a. The extra embryonic coelom obliterates.
    b. The amnion fuses with chorion.
    c. The amniochorionic membrane (chorion laeve) fuses with decidua capsularis.
  C. The decidua capsularis disintegrates and fuses with decidua parietalis and obliterates the uterine cavity.

    At the time of delivery, placenta separates with decidua basalis and parietalis and is delivered.

SN-11	**Amnion**

(*Amnion* bowl)

1. **Introduction:** It is the thin but tough extraembryonic membrane derived from amniogenic cells. It forms the wall of the amniotic cavity, which exclude the cells of the ectoderm. It form the hydrostatic bag containing fluid which envelopes the embryo, umbilical cord and foetal part of placenta.

2. **Chronological age:** Second week after fertilization.

3. **Responsible cells** are aminogenic cells. They are derived from the trophoblast cells which are present on the roof of ectoderm cells.

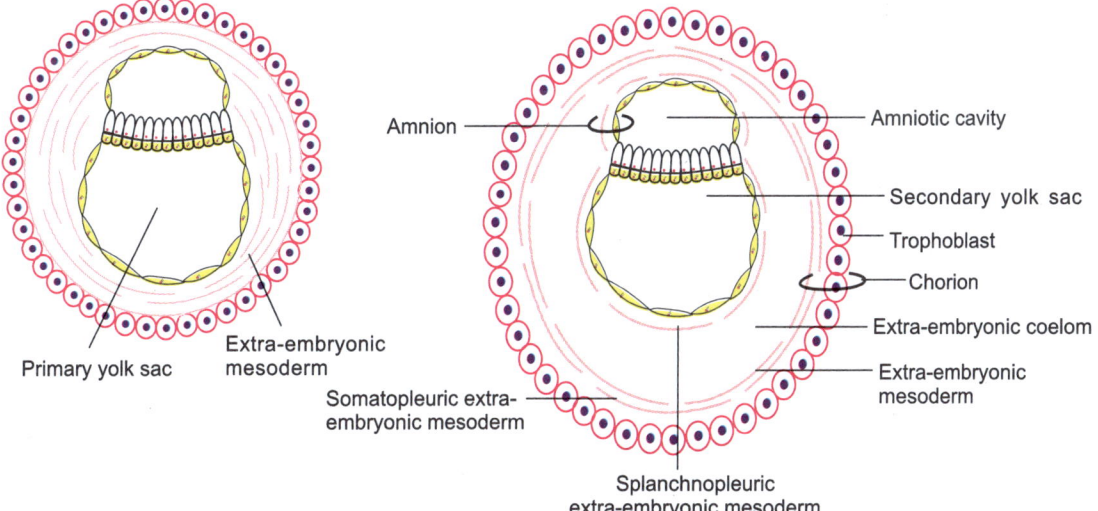

Fig. 4.24 Formation of extraembryonic mesoderm and extraembryonic coelom and structures forming amnion and chorion

4. **Sources of amniotic fluid** are mainly from
    A. Maternal blood,
    B. Amniotic cell &
    C. Urine secreted by foetus.

5. **Volume of amniotic fluid:**
    A. At 10 weeks of gestation, it is 30 ml.
    B. At 20 weeks of gestation, it is 350 ml.
    C. At 37 weeks of gestation, it is 800 to 1000 ml.

6. **Circulation of amniotic fluid:**
    A. Part of fluid goes into maternal blood.
    B. Part of it, is swallowed by foetus.
    C. Excess of water in fetal blood is excreted by urine and to the amniotic cavity.

7. **Composition of amniotic fluid:**
    A. Desquamated fetal epithelial cells,
    B. Water,
    C. Fats,
    D. Enzymes,
    E. Pigments &
    F. Hormones.

8. **Significance of fluid:**
    A. It allows free movement of fetus which helps in the development of musculo skeletal system.
    B. It permits symmetrical external growth of the embryo.
    C. It prevents adherence of amnion to the embryo.
    D. It protects embryo against injuries.
    E. It regulates the body temperature of the embryo.
    F. It dilates cervix during the act of parturition along with chorionic membrane.

9. **Anomalies:**
    A. Oligohydramnios: The amniotic fluid is less than 400 ml. The complications of the oligohydramnios include foetal abnormalities. These are
        a. Pulmonary hypoplasia,
        b. Facial defects,
        c. Limb defects,
        d. Urinary agenesis &
        e. Compression of the umbilical cord.
    B. Polyhydramnios: The amniotic fluid is more than 2000 ml. It is associated with the
        a. Severe anomalies of central nervous system &
        b. Oesophageal atresia.

10. **Applied anatomy:**
    A. Amniocentesis: It is a process by which amniotic fluid is removed and studied for the cells by 16 to 20 weeks.
    B. Detection of abnormal foetus e.g. encephalitis. It is detected by the estimation of alpha foetoprotein. The level is increased in neural tube defect like encephalitis.
    C. Determination of the sex.

SN-12   Yolk sac

1. **Introduction:** *The inner wall of the cavity of blastocyst is lined by flattened cells called Heuser's membrane (future endodermal cells).* Such structure is called primary yolk sac. It is described in three stages.

   A. Primary yolk sac: During the ninth day of development, flattened cells origination from endoderm form a thin membrane called Heuser's membrane. This membrane together with the cells of endoderm forms the primary yolk sac.

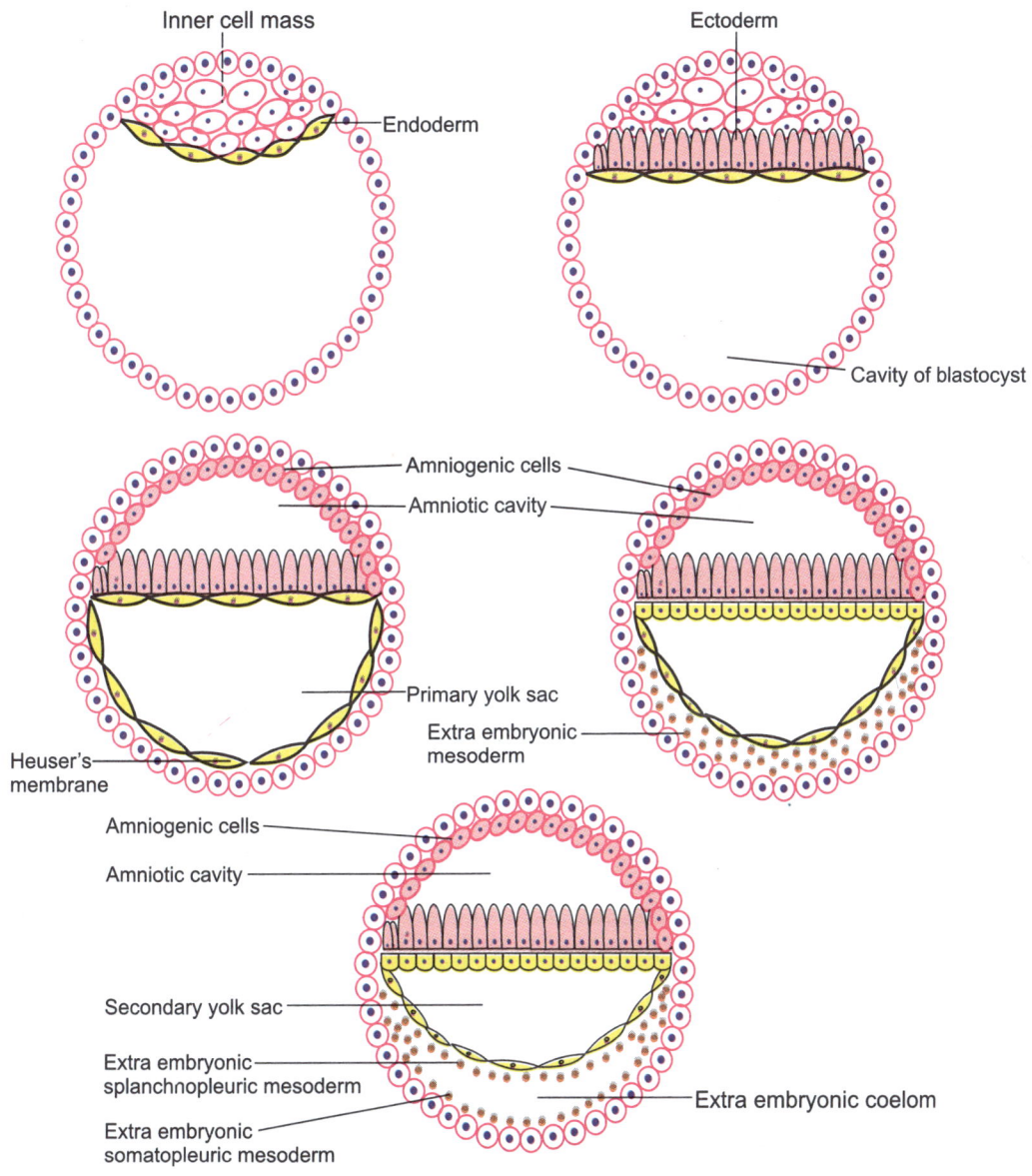

Fig. 4.25 Formation of different yolk sac

B. Definitive or secondary yolk sac: By thirteenth day, the extra embryonic mesoderm and it is filled by the cavity called extra embryonic coelom. This is much smaller than the primary yolk sac cavity. The decrease in the size is accompanied by the change in nature of lining cells. They are no longer flattened but becomes cubical.

C. Tertiary yolk sac: It is remnant of secondary yolk sac. It is divided into following parts.
   a. Intraembryonic part: It gives rise to foregut, midgut and hindgut.
   b. Intermediate or connecting part: It is also called vitellointestinal duct.
   c. Extraembryonic part: This is called tertiary yolk sac.

2. **Chronological age:** <u>Second week</u> after fertilization.

3. **Functions:**
   A. Nutrition to the embryom.
   B. Haemopoisis.
   C. Formation of
      a. Epithelium of
         I. Gastro intestinal,
         II. Respiratory tract &
         III. Urinary bladder.
      b. Male and female primordial germ cell.

4. **Fate:**
   A. Usually the yolk sac detaches from the midgut loop but its stalk (vitello-intestinal duct) may remain in continuation with midgut loop which persists as a **<u>diverticulum-called Meckel's diverticulum.</u>**
   B. **<u>Allantois</u>** in its distal part form a remnant called urachus, which extends from apex of bladder to umbilicus. With folding of embryo -
      a. The yolk sac incorporates into the developing gut tube and is reduces considerably,
      b. It lies in connecting stalk.

SN-13   Primitive streak

1. **Introduction:** It is a thickened band of ectodermal cells at the caudal end of embryo in the midline.

2. **Cells involved:** the pluripotent cells i.e. ability to transform into any type of the cells.

3. **Chronological age:** Third week of intrauterine life.

4. **Description:**
   A. It continues laterally upto the margins of the embryonic disc.
   B. It continues caudally upto the cloacal membrane and goes into connecting stalk.
   C. The cells of primitive streak fail to reach or they are absent at prochordal plate and cloacal membrane.
   D. The cells passing beyond the prochordal plate form cardiogenic area.

5. **Functions:**
   A. It organizes intra embryonic mesoderm (i.e. third germinal layer).
   B. It confirms the future cranio caudal axis of the embryo.
   C. It divides into left and right half of the embryo.
   D. It differentiates into notochord.

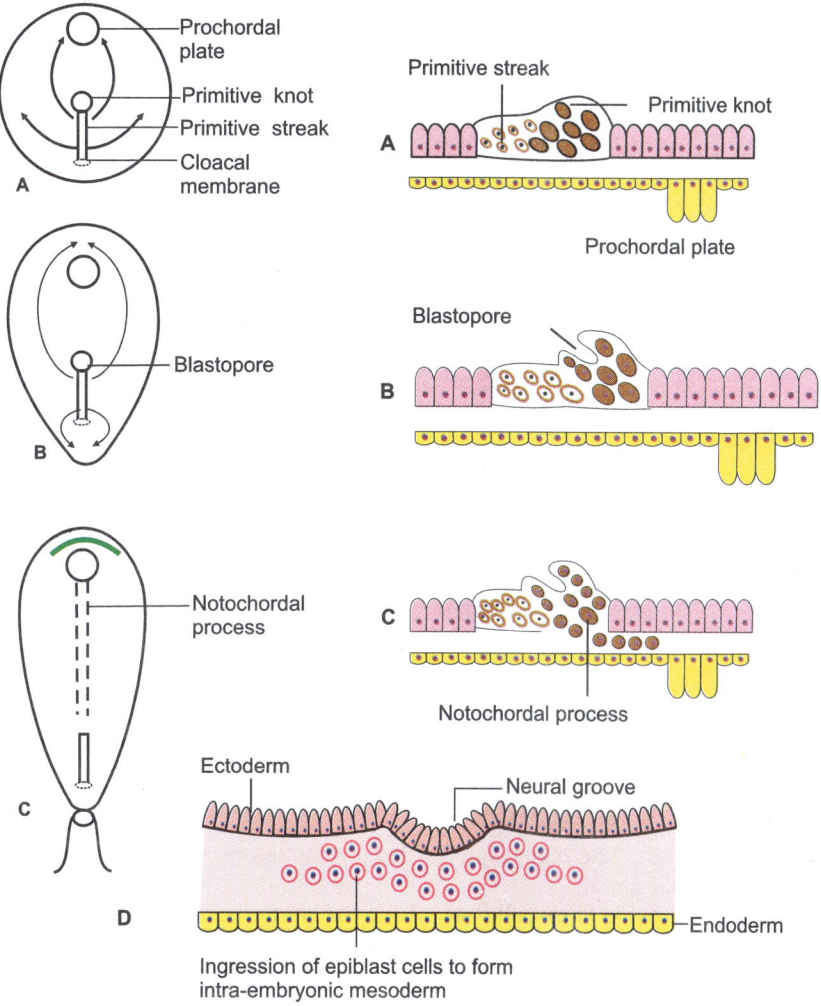

Fig. 4.26 Formation of the primitive streak

6. **Fate:** Cells of primitive streaks are continuously formed up to third week and then regresses but may remain up to fourth week. Cells of primitive streak give rise to:
   A. Lateral part of paraxial mesoderm,
   B. Primordial germ cells,
   B. Intra embryonic mesoderm and
   C. Extra embryonic mesoderm.

7. **Applied:** If the cells of the primitive streak remain after fourth week they give rise to teratogenic tumour at sacro coccygeal region.

8. **Recent view:** Primitive node gives rise to
   A. Notochord,
   B. Medial part of paraxial mesoderm and
   C. Endoderm.

SN-14   Notochord

(*Noto* relationship to back, *chord* rod shaped structure)

1. **Introduction:** It is a solid rod of cells which supports the embryo.

2. **Extent:** It extends from primitive node to prochordal plate.

3. **Situation:** Midline of the embryo.

4. **Source:** Cells of primitive node.

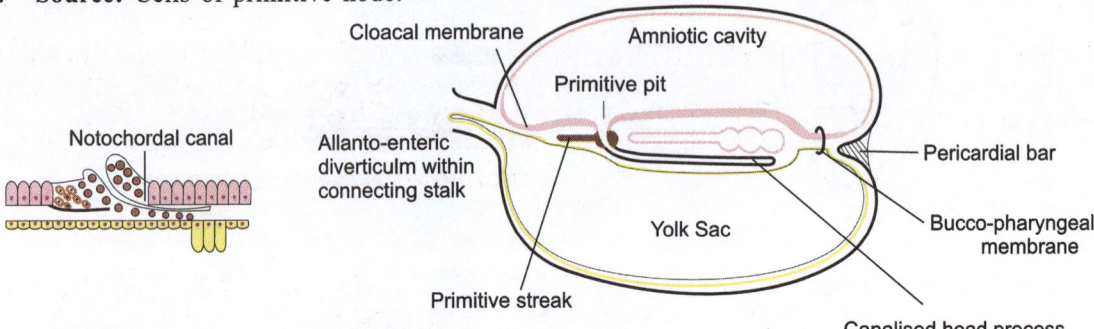

Fig. 4.27 Diagram showing the development of notochord

5. **Formation:**
   A. The cranial end of primitive streak (faint, white trace) becomes thick. This thickened part of primitive streak is called primitive node (knot or Hensen's node).
   B. A depression appears in the center of primitive knot, this depression is called blastopore.
   C. Notochordal process: The cells of primitive node present in the central axis migrates cranially towards prochordal plate.
   D. Notochordal canal: The canal arises from blastopore and extends into notochord is called notochordal canal.
   E. Neuroenteric canal: The cells at floor of notochordal canal break and form a communication between amnion and yolk sac through the canal.
   F. Notochordal plate: The cells in the floor of neuroenteric canal reappear and fills a gap at the floor and form a plate. Such plate is called notochordal plate.
   G. Solid notochord: The proliferation of cells of notochordal plate give rise to solid notochord, which extends from prochordal plate to primitive node.

6. **Functions:**
   A. It supports the embryo.
   B. It acts as a vertebral column in the embryonic life.
   C. It induces surface ectoderm to form neural plate.

7. **Fate:** Notochord do not have any contribution for formation of vertebra. It remains as
   A. Nucleus pulposus of the intervertebral disc.
   B. The apical ligament of dens.

8. **Applied anatomy:** Anomalies
   A. Neuroenteric canal: Notochord partly remains patent and is connected to lumen of intestine to central canal of spinal cord.
   B. Notocordal cells in body of vertebrae proliferate to form chordoma.

SN-15   Connecting stalk

1. **Introduction:** It is a part of extraembryonic mesoderm which is not encroached by extraembryonic coelom.

2. **Formation:**
   A. As the embryo grows, size of stalk becomes relatively small.
   B. Gradually the attachment is shifted to the caudal end of embryonic disc.
   C. With the rotation of tail fold, attachment of the stalk moves and gets attached to region of umbilical opening.
   D. The blood vessels start developing in embryo and placenta.
   E. The blood vessels of the placenta, communicates with the blood vessels of the mother.

3. **Contents:**
   A. Two umbilical arteries and one umbilical vein.
   B. The vitello intestinal duct may remain as remnants of yolk sac.
   C. The mesoderm of connecting stalk forms a gelatinous substance called Wharton's jelly.

4. **Functions:**
   A. It protects umbilical vessels.
   B. It forms small part of the extraembryonic coelom.
   C. It increases the length of the umbilical cord to allow free movement of the embryo.
   D. It suspends embryo.
   E. It nourishes embryo.
   F. It provides space for physiological hernia.

5. **Fate:** It gets converted into umbilical cord.

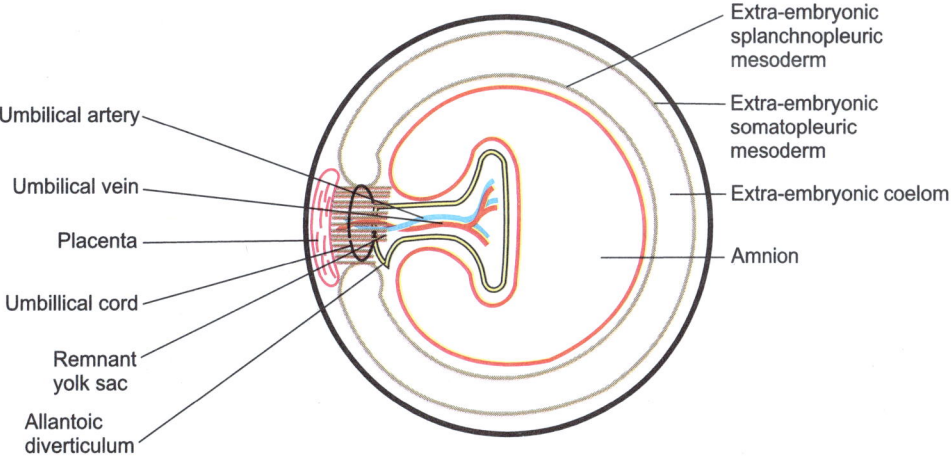

Fig. 4.28 Structures forming the umbilical cord.

SN-16   Somites

1. **Introduction:** The solid segmentation of paraxial intraembryonic mesoderm on either side of notochord is called somites.

2. **Extent:** It extends from cranial end of notochord to the coccygeal end.

3. **Chronological age:** <u>Twenty to thirty day.</u>

4. **Total number of somites:**
   42 - 44
   4 - Occipital
   8 - Cervical
   12 - Thoracic
   5 - Lumbar
   5 - Sacral
   8-10 Coccygeal

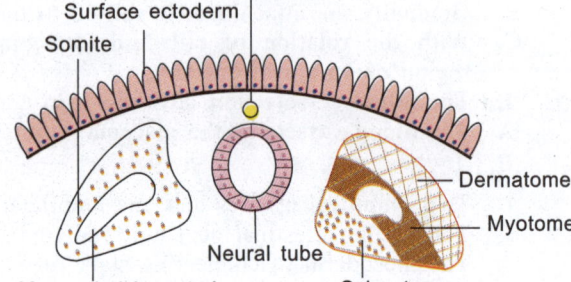

Fig. 4.29 Derivatives of somites

5. **Derivatives:**
   A. Sclerotome: Axial skeleton, ribs and sternum.
   B. Myotome: Muscles of back, front and limbs.
   C. Dermatome: Dermis of skin of the back and front.

6. **Nerve supply:** Mesodermal somites are supplied by corresponding segments of the spinal cord.

7. **Applied anatomy:**
   A. The age of the foetus can be determined by counting the number of somites.
   B. Spina bifida: The two halves of the neural arch may fail to fuse in the midline.
   C. Hemivertebrae: Incomplete development of one half of a vertebra.

SN-17   Umbilical cord

1. **Introduction:** It is a cord extending from umbilicus of foetus to the placenta.

2. **Embryonic tissue:** After folding of embryo connecting stalk elongates and forms umbilical cord .

3. **Dimensions:**
   A. Length: 50 cm
   B. Diameter: 1-2 cm

4. **Content:**
   A. Vessels
      a. Two umbilical arteries.
      b. One umbilical vein.
   B. Mesoderm: Intraembryonic mesoderm called Wharton's jelly.
   C. Remnant structures: Vitello intestinal duct and allantois.
   D. Layer of amnion.

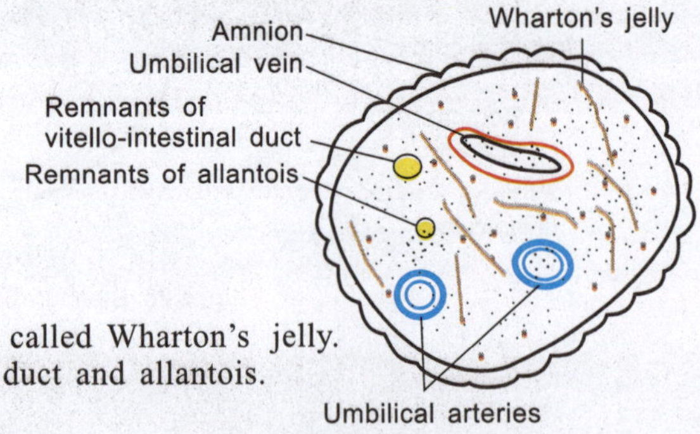

5. **Functions:**
   A. It suspends fetus into amniotic cavity.

Fig. 4.30 Structures in the umbilical cord

B. It transfers nutrients.

6. **Knots of umbilicus:** These are
    A. True knots of umbilicus: These are due to excessive movements.
    B. False knots of umbilicus: These are due to sharp bend of the cord.

| SN-18 | **Intra embryonic mesoderm (secondary mesoderm)** |

1. **Introduction:**
    A. It forms the third germinal layer.
    B. It is present between ectoderm and endoderm.

2. **Chronological age:** It is formed in the third week of gestation.

3. **Sources:**
    A. The cells of primitive streak.
    B. The cells of prochordal plate.
    C. The cells of neural crest.

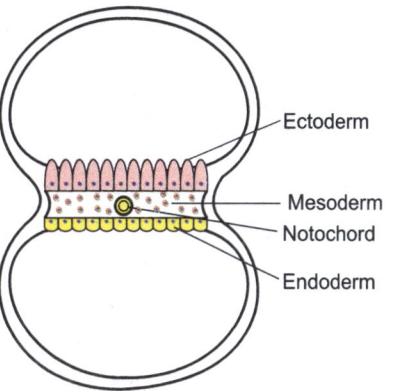

Fig. 4.31 Formation of intra embryonic mesoderm

4. **Derivatives of mesoderm:**
    A. Paraxial mesoderm
        a. Somites
            I.   Sclerotome
                  i.   Vertebrae,
                  ii.   Portions of the neurocranium and
                  iii. Axial skeleton.
            II.   Myotome: All voluntary muscles of the head, trunk and limb.
            III. Dermatome - dermis of skin over the dorsal region.
        b. Neuromeres (head mesoderm): Endosteal layer of dura mater.
    B. Intermediate cell mass or column.
        a. Connective tissue of the gonads.
        b. Mesonephric and metanephric nephrons.
        c. Smooth muscles and connective tissues of the reproductive system.
    C. Lateral plate or column
        a. Septum transversum
            I.   Epicardium,
            II.   Fibrous pericardium,
            III. The diaphragm,
            IV.   Oesophageal mesentery,
            V.   Sinusoids of liver and
            VI.   Falciform ligament.
        b. Splanchnopleuric layer
            I.   Smooth muscle and connective tissues of the intestinal tract and associated glands.
            II.   Smooth muscles and connective tissues of respiratory tract and associated glands.
        c. Somatopleuric layer
            I.   Appendicular skeleton,

II. Connective tissue of limbs and trunks including cartilage, ligament and tendons.
III. Dermis of the ventral part of the body and limbs.
IV. Mesenchyme of external genitalia.
d. Angiogenic mesoderm
I. Endocardium of the heart.
II. Endothelium of the blood and lymphatic vessels.

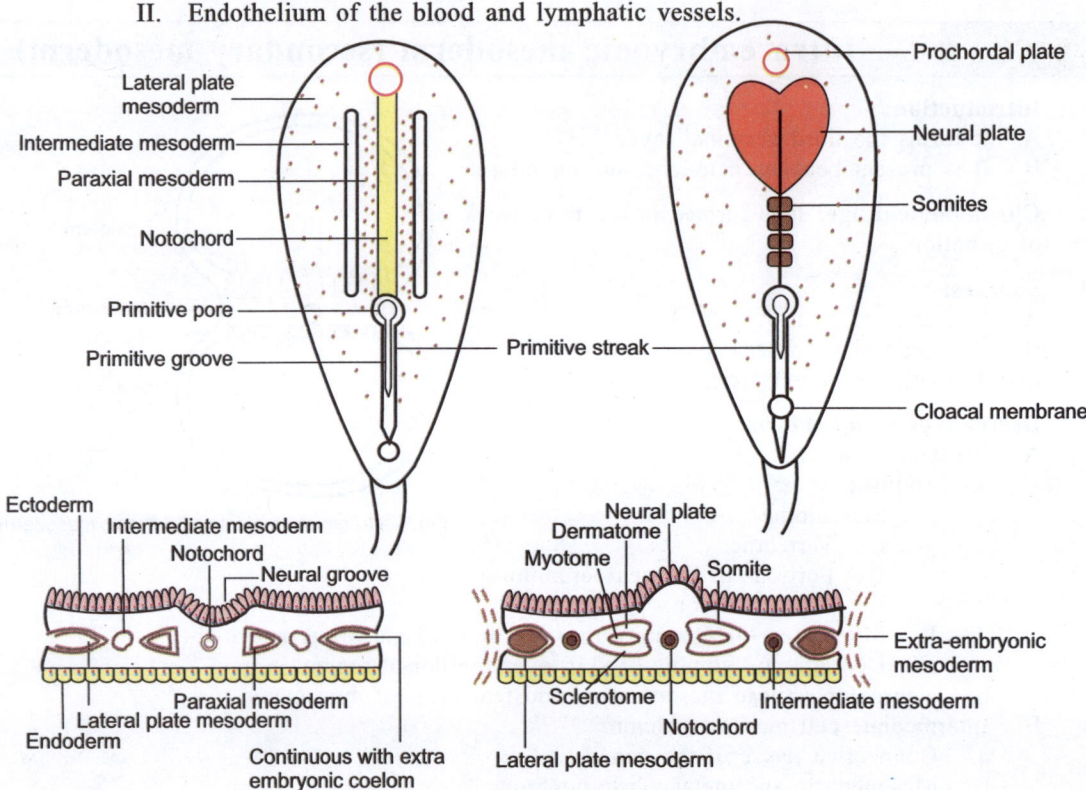

Fig. 4.32 Fate of intra embryonic mesoderm

SN-19 Allantois

1. **Introduction:** It is the diverticulum developing from the hind gut of the foetus.

2. **Evolution:** In ungulates and certain mammals allantois is large and is filled with fluid. In animals it act as a reservoir of the excretory products of urinary system. It is vestigial in man.

3. **Formation:** Before the formation of tail fold, a small endodermal diverticulum arises from the yolk sac near the caudal end of the embryonic disc. This diverticulum grows into the mesoderm of the connecting stalk. After the formation of the tail fold, part of this endoderm is absorbed into the hind gut. It now passes from the ventral side of the hind gut into the connecting stalk. The developing bladder is continuous with the allantois. The

allantois atrophies and is seen in post natal life as a fibrous band termed as urachus. The urachus extends from the apex of the bladder to the umbilicus as median umbilical ligament.

4. **Anomalies:**
    A. Patent urachus: Urachus may remain patent and urine may pass through the umbilicus.
    B. Urachal cyst: It results from partial persistence of the intraembryonic allantois. The secretory activity of the linings of allantois produces the dilatation (cyst).
    C. Urachal sinus: The persistence of the allantoic lumen in the lower part causes urachal sinus. The sinus is usually continuous with the urinary bladder.
    D. Urachal fistula: An abnormal passage resulting from a patent urachus communicating with the umbilicus and urinary bladder.

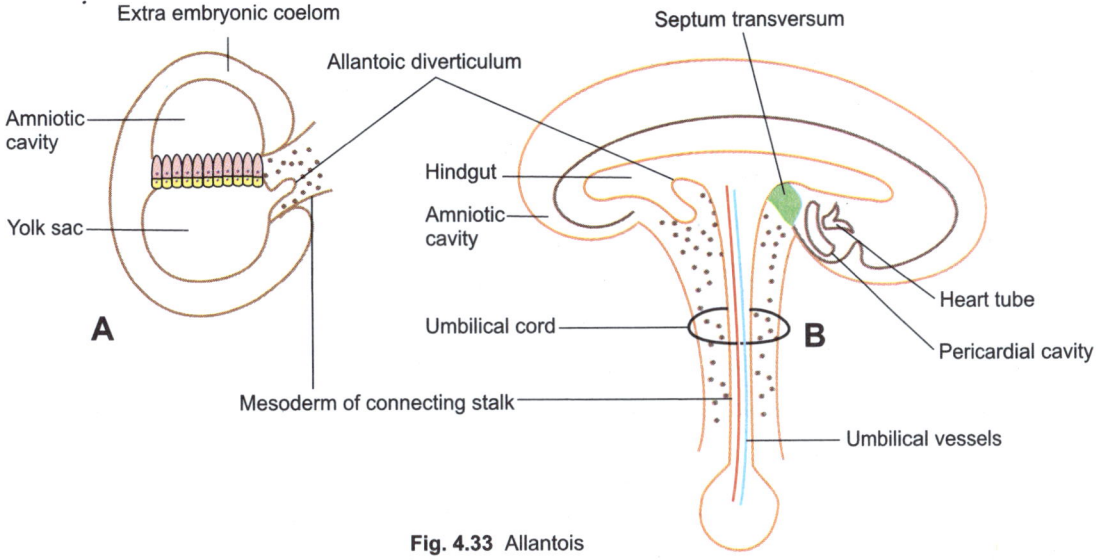

Fig. 4.33 Allantois

| SN-20 | **Trophoblast** |

Introduction: The cells lining the surface of the morula constitute the trophoblast

The trophoblast has a property of attaching itself to, and invading any tissue it comes in contact with. Once the zona pellucida disappears the cells of the trophoblast stick to the uterine endometrium. This is called implantation.

Villi are formed as offshoots from the surface of the trophoblast. As the trophoblast along with the underlying extra embryonic mesoderm constitutes the chorion, the villi arising form it are called chorionic villi.

The trophoblast is at first made up of a single layer of cells. As these cells multiply, two distinct layers are formed.

The cells that are nearest to the decidua (most superficial cells) loose their cell boundaries. Thus a continuous sheet of cytoplasm containing many nuclei is formed. Such a tissue is called a syncytium. Hence this layer of trophoblast is called syncytiotrophoblast or plasmodio trophoblast.

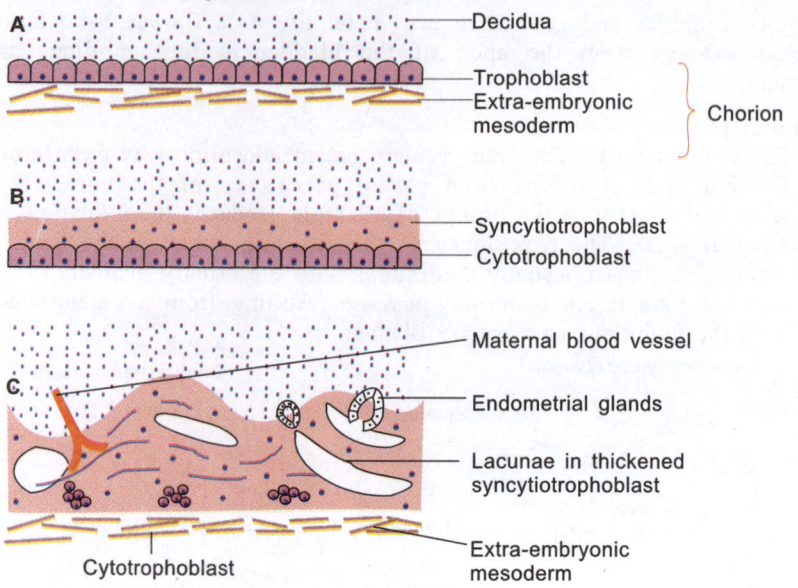

Fig. 4.34 Stages in the formation of chorionic villi.

Deep to the syncytium the cells of the trophoblast retain their cellwalls and form the second layer called cytotrophoblast [Langhan's layer].

SN-21	**Placenta**

1. **Introduction:** The placenta is an important foetal membrane. It acts as a temporary endocrine gland and maintains the pregnancy after first trimester.
   The placenta is a structure by which foetus is attached to mother and it gives nutrition to the embryo (or fetus) and excretes waste products from foetus to mother.

2. **Formation:** The placenta is formed from both fetal and maternal sources. Foetal source is chorion frondosum and maternal source is decidua basalis.
   A. Formation of chorion frondosum: It follows the following stages
      a. Primary stem villi: By the beginning of the third week, a cytotrophoblastic core is covered by a syncytiotrophoblastic layer and thus forms primary stem villi.
      b. Secondary stem villi: Mesodermal core penetrates the primary stem villi and thus forms secondary stem villi.
      c. Tertiary stem villi: The blood vessels appear in the mesoderm of secondary villi to form tertiary villi. These vessels establish contact with intra embryonic circulatory system.
      d. Cytotrophoblastic shell: The cytotrophoblast emerges through the syncytium of each villus until they reach the maternal decidua where it spreads out to form a layer. Thus the shell is formed. The cytotrophoblastic shell gradually surrounds the syncytiotrophoblast entirely and attaches the chorionic sac firmly to maternal endometrial tissue.

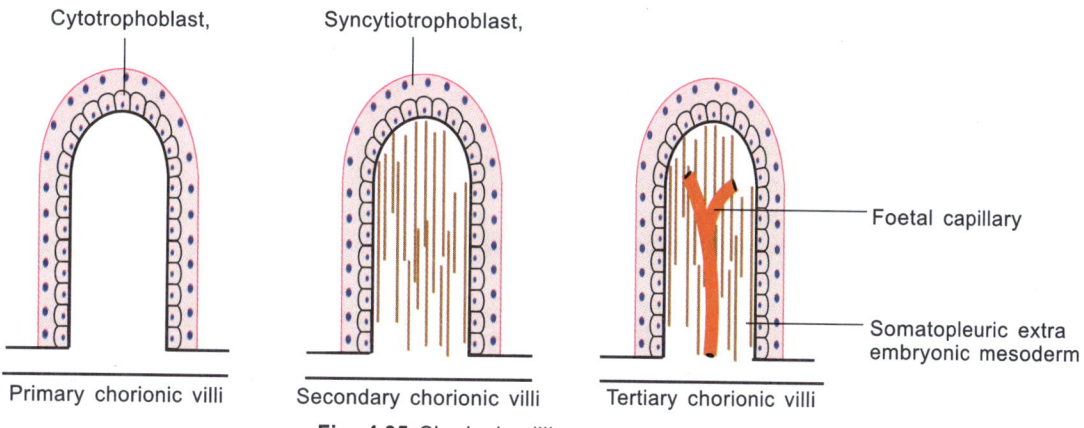

Fig. 4.35 Chorionic villi

e. Between the villi: Numerous intervillous spaces are formed. The villi on the embryonic pole continue to grow and expand and thus give rise to chorion frondosum. (The villi on the abembryonic pole degenerate and are called chorion laeve).

B. Decidua basalis: The decidua over the chorion frondosum is called decidua basalis. Chorion frondosum and decidua basalis together form the placenta.

C. The placenta becomes subdivided into a number of lobes by septa that grow into the intervillous spaces from the maternal side. Each of such lobe of placenta is often called as a maternal cotyledon. If the placenta is viewed from the maternal side, the bases of the septa are seen as grooves, while the cotyledons appear as convex areas bounded by the grooves.

Each lobe contains the number of anchoring villi and their branches. One such villi and its branches constitute fetal cotyledon. The placenta then forms a compact mass. Structures found in the cut section of placenta are

a. Amnion
b. Chorion
c. Chorio-decidual space
d. Cotyledons
e. Decidua

3. **Attachment:** The placenta is attached mostly in the upper part of the posterior wall of the uterus.

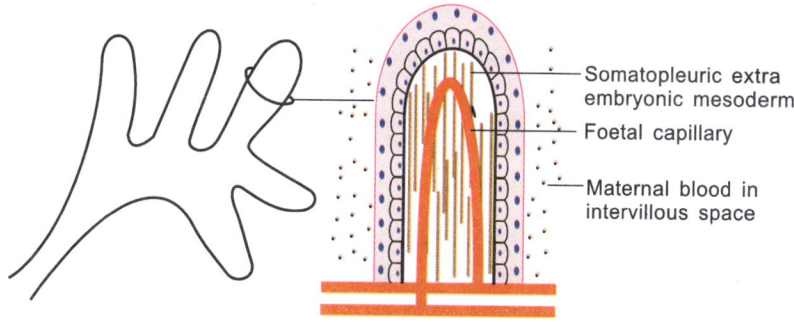

Fig. 4.36 Fundamental structure of placenta

4. **Dimensions:** At full term.
   A. Weight: 500-600 gms.
   B. Diameter: 15-25 cm.
   C. Thickness: 3 cm

5. **Functions of placenta:**
   A. It exchanges respiratory gases i.e. O_2 and CO_2 between foetal and maternal blood.
   B. It exchanges nutrients and metabolic waste products between foetus and the mother.
   C. It transfers maternal antibodies to the foetus.
   D. It transfers drug from mother to foetus.
   E. It synthesizes following hormones
      a. Human chorionic gonadotropin (HCG).
      b. Somatotropic hormone.
      c. Estrogen
      d. Estradiol.
      e. Progesterone
      f. Relaxin
   G. It detoxifies the toxic substances.
   H. It connects foetus to the mother.

6. **Types:** Placenta may be of following types
   A. According to the position of the placenta:
      a. Placenta parietalis: When placenta lies on the other walls of the uterus than the fundus.
      b. Placenta praevia.
   B. According to shape:
      a. Discoid,
      b. Bilobed,
      c. Multilobed,
      d. Circumvallate and
      e. Placenta succenturiate (*Succenturiate* substitute).
   C. According to attachment of the umbilical cord
      a. Marginal,
      b. Velamentous,
      c. Furcate and
      d. Central.

7. **Anomalies:**
   A. Hydatidiform or vesicular mole: It results from pathological overactivity of the trophoblast. It is simple, noninvasive new growth.
   B. Chorion epithelioma: It is highly malignant tumor. It results when endometrium is too resistant to blastocyst.

| SN-22 | Types of placenta depending upon shape |

1. **Lobed :** When the placenta is divided into lobes.

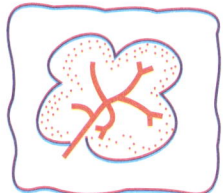

Fig. 4.37 Lobed

2. **Bidiscoidal :** It consists of the two discs.

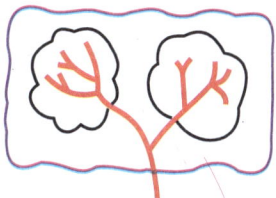

Fig. 4.38 Bidiscoidal

3. **Circumvallate :** The peripheral margin of placenta is surrounded by a sulcus and overlapped by circular fold of decidua.

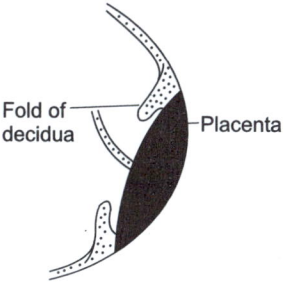

Fig. 4.39 Circumvallate

4. **Placenta succenturiate :** A small placenta is connected with main placenta by blood vessels and membranes.

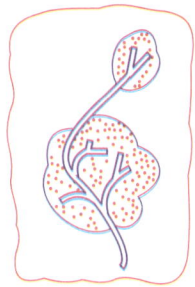

Fig. 4.40 Placenta succenturiata

| SN-23 | Types of placenta depending upon attachment |

According to attachment of the umbilical cord

1. **Marginal:** When the umbilical cord is attached close to the margin of placenta. This type of placenta is called battledore placenta. (Battledore racket used to strike the shuttle cock in play).

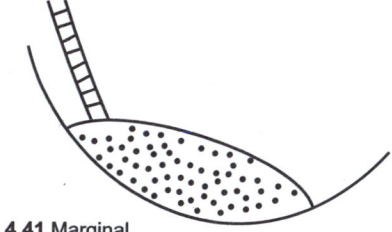

Fig. 4.41 Marginal

2. **Velamentous (membranous or veil like):** When the cord fails to reach the placenta and is attached to the fetal membrane close to the periphery of the organ.

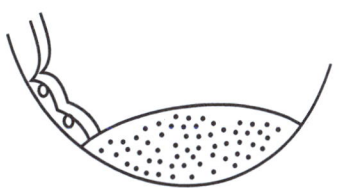

Fig. 4.42 Velamentous insertion

3. **Furcate (*furca* fork):** When the blood vessels divide before reaching the placenta.

4. **Central:** When the cord is attached nearer the centre. This is normal type.

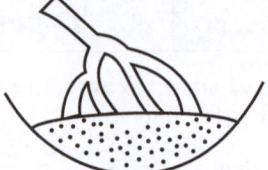

Fig. 4.43 Furcate

SAQ-3   **Placenta praevia**

1. **Introduction:** Implantation of placenta in lower uterine segment is called placenta praevia.

2. **Degrees of placenta praevia:**

   A. **First degree:** The attachment of placenta extends into lower uterine segment, but does not reach internal os.

   B. **Second degree:** The margin of the placenta reaches the internal os, but does not cover it.

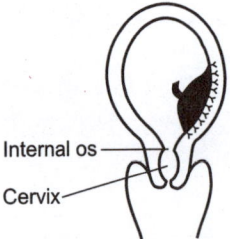

Fig. 4.44 First degree

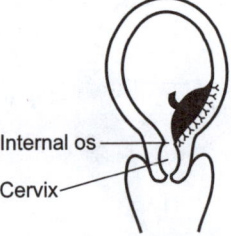

Fig. 4.45 Second degree

   C. **Third degree:** The edge of the placenta covers the internal os, but when the os dilates during child-birth, the placenta does not occlude it.

   D. **Fourth degree:** The placenta completely covers internal os and occludes the os even after it has dilated.

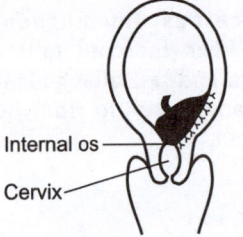

Fig. 4.46 Third degree

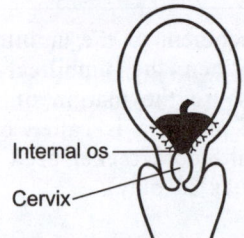

Fig. 4.47 Fourth degree

3. **Incidence:** 1:200

4. **Clinical features:** Painless haemorrhage in the last trimester particularly in the eighth month is a diagnostic feature of placenta praevia. It is common in the third and fourth degree of placenta praevia.

SN-24   Chorion

(*Chorion* skin)

1. **Introduction:** The structures which cover the conceptus is called chorion. It resembles skin. It develops from the cells of the trophoblast.

2. **Formation:** It is formed by
   A. Trophoblast
   B. Somatopleuric extraembryonic mesoderm.

3. **Villi:** Are formed as offshoots from the surface of the trophoblast. Villi arising from chorion are called chorionic villi. They grow into the surrounding decidua. They are of two types
   A. Temporary: These are related to decidua capsularis and are called chorionic laevae.
   B. Permanent: They are present in the decidua basalis and are called chorion frondosum (bearing villi). They undergo considerable development and form a disc shaped mass called placenta.

4. **Chorionic villi can be subdivided into:**
   A. Depending upon the constituent of the villi
      a. Primary chorionic villi consist of
         I. Cytotrophoblast.
         II. Syncytiotrophoblast.
      b. Secondary chorionic villi consist of
         I. Cytotrophoblast.
         II. Syncytiotrophoblast.
         III. Primary extraembryonic mesoderm.
         At the end of third week secondary villi are converted into tertiary villi.
      c. Tertiary chorionic villi consist of
         I. Cytotrophoblast.
         II. Syncytiotrophoblast.
         III. Primary extraembryonic mesoderm.
         IV. Foetal blood capillaries.
   B. According to the branching pattern the villi may be
      a. Truncus chorii: Stem
      b. Rami choric: Branches
      c. Ramuli chorii: Finer branches - Ramuli are attached to the cytotrophoblastic shell.

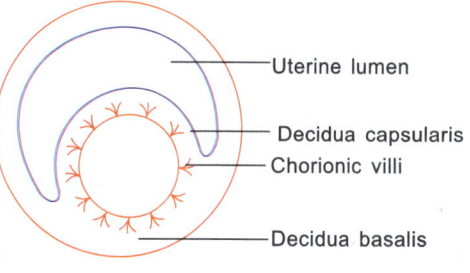

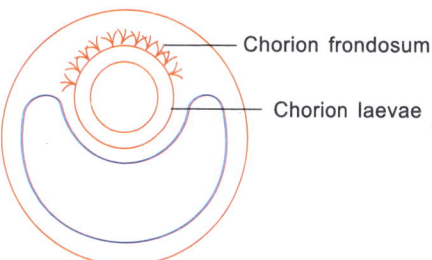

Fig. 4.48 Chorion

5. **Anomalies:**
   A. Hydatiform or vesicular mole (hydatidiform resembling hydatid cyst, hydatid a drop of water) result from pathological overactivity of the trophoblast. It is simple, non-invasive new growth. This is because of failure of vascularization of placental villi.
   Most moles are benign but 15% invade and destroy myometrium.
   Incidence 1:2000
   The diagnosis of the hydatiform mole is made by
      a. The estimation of high level of chorionic gonadotrophin hormone and
      b. Ultra sonography which reveals absence of embryo.
   Treatment: It doesn't abort spontaneously. It must be removed surgically.

B. Chorio epithelioma: It is highly malignant tumor. It results when endometrium is too resistant to blastocyst.

It consists of uncontrolled proliferation of cytotrophoblastic cells result in disorganized masses of invasive tissue. There is rapid metastasis to many other organs, including the lungs and brain.

SN-25   The maternal-foetal barrier

1. **The maternal-foetal barrier consists** of several structures separating maternal and foetal blood. The structures forming placental barrier are:
   A. Maternal erythrocyte membrane,
   B. Maternal blood,
   C. Syncytiotrophoblast,
   D. Cytotrophoblast,
   E. Cytotrophoblast basement membrane,
   F. Villous connective tissue,
   G. Foetal capillary basement membrane,
   H. Foetal capillary endothelium,
   I. Foetal blood and
   J. Foetal erythrocyte membrane.

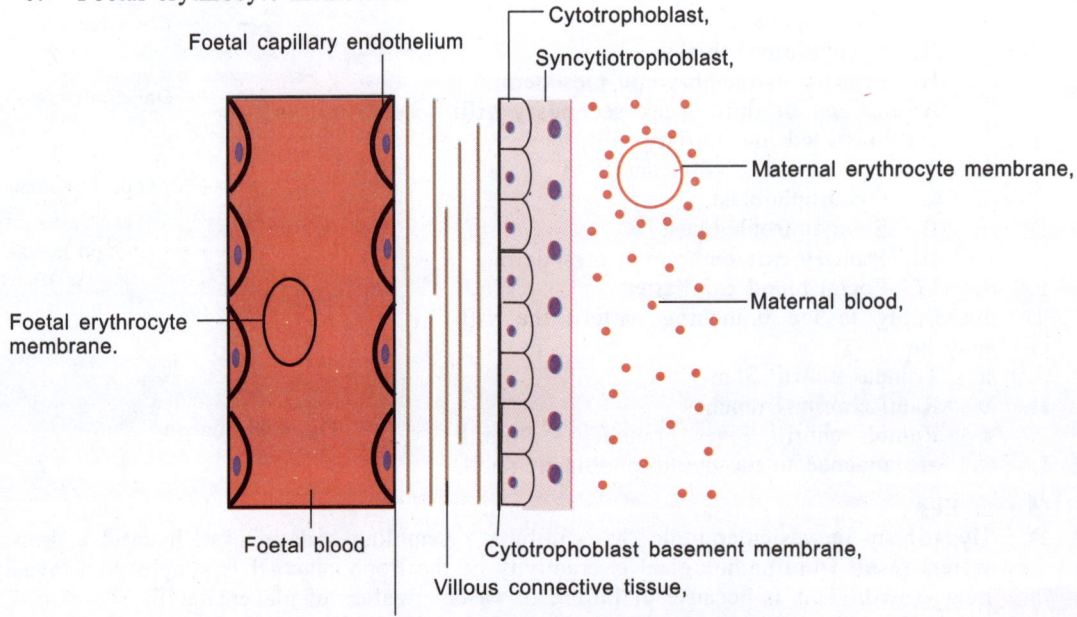

Fig. 4.49 Structures forming placental barrier

2. As the placenta grows, the nature of the barrier between maternal and fetal blood also changes.
   This barrier becomes reduced in several different ways:

A. The cytotrophoblast, by continuously dividing and fusing to form the syncytiotrophoblast, in effect proliferates itself out of existence, so that it is no longer present as a barrier to diffusion.

B. The connective tissue stroma becomes more spongy.

C. The foetal blood vessels migrate from the center of villi toward the periphery, displacing intervening connective tissue elements.

3. **The end result** of these changes is a barrier between fetal and maternal blood that is often only a micrometer or less in thickness.

4. **Applied anatomy:**
   A. Immunity from mother to foetus.
   B. Protection of foetus from syphilis in first trimester.

SN-26   Coelomic wall epithelium

1. **Introduction:** Walls of intraembryonic coelom.

2. **Derivative of coelomic wall epithelium:**
   A. Primitive pericardium: Myocardium, parietal pericardium.
   B. Pericardio peritoneal canals: Visceral, parietal and mediastinal, pleuro-peritoneal membrane contributing to diaphragm.

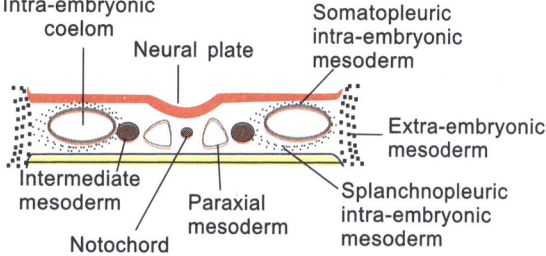

Fig. 4.50 Coelomic wall epithelium

   C. Splanchnopleuric epithelium: Visceral peritoneum of stomach, peritoneum of lesser and greater omenta, falciform ligament, lienorenal and gastrosplenic ligaments.
   D. Somatopleuric epithelium: Parietal peritoneum.
   E. Primitive peritoneal cavity.
   F. Spanchnopleuric epithelium: Visceral peritoneal covering of mid and hind gut, the mesentery, transverse and sigmoid mesocolon.
   G. Pronephros: Epithelial lining of mesonephric ducts, ductus deferens, epididymis, seminal vesicles, ejaculatory duct, ureters and vesical trigone.
   H. Mullerian ducts: Epithelial lining of uterine tubes, body and cervix of uterus, vagina, broad ligament of uterus.
   I. Germinal epithelium of gonad .
   J. Germinal epithelium forming cortex of adrenal gland.
   K. Somatopleuric epithelium: Parietal peritoneum, tunica vaginalis of testis.

SAQ-4   Surface ectoderm epithelium

1. **Introduction:** It is the epithelium lining the ectoderm.

2. **Derivatives:**
   A. Ectodermal placodes and
   B. Adenohypophysis.
   C. Cranial sensory ganglia of nerves V, VII, IX and X.

D. Olfactory receptor cells and olfactory epithelium.
E. Epithelial walls of the membranous labyrinth, organ of Corti.
F. Lens of the eye.
G. Enamel of the teeth.
H. Cranial structures
I. Secretory and duct lining cells of the lacrimal, nasal labial, palatine, oral and salivary glands.
J. Epithelia of the cornea and conjuctiva.
K. Epithelial lining of the external acoustic meatus and external epithelium of the tympanic membrane.
L. Epithelial lining of the paranasal sinuses, lips, cheeks, gums and palate.

SAQ-5 Septum transversum

1. **Introduction:** It is unsplit part of lateral plate mesoderm cranial to the prochordal plate and intraembryonic coelom.

2. **Derivatives of septum transversum:**
   A. Epicardium, fibrous pericardium,
   B. Portion of diaphragm,
   C. Oesophageal mesentery and
   D. Sinusoids of liver, tissue within lesser omentum and falciform ligament.

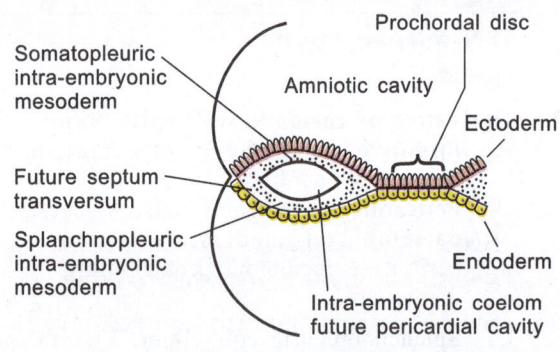

Fig. 4.51 Surface ectoderm epithelium

SN-27 Neural crest

1. **Introduction:** It is ectoderm present at the junction of neural tube & rest of the ectoderm.

2. **Neural derivatives:**
   A. Sensory neurons of the cranial ganglia V, VII, VIII XI and X.
   B. Sensory neurons of the spinal dorsal root ganglia and their peripheral sensory receptors.
   C. Satellite cells in all sensory ganglia.
   D. Sympathetic ganglia and plexuses: Neurons and satellite cells.
   E. Parasympathetic ganglia and plexuses: Neurons and satellite cells.
   F. Enteric plexuses: Neurons and glial cells.
   G. Schwann cells of all the peripheral nerves.
   H. Medulla of the adrenal gland, chromaffin cells.
   I. Carotid body type I cells (type II, satellite type cells).
   J. Calcitonin: Producing (C - cells)
   K. Melanocytes.
   L. Odontoblast.
   M. Leptomeninges.
   N. Head mesoderm etc.

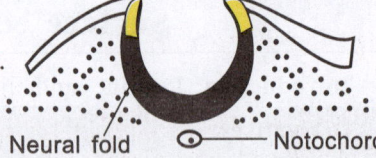

Fig. 4.52 Neural crest

GENERAL ANATOMY

SECTION FIVE

SN-1	Long bone	243
SAQ-1	Short bone	243
SN-2	Pneumatic bone	244
SN-3	Sesamoid bone	244
SAQ-2	Growing end	245
SAQ-3	Primary centre	246
SAQ-4	Secondary centre	246
SN-4	Metaphysis	246
SN-5	Diaphysis	247
SN-6	Epiphysis	247
SN-7	Blood supply of the long bone	248
SN-8	Suture	250
SN-9	Syndesmoses	251
SN-10	Primary cartilaginous joint	252
SN-11	Secondary cartilaginous joint	252
SN-12	Pivot joint	253
SN-13	Typical synovial joint	253
SN-14	Prime movers	255
SN-15	Antagonist	256
SN-16	Synergist	256
SN-17	Fixators	257
SN-18	Bursa	257
SN-19	Anastomosis	258
SN-20	End arteries	258

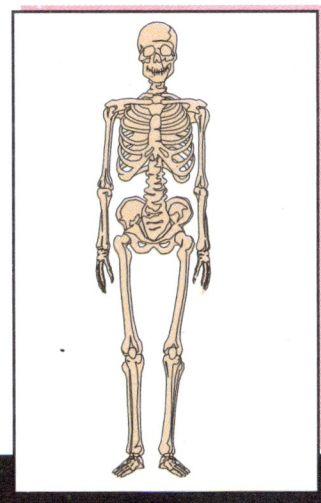

SN-1   Long bones

1. They are placed vertically in the body.

2. They have shaft with 2 expanded ends.

3. Their length is more than breadth.

4. They have three surfaces and three borders.

5. They contain medullary cavity.

6. They have one diaphysis and at least 2 epiphysis.

7. They develop in cartilage.

8. They act as lever for muscles.

9. They transmit weight, from axial to appendicular skeleton.
   - A. Typical long bones: Humerus, radius, ulna, femur, tibia, and fibula.
   - B. Modified long bone: Some of the characters of typical long bones are modified namely
     - I. It does not have medullary cavity
     - II. It ossifies in membrane
     - III. It transmits the weight from appendicular skeleton to axial skeleton.
       e.g. - Clavicle
   - C. Miniature long bones (mockery of long bone) Long bones are smaller in dimensions and have only one epiphysis e.g.
     - a. Metacarpals,
     - b. Metatarsals and
     - c. Phalanges.

SAQ-1   Short bones

1. **Introduction:** The bones which are not long, which are cubical in shape and present six surfaces are called short bones.

2. **Features:** Out of the six surfaces 4 are articular and remaining 2 are non-articular.
   Articular surfaces give attachment to muscles and ligaments.
   They are pierced by blood vessels.

3. **Examples:**
   - A. Carpal bones: She look too pretty, try to catch her.
     - a. Scaphoid,
     - b. Lunate,
     - c. Triquetral,
     - d. Pisiform,
     - e. Trapezium,
     - f. Trapezoid,
     - g. Capitate and
     - h. Hamate.
   - B. Tarsal bones:
     - a. Calcaneus,

    b.   Talus,

    c.   Cuboid,

    d.   Navicular &

    e.   Cuneiform.

4. Ossification:

    A.   They ossify in cartilage.

    B.   They ossify after birth except talus, calcaneus and cuboid which ossifies in intra uterine life.

SN-2   Pneumatic bone

(*Pneuma* air)

1   Introduction: Bones have outer and inner table and are lined by mucoperiosteum and contain air.

2   Site: Cranium (bones of facial skeleton. surrounding the nasal cavity.)
e.g. maxilla, frontal, ethmoid and sphenoid.

3.   Functions:

    A.   They act as air conditioning chamber. They change humidity and temperature of the inspired air and makes the air free from foreign particles.

    B.   They improves timber (quality) of the voice.

    C.   They provide insulation.

    D.   They reduce the weight (200 - 300 gms.)

    E.   They act as resonance (prolongation and intensification of sound) of the voice

4.   Development:

    A.   They develop in membrane due to differential growth of two tables.

    B.   Inner table breaks up and penetrates into neighboring mucosa and forms the pneumatic bone.

SN-3   Sesamoid bone

1.   Nomenclature: (Arabic term) sesame - seed like, oid - resemblance.

2.   Introduction: Oval shaped nodules, a few millimeters in diameter varying in shape and size which develop in tendons or and joint capsule.

3.   Evolution: Phylogenetically part of skeleton.

4.   Formation: Separate cartilaginous centres in certain tendons

5.   Structure: Fibrous tissue, cartilage or bone which develops in tendon.

6.   Ossification: They ossify in second decade except patella which ossifies in the first decade.

7.   Characters:

    A.   No Primary centre.

    B.   No periosteum.

    C.   No Haversian system.

D. It is related to articular or non - articular bony surface.
E. It is covered with hyaline cartilage.
F. It is lubricated by bursa or synovial fluid.

8. **Functions:** The exact function is not definitely known. However the following functions are attributed.   SESAMOID
    A. **S**erves as a mechanical advantage to the tendon.
    B. **E**nsures the prevention of wear and tear of the tendon.
    C. **S**tabilises the local circulation.
    D. **A**lters the direction of pull of the muscle.
    E. **M**aintains the local circulation.
    F. **O**vercomes the pressure.
    G. **I**nsures the vessels and nerves.
    H. **D**iminishes the friction.

9. **Site:** Following are the sesamoid bones related to tendons

Tendon		Bone	
A.	Quadriceps femoris	a.	Patella
B.	Flexor carpi ulnaris	b.	Pisiform
C.	Gastrocnemius (lateral head) (articular sesamoid bone)	c.	Fabella (beans)
D.	Adductor longus	d.	Riders bone

Table 5.1 Showing sesamoid bones related tendons

10. **Applied anatomy:**
    A. Failure of ossification is mistaken for fracture of bone e.g. patella.
    B. Stress fracture occurs in ballet dancers and long distance runners.

SAQ-2	Growing end

The active end of the long bone is called growing end. It appears first and fuses last.
e.g. All long bone except fibula.
The growing end is opposite to the direction of nutrient foramen. The direction of nutrient foramen is decided by jiggle.
"Towards the elbow I go, and away from the knee I flee".
The following table shows the growing end of different long bones.

Table 5.2 Showing the direction of nutrient foramen and growing end of long bones.

Bone	Direction of nutrient foramen	Growing end
Humerus	Lower end	Upper end
Radius, ulna	Upper end	Lower end
Femur	Upper end	Lower end
Tibia, fibula	Lower end	Upper end

Applied anatomy: The knowledge of growing end is important in keeping additional space for the growth of the bone especially in young person.

SAQ-3 Primary centre

1. **Introduction:** It is the centre from which the main part of the bone ossifies.

2. **Appearance:** The primary centre appears before birth.

3. **Examples:**
   A. Shaft of all long bones and
   B. Short bones like talus, calcaneus and cuboid.

4. **Exception:** Carpal and tarsal bones, the centre for which appears after birth.

SAQ-4 Secondary centre

1. **Introduction:** Centre which appears after birth

2. **Example:** Ends of all long bones.
   A. Greater tronchanter of femur.
   B. Greater tubercle of humerus.

3. **Exception:**
   A. Lower end of femur and
   B. Upper end of tibia, the centre for these bones appear at birth.

4. **Applied anatomy:** Presence of secondary centre at lower end of femur or upper end of tibia confirms viability. Absence of secondary centre does not exclude viability.

SN-4 Metaphysis

(*Meta* end, *physis* growth)

1. **Introduction:** It is the epiphyseal end of diaphysis. It is the peripheral part of the shaft which is in contact with epiphyseal plate of cartilage.

2. **Characters:**
   A. It is most active part of bone.
   B. It is most vascular part of bone, flooded in the lake of blood.
   C. It is the site of attachment of tendons, and ligaments.
   D. It is the site of maximum pull, stress, strain and tension.

3. **Blood supply:** It is by following arteries
   A. Nutrient artery,
   B. Periosteal artery and
   C. Juxta epiphyseal artery.

4. **Applied anatomy:**
   A. Site of osteomyelitis
   B. Medicolegal importance.
      e.g. Lower end of femur, upper end of tibia
      Note: Presence of centre at the lower end of femur confirms viability and absence of centre not exclude viability.

C. Infection of long bone primarily affects metaphysis because nutrient arteries form hair pin bend and may get blocked by thrombus and undergoes necrosis.

D. Since muscles, ligaments and joint capsules are attached close to metaphysis. This is likely to be damaged by sheering strain of the muscle.

SN-5   Diaphysis

(*Dia* in between, *physis* growth)

1. **Introduction:** It is the part of long bone present between two growing ends. It develops from one primary center and forms the shaft of long bone.

2. **Blood supply:** Is mainly by nutrient artery - (branch of regional artery) Direction of nutrient artery is opposite the direction of growing end.

3. **Structure:** It is described as-
   A. Outer: It is compact and strong.
   B. Inner: It is spongy and site of erythropoiesis.

4. **Growth:**
   A. Height by interstitial growth.
   B. Thickness by appositional growth.

5. **Applied anatomy:** Infection of the bone causes osteomyelitis.

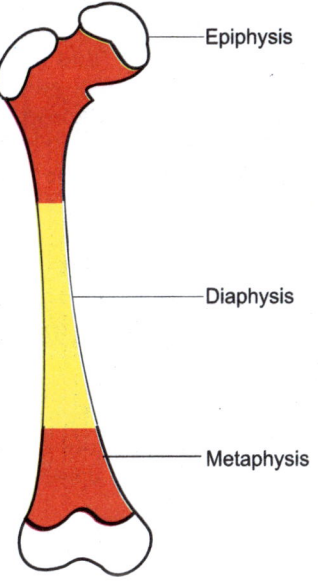

Fig. 5.1 Parts of a young long bone.

SN-6   Epiphysis

(*Epi* above, *physis* growth)

1. **Introduction:** Part of bone which develops from secondary centre. Secondary centre is one which develops after birth.

2. **Number:** The number of epiphysis is more than one except metacarpal, metatarsal and phalanges.

3. **Classification:**
   A. Based on number of epiphysis (structurally).
      a. Simple: Ends of long bone fuses independently with shaft e.g. femur.
      b. Compound: Ends of bone develop from many centers and these centers unite to form a single epiphysis which subsequently fuses with shaft.
         e.g. head of humerus.
   B. Based on functions
      a. Pressure epiphysis

Characters:

I. Takes part in weight transmission and articulation

II. The centre of ossification in bones of pressure epiphysis appears earlier than the centre of ossification occurring in traction epiphysis
e.g. head of femur, medial end of clavicle

b. Traction epiphysis
   I. Does not transmit weight
   II. Does not take part in articulation
   III. e.g. greater trochanter

c. Atavistic (grand father) epiphysis: In the early part of evolution, such part of the bone were separate bones but they were deriving nutrition from the neighboring bone and later they fuse with host bone and forms part of the bone.
   I. Coracoid process of scapula
   II. Os trigonum: Triangular bone at the back of talus, sometimes it occurs as independent bone.

d. Aberrent epiphysis (wandering): It is not always present.
   e.g. The metacarpals have only one epiphysis. The epiphysis of the first m etacarpal is at head and the epiphyses of the other metacarpals appear at the base. Such epiphysis is called aberrent epiphysis.

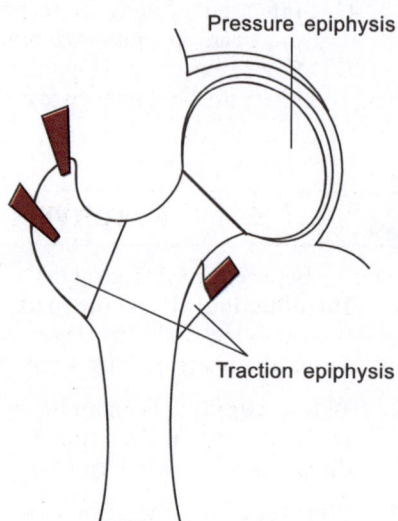

Fig. 5.2 Pressure & traction epiphysis

4. **Applied anatomy:**
   A. The head of the femur receives blood supply from the epiphyseal artery, which pierces the epiphyseal cartilage. In case of separation of epiphyseal plate, from the neck of femur, there is a necrosis of head due to loss of blood supply.
   B. The artery supplying the upper end of the tibia do not pierce the epiphyseal plate. Hence separation of the upper end will not result in loss of blood supply in the upper end.

SN-7   Blood supply of the long bone

The blood supply of long bone is by following arteries:

1. **Nutrient artery:** It is a branch of regional artery.
   Its direction is away from growing end.
   The direction of the nutrient foramen is decided by the jiggle.

Table 5.3 Showing direction of the nutrient foramen and growing end of long bone

Bone	Direction of nutrient foramen	Growing end
Humerus	Lower end	Upper end
Radius, ulna	Upper end	Lower end
Femur	Upper end	Lower end
Tibia, fibula	Lower end	Upper end

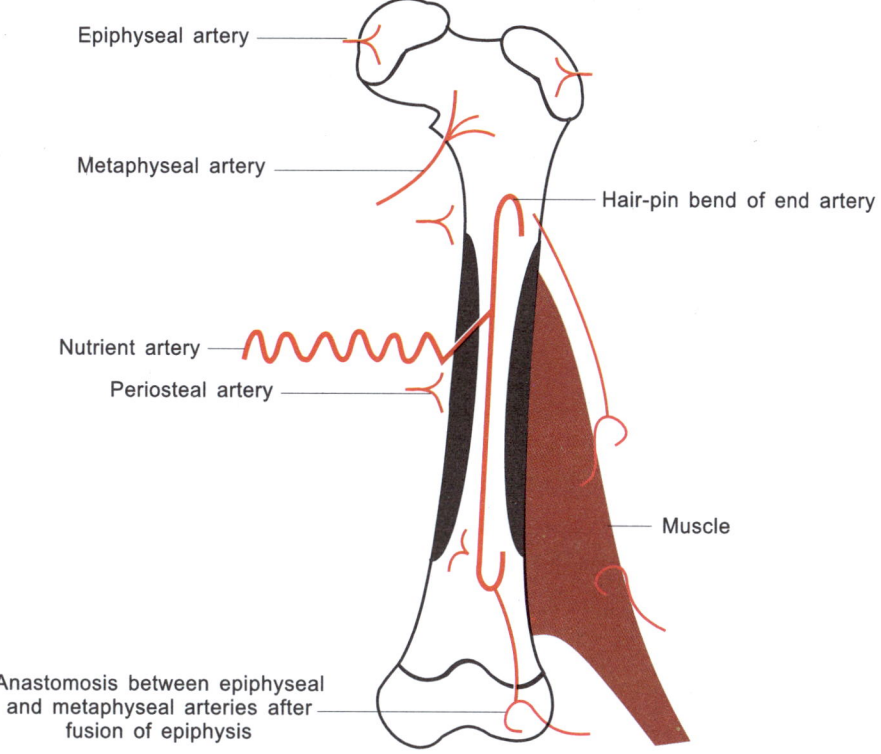

Epiphyseal artery

Metaphyseal artery

Hair-pin bend of end artery

Nutrient artery

Periosteal artery

Muscle

Anastomosis between epiphyseal and metaphyseal arteries after fusion of epiphysis

Fig. 5.3 Blood supply of long bone

A. Peculiarities: It is tortuous before it enters the nutrient foramen for following reason:
   a. For the uniform distribution of blood and
   b. To avoid rupture during contraction and relaxation of the muscle.
B. Number: It is usually one except in femur which has two nutrient foramina which transmits arteries.
C. Course:
   a. It enters the compact bone through nutrient foramen situated in the middle of shaft.
   b. It divides into ascending and descending branches in to the medullary cavity.
   c. Each ascending or descending branch divides into many small branches which turns down to form a hair pin loop.
D. It anastomoses with:
   a. Periosteal artery
   b. Metaphyseal artery and
   c. Epiphyseal artery.
E. Distribution: It supplies
   a. The inner 2/3rd of compact bone,
   b. The spongy bone &
   c. Haversian system of less than 2 mm diameter.

2. **Metaphyseal artery:**
    A. Arises from anastomosing arteries around joint.
    B. Enters metaphysis through joint capsule.

3. **Epiphyseal artery:** Divides into two types - depending upon mode of blood supply.

Table 5.4 Showing the course of the epiphyseal artery at the upper end of femur and tibia

Particulars	Articular cartilage and epiphyseal cartilage are continuous	Articular cartilage and epiphyseal cartilage are not continuous
A. Mode of distribution	Supplies epiphysis after piercing the epiphyseal cartilage	Supplies epiphysis without piercing epiphyseal cartilage.
B. Example	Upper end of femur	Upper end of tibia.
C. Applied	Artery is vulnerable for injury in epiphyseal separation. It produces avascular necrosis in epiphyseal separation.	Artery is not vulnerable for injury in epiphyseal separation. No vascular necrosis.

4. **Periosteal artery:** It enters bone through Volkman's canal and supplies Haversian system in outer one third of the compact bone.

5. **Muscular artery:** It is a branch of muscular artery supplying adjacent muscles.

6. **Endosteal artery:** It supplies the inner surface of the bone.

7. **Applied anatomy:**
   A. Osteomyelitis: The small emboli blocks the nutrient arteries at the site of hairpin bend. The distal part of the bone results into avascular necrosis. This condition is called osteomyelities.
   B. Shaft of long bone is affected in congenital syphilis.

SN-8	**Suture**

(*Suture* stitch, seam)

1. **Introduction:** Joints of skull are connected by   fibrous tissue.

2. **Movement:** Slight or no movement.

3. **Types:** Depending upon articular margin they are subdivided into
   A. Plane: Margins are straight e.g.
      a. Interpalatine,
      b. Intermaxillary,
      c. Palatomaxillary.

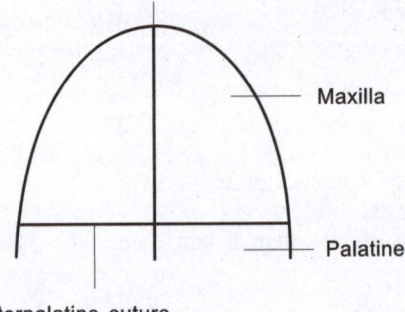

Fig. 5.4 Suture

B. Serrate (saw): Margins are wavy (saw like) e.g.
   a. Sagittal suture,
   b. Coronal suture.
C. Denticulate: The articulating margins resemble teeth. The tips are border than the roots to have effective inter locking e.g. lambdoid suture (suture between parietal and occipital bone)
D. Squamous: The articulating margins are bevelled e.g. Temporoparietal
E. Schindylesis (splinting = piece of wood): The ridged bone fits into a groove e.g.
   Rostrum of sphenoid overlapped by ala of vomer.

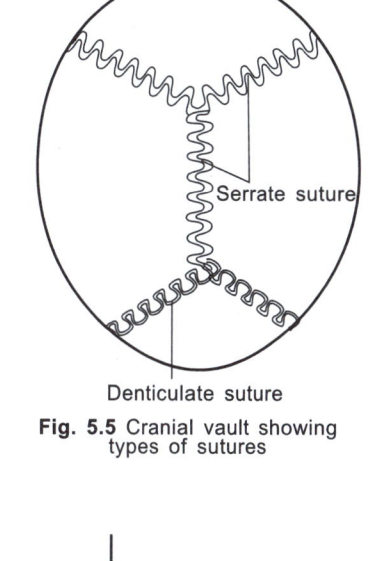

Fig. 5.5 Cranial vault showing types of sutures

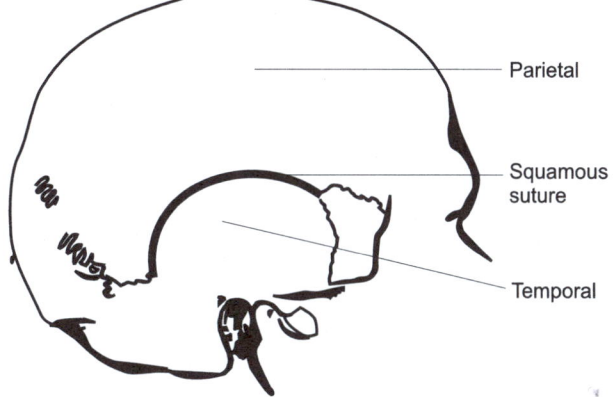

Fig. 5.6 Squamous suture

Fig. 5.7 Schindylesis (Wedge and groove suture)

F. Limbus (border) borders are mutually ridged or serrated.

4. **Age changes:**
   A. Ossification of sutural membrane starts at the age of 20 years and is slow.
   B. Ossification completes at late twenties.

SN-9   Syndesmoses

(*Syn* fusion, *desmos* band)
1. **Introduction:** Bony surfaces are joined together by interosseus membrane or ligament.

2. **Characters:**
   A. It is a type of fibrous joint.
   B. The bones are kept together at a distance by interosseus membrane.
   C. The interosseus membrane persist throughout life.

3. **Movement:** Slight degree of movement is possible. e.g. 🔑 **IMP**
   A. **I**nferior tibiofibular joint,
   B. **M**iddle radioulnar joint and
   C. **P**osterior sacroiliac joint.

SN-10   Primary cartilaginous joint (Synchondrosis)

1. **Characters:**
   A. The articulating surfaces are covered by a hyaline cartilage.
   B. They are immovable and strong.
   C. They are temporary in nature.
   D. cartilaginous plate is replaced by bone synostosis.

2. **Example:** 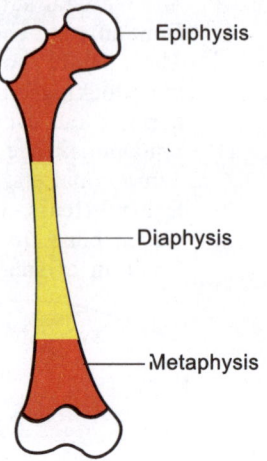 First, Second, Third & fourth letter in alphabet.
   A. **F**irst condrosternal joint.
   B. **S**pheno-occipital.
   C. **C**osto-chondral.
   D. **D**iaphysis and epiphysis of long bone.
   E. **S**terno - xiphisternal.

Fig. 5.8 **Parts of a young long bone.**

SN-11   Secondary cartilaginous joint (Symphysis)

1. **Introduction:** The articulating surfaces of bones are covered by hyaline cartilage and separated by a fibrocartilage.

2. **Characters:** The thickness of fibro cartilage is Directly related to range of movements.

3. **Site:** All midline joints of body except.
   A. Symphysis menti (atypical and temporary).
   B. Joint between sternum and xiphoid.

4. **Fate:** Limited movement is possible.

5. **Duration:** Persists throughout life.

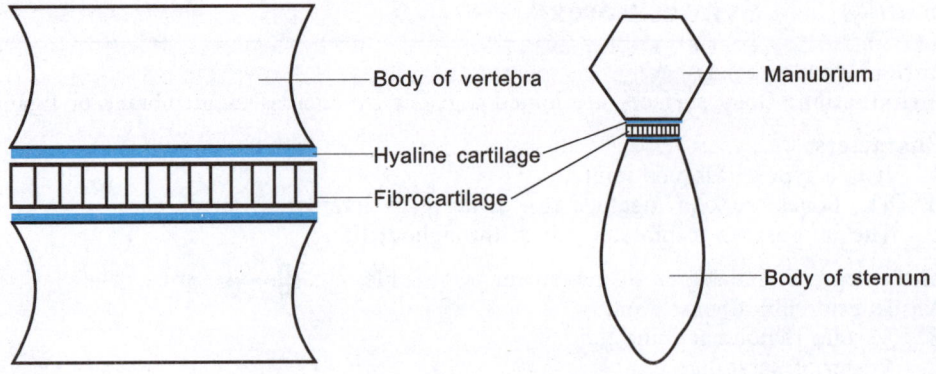

Fig. 5.9 Examples of secondary cartilaginous joint

6. **Example:** 🔑 **IMP**
   A. **I**ntervertebral joint.
   B. **M**anubrio sternal.
   C. **P**ubic symphysis.
   D. Sacral joint.

SN-12   Pivot joint

(*Pivot* a pin on which anything turns)
Introduction: It is an uniaxial (transverse axis) synovial joint.

Table 5.5 Showing comparison of superior and inferior radioulnar joint with median atlantoaxial joint

Joint	Superior and inferior radio ulnar joint	Median atlantoaxial joint
Bones	Radius and ulna.	Atlas and axis vertebra.
Articulating surfaces	Head of radius and radial notch on ulna.	Posterior surface of body of atlas and anterior surface of odontoid process of axis.
Axis (vertical)	Radius.	Odontoid process of axis vertebra.
Ring A. Formation	Annular ligament.	Posterior arch of atlas.
B. Structure	Bone and fibrous tissue.	Bone.
Mechanism during movement Ring	Fixed.	Moving.
Axis	Moving.	Fixed.
Movement	Supination, pronation.	Side to side movement (no movement).
Range of movement	More.	Less.
Applied	In children subluxation of superior radio ulnar joint is common.	Death in hanging is due to rupture of transverse ligament of atlantoaxial joint.

SN-13   Typical synovial joint

1. **Introduction:** The joints with free movement where bones are not directly connected by any tissue are called synovial joint.

2. **Characters:** Synovial joints are characterized by six features.
   A. Articular cartilage: Articular surfaces are covered by a layer of hyaline cartilage which is devoid of pericondrium.

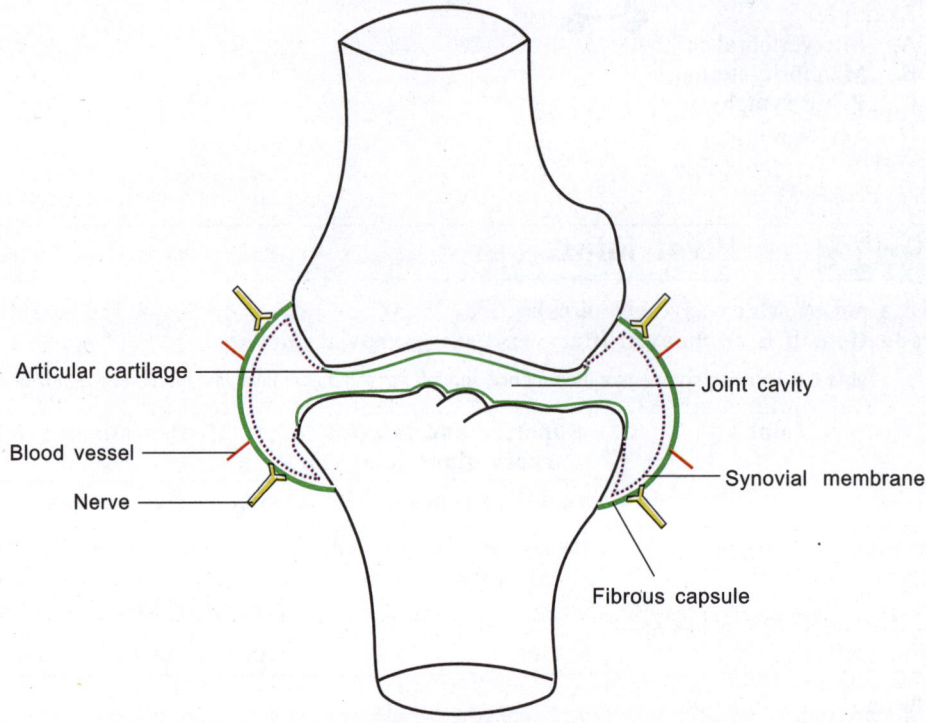

Articular cartilage

Joint cavity

Blood vessel

Synovial membrane

Nerve

Fibrous capsule

Fig. 5.10 Structure of a synovial joint

B. Fibrous capsule:
  a. It consists of longitudinal and interlacing bundles of white connective tissue fibers. It is attached to articulating ends of the bones and forms as a cuff. It encloses a joint cavity.
  b. It is pierced by blood vessels and nerves.
  c. It acts as watch dog i.e. it prevents the excessive movement and protects the joint from dislocation.
  d. It has rich nerve supply hence it is highly sensitive.
  e. It is strengthened by
     I. Accessory ligaments and
     II. Muscles surrounding the joint.
C. Synovial membrane:
  a. Characters:
     I. It lines the inner surface of fibrous capsule.
     II. It is deficient at articular surfaces.
     III. It secrets hyaluronic acid which is responsible for viscosity of the synovial fluid.
     IV. The viscosity of the fluid varies with the movements.
     V. The quantity of the fluid also varies. The knee which is the largest joint contains 0.5 ml.
  b. Functions:
     I. Lubrication and
     II. Nutrition.

D. Joint cavity: All synovial joints are enclosed a joint cavity.

E. Ligaments: The capsule is reinforced externally or internally or both by ligaments.

F. Movements: The joint is capable of varying degrees of movement.

3. **Functions:** Varying degrees of movements.

4. **Classification:** The synovial joints are sub-classified depending upon
   A. Articular surfaces,
   B. Depending upon the axis,
   C. Depending upon the number of bones and
   D. Depending upon the presence of interarticular disc.

5. **Applied anatomy:**
   A. Tuberculosis and gonococcal arthritis affects synovial joint.
   B. More than one joint may have same nerve supply e.g.
      Hip and knee joint supplied by obturator nerve. Thus disease of one joint may cause referred pain to other joint.

| SN-14 | **Prime movers (Agonists)** |

1. **Introduction:** The muscles which initiate and carry out the desired action by active contractions (shortening) are called prime movers.
   e.g. In the flexion of elbow joint, the biceps is prime mover.
   A muscle may perform all the four roles under different situations. Flexor carpi ulnaris is a prime mover in flexion at the wrist and an antagonist in extension. It acts as a fixator in flexion of the thumb and is a synergist in extension of the thumb.

2. **Contraction of muscle** may be   **Table 5.6** Showing types of contraction of the muscle

Type of contraction	Tone	Length	Movement
Isotonic	Equal	Changes	Yes
Isometric	Changes	Equal	No

   A. Isotonic (*Iso* equal, *tonic* tone): During contraction, the length of the muscle decreases to one third and the tone of the muscle remains unchanged. It is associated with the movement e.g. In flexion of the elbow joint, length of biceps is decreased but the tone remains unchanged.

   B. Isometric (*Iso* equal, *metric* measurement): During contraction, the length of muscle fibre remain unchanged but the tone of the muscle tone is changed.
      e.g. After semi flexion of the elbow joint against resistance, the length is not decreased but tone is changed.

3. **Following are the forces opposing the action of the muscle**
   A. Antagonist
   B. Gravity: It is a valuable aid to some movements, depending upon the position of the limb of the body.
      e.g. On raising the arm from the side, the deltoid is a prime mover at the shoulder & the gravity (certainly if there is a weight in the hand) is sufficient to lower the arm.
   C. Connective tissue resistance.
   D. Active resistance.

4. **The range and force of movement depend upon**
    A. Length of the fibres.
    B. Number of the fibres.

5. **Law of Sherrington:** When the agonists or prime movers are active, antagonists are inhibited by reciprocal innervation. When a muscle receives a nerve impulse to contract, its antagonist muscle receives simultaneously an impulse to relax.
    e.g. Flexion of wrist joint is opposed by the extensor.

6. **Action of paradox:** When a prime mover helps opposite action by active controlled lengthening against gravity, it is known as action of paradox.
    e.g. Putting a glass on a table is assisted by gravity but controlled by gradual, active lengthening of biceps.

SN-15   Antagonist

1. **Introduction:** They oppose the prime movers. They help the prime movers by active controlled fractional relaxation, so that the desired movement is smooth and precise. Thus, the antagonists cooperate rather than oppose the prime movers. This is due to reciprocal innervation of the opposite groups of muscles, regulated by the spinal cord through stretch reflex. Antagonist muscle pass over the opposite side of the axis of rotation.
    A. Flexion of wrist joint is done by flexor carpi radialis and ulnaris, which is opposed by extensor carpi radialis longus, brevis and extensor carpi ulnaris.
    B. Flexion of digit is done by efficient extension of wrist joint. This is done by flexor digitorum superficialis and profundus helped by extensor digitorum, which is antagonist.
Note: In addition to the above description, please add points 2,3,4,5 & 6 of Prime Movers.

SN-16   Synergist

(*Syn* together, *ergon* work)
Introduction: Muscles that assist prime movers are called synergists. When a prime movers passes over more than one joint, certain muscles are required to steady the unstable joint such muscle are called synergists. Muscles cross the same site of axis of rotation.

1. During flexion of elbow, biceps brings flexion of elbow assisted by branchialis which synergist.

2. Flexion of digit is efficiently done by efficient extension of wrist joint. This is done by flexor digitorum superficials & profundus helped by extensor digitorum which is antagonist.

3. In most intances, motion at a joint is initiated by one set of synergistic muscles and brought to a close by the antagonists. For example, controlled flexion of the forearm at the elbow joint is initiated by flexor muscles and slowed or stopped at any desired position by extensor muscles.

4. Simultaneous contraction of both synergists and antagonists produces maximal joint stability (dynamic stability) with little or no movement.

Note: In addition to the above description, please add points 2,3,4,5 & 6 of Prime Movers.

SN-17   Fixators

Introduction: The accessory muscles which steadies the proximal joint to bring the desired action on the joint under consideration.

In flexion of wrist joint, the rotator cuff (subscapularis, infraspinatus and teres minor) fixe the shoulder joint, to have the smooth movement at wrist joint.

Note: In addition to the above description, please add points 2,3,4,5 & 6 of Prime Movers.

SN-18   Bursa

(*Bursa* purse)

1. **Introduction:** Bursa is collapsed sac containing small amount of fluid.

2. **Types:**
   A. Communicating: Some bursa communicates with joint cavity.
      e.g. Subscapular bursa of shoulder joint.
   B. Non communicating: e.g. Infrapatellar bursa of knee joint.

3. **Functions:**
   A. It reduces the friction between two mobile and tightly opposed surface.
   B. It permits complete freedom of movement within limited range.

4. **Classification:** It is classified depending upon the situation
   A. Subcutaneous: Deep to the skin.
   B. Subtendinous: Deep to the tendon.
   C. Submuscular: Deep to the muscle.
   D. Subfascial: Deep to the fascia.

5. **Examples:**
   A. Subscapular bursa: It communicates with the shoulder joint. It lies deep to scapula and present between superior and inferior glenohumeral ligament.
   B. Semimembranosus bursa: Deep to semimembranosus muscle.

6. **Applied anatomy:**
   Bursitis: Inflamation of bursa e.g.
   A. Clergyman's knee: It is superficial infrapatellar bursa.
   B. Olecranon bursitis (Miner's elbow, students elbow): Inflammation and enlargement of the bursa over the olecranon process of ulna. This bursa lies between olecranon process and the overlying skin.
   C. Morrant Baker's cyst: The swelling behind the knee is caused by escape of synovial fluid which lies in space or membrane. It is prominent during extension and disappears during flexion. It is associated with the tendons of semimembranosus or gastrocnemius.
   D. Housemaid's knee: The bursa between the skin and anterior surface of patella is called prepatellar bursa and it is inflammed in housemaid.
   E. Weavers bottom: The bursa over ischial tuberosity is inflammed in weavers.

SN-19   Anastomosis

1. **Introduction:** It is a precapillary or/and postcapillary communication of vessel. The blood passing through these communication is called collateral circulation.

2. **Types:** The anastomosis may be following types
   A. Arterial anastomosis: Anastomosis between the two arteries or branches of the two arteries. It is further divided into
      a. Actual arterial anastomosis: Main arteries communicate with each other. In this the blood spurts through the cut ends on both the sides.
         e.g. Circle of Willis, palmar arches, labial artery (branch of facial artery).
      b. Potential arterial anastomosis: Communication takes place between the terminal arterioles. Such communication is gradually through collateral circulation.
         Blockage of main artery may fail to compensate the blood.
         e.g. Coronary arteries, cortical branch of cerebral arteries.
   B. Venous anastomosis: It is the communication between veins or tributaries of veins.
      e.g. Dorsal venous arch of foot and hand.
   C. Arteriovenous anastomosis (shunt): It is the communication between an artery and a vein. When an organ is active these shunts are closed, and the blood circulates through capillaries. It divided into
      a. Simple shunts e.g. Skin nose, lips and external ear.
      b. Specialized e.g. Skin of digital pads and nail beds. These form number of small units called glomeruli.
      c. Preferential through channels: The blood passes through the capillary network and they form microcirculatory units.

3. **Functions:** The nutrition of the organ is maintained, in case of blockage of the artery.

SN-20   End arteries

1. **Introduction:** The arteries which do not communicate with neighbouring arteries are called end arteries.

2. **Types:** They are of following types
   A. Functional end arteries.
      a. These are not true end arteries.
      b. There is a structural communication between these arteries.
      c. But these communications fail to meet the required demand e.g. Coronary arteries.
   B. Structural end arteries:
      a. There is no structural communication between these arteries.
      b. These are true end arteries e.g.
         I. Central artery of retina,
         II. Central arteries of the cerebrum,
         III. Renal arteries &
         IV. Arteries of spleen.

3. **Applied anatomy:** Occlusion of an end artery causes serious nutritional disturbances resulting in death of tissue supplied by it. e.g. In case of blockage of right coronary artery, the muscles of the heart undergo ischaemia and results into myocardial infarction.

GENETICS

SECTION SIX

SN-1 Gene   261

SN-2 Barr body   262

SN-3 Structure of chromosome   263

SN-4 Classification of chromosomes   264

SN-5 Chromosomal aberrations   264

SN-6 Chromosome banding   266

SN-7 Trisomy 21   266

SN-8 Autosomal dominant inheritance   267

SN-9 Autosomal recessive inheritance   267

SN-10 X' linked recessive traits   268

SN-11 Turner's syndrome (45 X)   270

SN-12 Klinefelter syndrome (47 XXY)   270

SN-13 Cru - de - chat syndrome 45 5p   271

SN-14 Non disjunction   271

SN-15 Aneuploidy   272

SN-16 Karyotyping   273

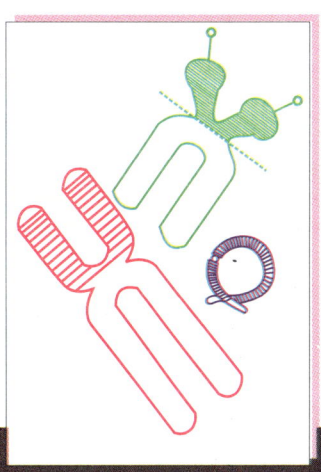

SN-1   Gene

1. **Introduction:** It is the hereditary unit formed by segments of DNA (Deoxyribonucleic acid).

2. **Function:** It synthesises the polypeptide.

3. **Number:** There are about 80,000 genes in a human cell.

4. **Composition:**
   A. Deoxyribose sugar,
   B. Nitrogen bases and
   C. Phosphates.

5. **Parts:**
   A. The functional part is called exon.
   B. The silent part is called intron.

6. **Position:**
   A. Locus: It is the position of the genes on chromosome.
   B. It is described in relation with centromere.
   C. Alleles genes at some locus of homologous pairs are called allelomorphs or alleles.

7. **Types:**
   A. Regulator gene.
      a. It represses the activities.
      b. It inhibits protein synthesis.
   B. Operative gene.
      a. Site: It is present at one end of particular gene.
      b. Function: It allows transcription.
   C. Dominant gene: It expresses its physical or biochemical trait, when allelic genes are either homozygous or heterozygous e.g.
      a. The person showing brachydactyly, the prominent genes are NB, BB
      b. The tallness is caused by dominant gene, the genotype of the tall individual is T:T, T:t
   D. Co-dominant gene: When both allelic genes are dominant but of two different types, both traits may have concurrent expression.
   E. Recessive gene: It expresses its biochemical and physical traits only in homozygous state. e.g. Albinism which is recessive.
   F. Sex linked gene:
      a. Abnormal gene located on X or Y chromosome.
      b. 'X' linked inheritance are more common and is mostly expressed by recessive gene.
   G. Sex limited gene: Born by autosomes but trait is expressed in one of the sex. e.g. Gout, Baldness.
   H. Carrier gene: Heterozygous recessive gene act as carrier gene. It may be expressed in subsequent generation.

SN-2   Barr body (Sex chromatin)

1. **Introduction:** It is an inactivated X chromosome attached to nuclear membrane. It is found by Barr and Bertram in 1949.

2. **Morphology:**
    A. Site: It is attached to nuclear membrane.
    B. Nature: Heterochromatin.
    C. Shape: Planoconvex .
    D. Dimension: 1µ
    E. Staining: Darkly stained
    F. In female ⟶ chromosomes XX
    G. In male (XY) ⟶ There is only one X chromosome which is for cellular function. Y chromosome is for the determination of sex. Hence there is no Barr body.

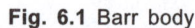

Nuclear membrane — Barr body

Fig. 6.1 Barr body

3. Person with XO will be female as the Y chromosome is absent. The only X chromosome that is present will be in an extended stage and no Barr body is seen.
    The inert X chromosome (Barr body) also divide during cell division. This Barr body is also known as sex chromatin.
    Cell + Barr body = Chromatin positive
    Cell - Barr body = Chromatin negative

4. **Appearance:** It appears by second week of gestation.

5. **Lyon's Hypothesis:** The number of Barr bodies is less than the total number of X chromosome.

    🔑 Number of chromosome - One = Number of Barr bodies. e.g.
    A. In female with XX chromosome, there is a Barr body.
    B. In male with XY chromosome, there is no barr body.
    The absence of Barr body is not enough to prove that cell is from female.

Table 6.1 Showing number of barr bodies in different syndromes

Name of chromosomes	Number of Barr bodies	Syndrome
XX	One	-
XY	No Barr body	-
XXX	2	Triple XXX
XXY	1	Klinefelter's
X	0	Turner's
XO	-	-

5. **Applied anatomy:**
    A. It is helpful for the determination of sex in case of genital ambiguity.
    B. It is a supplementary test in chromosomal aberrations.

SN-3   Structure of chromosome

All chromosomes consists of two parallel identical filaments called chromatids joined together at narrowed construction called primary constriction. Inside the primary constriction there is a pale staining region called centromere. Free ends of chromatids are called as telomeres. Each chromatid is divided by centromere in two arms. In certain chromosomes there is another narrowing (constriction) near one end of each chromatid called as secondary constriction. It is stained faintly. If secondary constriction is close to telomere then the terminal knob of chromosome is termed as satellite. As per the position of centromere, chromosomes are grouped in 4 types.

Table 6.2 Showing types and position of chromosome

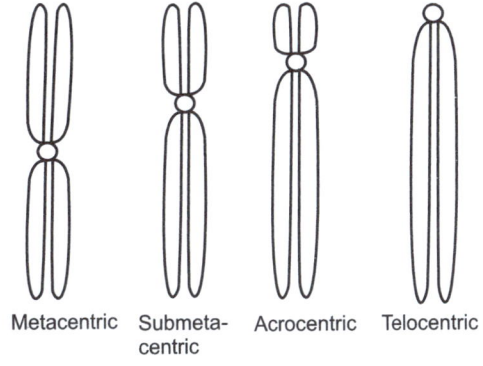

Type	Position of centromere in chromosome
Metacentric	Middle.
Acrocentric	Near one end.
Submetacentric	Between midpoint and end of the chromosome.
Teleocentric	At one end not seen in humans.

Metacentric   Submeta-centric   Acrocentric   Telocentric

Fig. 6.2 Types of chromosomes

The chromosome arranged in descending order of length. The pair No.1 is longest and the pair No. 22 is shortest. They are grouped into 7 groups. They are denoted as A to G.

Table 6.3 Showing classes of the chromosome

Group	Chromosome number	Features
A	1 to 3	Large, metacentric
B	4 & 5	Large, submetacentric
C	6 to 12	Medium sized, submetacentric
D	13 to 15	Medium sized acrocentric with satellite
E	16 to 18	Short submetacentric
F	19 & 20	Short metacentric
G	21 & 22	Very short acrocentric

Sex chromosomes are X & Y, X belongs to C group and Y belongs to G group.

Each cell contains fixed number of chromosomes, which is characteristic of that species or organism.

1. In somatic cell (Body cell) of man the number is 46, which is diploid number.
2. In germ cell i.e. ova & sperms the number is 23, called haploid number. When fertilization takes place, union of two haploid cells restores diploid number of fertlized ovum. The number of sets is termed as ploidy. If more than two sets are present the cell is said to be polyploid. Chromosomes are in multiples of haploid number that is tetraploid (*tetra* 4) it has 4 times haploid number of chromosomes. Triploid (*tri* 3) number of chromosomes will be 69 i.e. three times the haploid number.

SN-4   Classification of chromosomes

(*Chrom* colour, *soma* body)

1. **Structure:** Each chromosome is made up of two identical parallel filaments called chromatids, which are held together at a narrow constricted region, usually pale staining, known as primary constriction, or centromere or kinetochore. This structure is visible only during metaphase stage of cell division.

   Chromosome consists of
   A. Centromere: The constricted part is called chromosome.
   B. Telomere: Free ends (arms) of chromosome.
   C. Satellite body: Part distal to secondary construction.

2. **Function of chromosome** is for perpetuation of species.

3. **Classification:**
   A. According to functions
      a. Autosomes: 22 pairs in human.
      b. Sex chromosomes decides the sex of a person.
         I. Male - XY
         II. Female - XX
   B. According to the positions of the centromere (Denver's classification).

Table 6.4 Showing positions of the centromere

No.	Particulars	Metacentric	Submetacentric	Acrocentric	Telocentric
1	Centromere	Centrally	Subcentrally	Near one end	At one end so that chromatid has only one arm.
	Arms	Equal	p arm (short) q arm (long)	p arm shortest q arm long	One side arms.
	Satellite body	-	-	May present	-
	Secondary construction	-	-	May present	-
	Remark				Not found in human being.
2	Chromatid				Only one arm.

4. **Applied anatomy:** Chromosomes are mapped according to length of arm and position of centromere and it is called karyotyping.

SN-5   Chromosomal aberrations

1. **Introduction:** It is the change in the structural component or number of chromosome. The deletion of a segment or addition of a segment from other chromosomes results in structural aberration while change in number leads to numerical aberration.

2. Factors: Following are the factors for the chromosomal variations

A. Late age of parents for conception.

B. Genes predisposing to non-disjunction.

C. Viral infection during pregnancy.

D. Exposure to radiation.

E. Autoimmune disease of parents.

3. Type:

A. Numercial

    a. Aneuploidy: 2n+1, 2n - 1

    b. Polyploidy: Multiple of n except 2n, e.g. triploidy.

B. Structural: Cause change in number or sequence of genes.

    a. Inversion - Paracentric - Pericentric

    b. Deletion - Termination - Interstitial

    c. Translocation: They are of two types

        I. Robertsonian translocation and

        II. Resiprocal translocation.

    d. Insertion:

    e. Ring chromosome

    f. Isochromosome

    g. Duplication

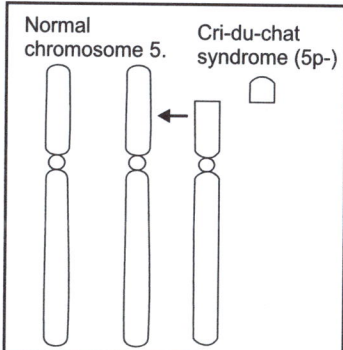

Fig. 6.3 Deletion

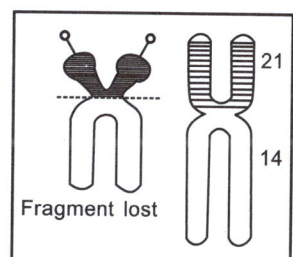

Fig. 6.4 Robertsonian

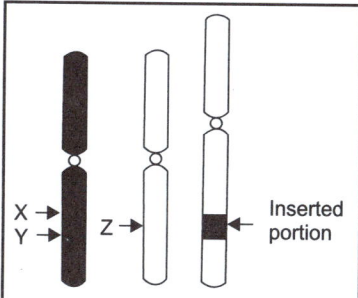

Fig. 6.5 Insertion

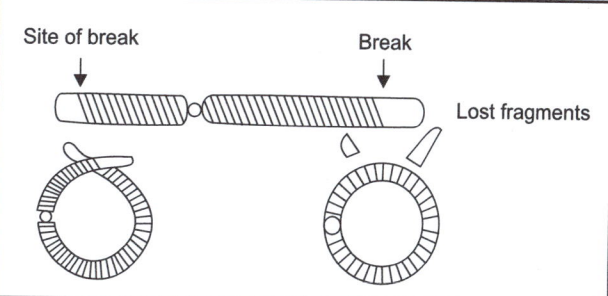

Fig. 6.6 Ring Chromosome

SN-6   Chromosome banding

1. **Introduction:** The chromosomes are identified by banding technique.

2. **Procedure:** The chromosomes are treated first with trypsin and then stained. All the chromosomes are stained with dark and light regions. The dark regions are known as bands. Position of bands in normal chromosome remains fixed and is different for different chromosomes.

3. **Types of banding:** Banding can be of different types.
   A. GTG = Giemsa Trypsin Giemsa banding.
   B. ASG = Acetic saline Giemsa banding.
   C. Q = Quinacrine mustard banding.

4. **Importance of banding:** It helps in:
   A. Identification of individual chromosome.
   B. Confirmation of deletion and inversion.

SN-7   Trisomy 21

1. **Introduction:** It is most common autosomal abnormality syndrome described by Dr Langdon Down's in 1866.

2. **Genotype:** Trisomy 21 (Down's syndrome, Mongolism) 47 XX (+ 21) or 47 XY (+21).

3. **Phenotype:** It is most common autosomal abnormality.

4. **Incidence:** One in 650 to 700 new born.

5. **Factors for chromosomal variations are**
   A. Advanced maternal age.
   B. Genes predisposing to non-disjunction.
   C. Viral infection during pregnancy.
   D. Exposure to radiation.
   E. Autoimmune disease of parents.

6. **Risk factors:** It increase with increasing mother's age. Majority of Down syndrome are found in infants born to mothers above 35 years of age. Probable reason is aging of ova. Sperms are formed fresh every time, hence aging factor is not applicable for sperms.

7. **Clinical Features:**
   A. Affected individual is mentally retarded.
   B. Nasal bridge is flat.
   C. Palpebral fissure is slanting upwards at lateral end.
   D. Epicanthic fold of eyes.
   E. Maxilla is small,
   F. Palate is narrow, so the oral cavity cannot accommodate tongue.
   G. The tongue protrudes out of mouth.
      In about 50 percent of the cases congenital heart disease is present.

SN-8 Autosomal dominant inheritance

1. **Characters:** Commonest mating normal with heterozygote,
   A. The parents show the trait.
   B. There is horizontal and vertical transmission (50% affected)
   C. The trait appears in each generation with no skipping.
   D. Normal (Unaffected) individual does not carry the gene and does not transmit the trait.
   E. No sex predilection.

2. **Autosomal dominant traits:**
   A. Achondroplasia
   B. Brachydactyly

a.

1:	NN x NB	
	N	N
N	NN	NN
B	NB	NB

50% Affected
50% Normal

b.

	NB x NB	
	N	B
N	NN	NB
B	NB	BB

75% Affected
25% Normal

c.

	NN x BB	
	N	B
B	NB	NB
B	NB	NB

100% Affected

d.

	NB x BB	
	N	B
B	NB	BB
B	NB	BB

100% Affected

   C. Huntington's Chorea - Late expression.
   D. Osteogenisis imperfecta.
   E. Syndactyly.

SN-9 Autosomal recessive inheritance

1. **Characters:**
   A. Common mating: Two carriers 25% affected i.e. No horizontal transmission.
   B. The trait seen only in sibs, not in parents.
   C. There is vertical transmission with skipped generation.
   D. The carriers look normal.
   E. There is no sex predilection.
   F. Parents are from consanguineous marriage.
   Commonest mating NA x NA

1:	NA	x NA
	N	A
N	NN	NA
A	NA	AA

25% Affected (AA)

25% Normal (NN)

75% Carriers, 75% Phenotypically normal

2:	NA	x NN
	N	A
N	NN	NA
N	NN	NA

50% Normal

50% Carriers

100% Phenotypically Normal
Skipped Generation

3:	NA	x AA
	N	A
A	NA	AA
A	NA	AA

50% Affected

50% Carriers

50% Phenotypically Normal

Autosomal Recessive traits:

2. **Many inborn errors of metabolism**
   A. Phenyl Ketonuria.
   B. Albinism.
   C. Deaf mutism.
   D. Infantile spastic paraplegia.

SN-10   X' linked recessive traits

1. **The X' linked recessive traits are**
   A. Haemophilia.
   B. Colour blindness.
   C. Duchenne muscular dystrophy.
   D. Hydrocephalus.

2. **Characters:**
   A. The females are carriers and the males are sufferers.
   B. There is no direct transmission from father to son
   C. Zigzag transmission i.e. one generation escapes and trait appears in next generation
   D. The carriers show affection in milder form.

E. The females are rarely affected. Affected female is produced usually by consanguineous marriage between carrier female and affected male.

F. The carrier with Turner's syndrome will suffer.

a.

XhX x	XY	
	X	X
Xh	XhX	Xh
X	XX	XY

Female carrier

Male progeny likely to suffer

Daughter - carrier
Male - 50 % affected, 50 % normal
Female - 50 % carrier, 50 % normal

b. Normal female - Haemophilic male

XX x	XhY	
	X	X
Xh	XhX	XhX
Y	XY	XY

Both daughter - carrier

Both son - normal

Male - 100 % normal, Female - 100% carrier

c. Female carrier X male sufferer

XhX x	XhY	
	Xh	Y
Xh	XhXh	XhY
X	XhX	XY

Female - 50 % suffer, 50 % normal

Male - 50 % affected, 50 % carrier

d. Female Haemophilic X normal male

XhXh x	XY	
	X	X
Xh	XhX	XhY
Xh	XhX	XhY

Male - 100 % affected

Female - 100 % carrier,

SN-11   Turner's syndrome (45 X) 🔑

1. **Introduction:** Described by Turner in 1938.

2. **Aetiology:**
   A. Autoimmune disease of parents.
   B. Viral infection in pregnancy.
   C. Conception occurred late.
   D. Genes predisposing to non-disjunction.
   E. Exposure of radiation.

3. **Incidence:** 1:5000 new born.

4. **Genotype:** 45 X

5. **Phenotype:** In female Barr body is absent.

6. **Clinical Manifestations   :**
   A. Stature - small.
   B. Mouth - shark like.
   C. Lip:
      a. Upper - curved.
      b. Lower - straight.
   D. Chest: Shield like - breast under developed, widely placed rudimentary nipples.
   E. Genitalia: Small - Ovarian dysgenesis infertility, sterility.
   F. Low intelligence.
   G. Webbing of neck.

SN-12   Klinefelter's syndrome (47 XXY) 🔑

1. **Introduction:** Described by Klinefelter in 1942.

2. **Incidence:** 1:1000 live male birth.

3. **Phenotype:** Male.

4. **Genotype:** 44 XXY - Barr body present

5. **Aetiology:**
   A. Autoimmune disease of parents.
   B. Viral infection in pregnancy.
   C. Exposure of radiation.
   D. Conception occurred late.
   E. Genes predisposing to nondisjunction.

6. **Clinical manifestations:**
   A. Tall, long legged, fair intelligence.
   B. Body hair very less.
   C. Gynacomastia.
   D. Small testis, infertile, azoospermia.

SN-13   Cri-du-chat syndrome (5p-)

1. **Introduction:** It is an example of a condition caused by structural chromosomal aberration.

2. **Aetiology:**
   A. Autoimmune disease of parents.
   B. Viral infection in pregnancy.
   C. Conception occurred late.
   D. Genes predisposing to nondisjunction.
   E. Exposure of radiation.

3. **Genotype:** It is a microscopically detectable deletion of terminal portion of short arm of p of chromosome 5 (5p-).

4. **Clinical manifestations:**
   A. Microcephaly.
   B. Premature graying and hairs.
   C. Oblique palpebral fissure.
   D. Saddle nose.
   E. Cat like cry during infancy.
   F. Mental retardation and muscular hypotonia.

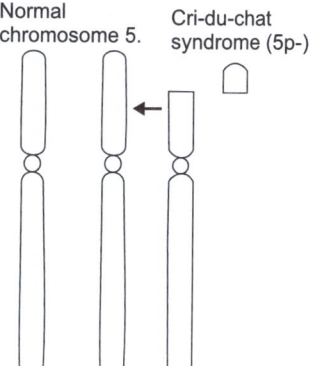

Fig. 6.7 Cri-du-chat syndrome

SN-14   Non disjunction

1. **Introduction:**
   A. Failure of normal migration of chromosome or chromosomes during anaphase of meiosis I.
   B. Failure of migration of chromatid or chromatids during meiosis II.

2. **Reason:** Factors responsible
   A. Faulty spindle formation.
   B. Slow movement of chromatid or chromsome during anaphase.
   C. Radiation, viruses, autoimmune disease -e.g. [Myesthinea Gravis, AIDS].

3. **Result:** Formation of abnormal gamets

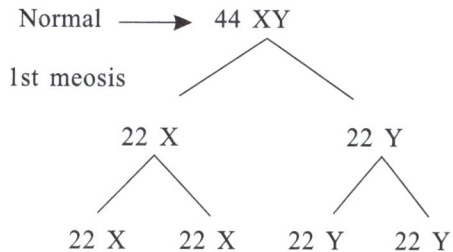

Normally each sperm has haploid number.

A. In non disjunction:

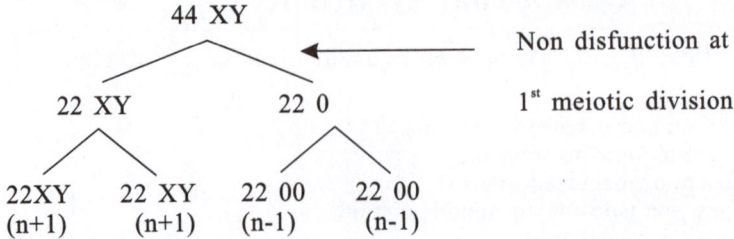

B. Non disjunction at second meiotic division

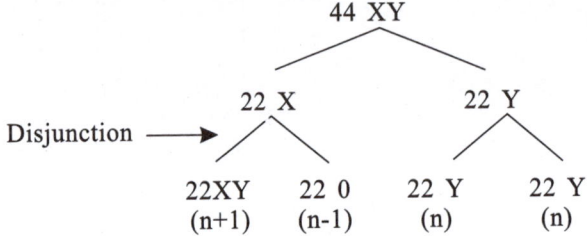

C. Change in number of chromosomes: It can occur in sex chromosomes and autosomes.
when (n+1) fertilized by n
⟶ result 2n+1 chromosomes (trisomy)
⟶ (N-1) fertilized by n
(2n-1) chromosomes (monosomy)
Effect of fertilization -------- abnormal gamet.

In meiosis II - if all chromatids go to one side. One daughter cell with 2n and other dies

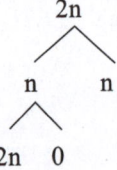

2n fertlises by n ⟶ 3n

| SN-15 | **Aneuploidy** |

(*An* not, *eu* good, *ploidy* multiplication)
If number of chromosomes in body cell is either
1. **More than diploid number** but not multiple of haploid number e.g. 47 chromosomes.
2. **Less than diploid number** but not haploid number e.g.
A. An abnormal X chromosome

B.   One more autosome goes in other cell during division

Each of 46 chromosomes is a member of homologous pair. One member of each pair being received from mother, one from father. The members of pairs are called homologues. 22 pairs are similar in males and females and are called as autosomes.

Chromosomes in remaining pairs are sex chromosomes. In female sex chromosomes (X and X) are identical so females are homogametes. In males one is X and other is Y which are unequal so males are heterogametic.

Homologous chromosomes in each pair of autosomes are indistinguishable i.e. Two chromosomes forming pair number 5 is not identified separately as they appear same.

SN-16   Karyotyping

1.   **Introduction:** Mapping of chromosomes depending upon length and position of centromere is called karyotyping.

2.   **Procedure:** It is done by the microculture of lymphosites. The cells are grown in culture media phytohaemagluttinin (PHA). The cell division is arrested in metaphase by adding colchicine. The spreads of the chromosome are counted and photographed. The images of the each chromosomes are cut out and arranged as per classification.

Karyo typing is done on the basis of

A.   Total length of chromosomes.

B.   Position of centromere.

C.   Relative length of two arms.

D.   Banding pattern.

The chromosomes are arranged according to their length in a descending order. Identical chromosomes are paired in Karyotyping. Then chromosomes paired are numbered 1 to 22 in descending order of length i.e pair No.1 is long, pair No. 22 is short. They are grouped into 7 groups. They are noted as A to G. The chromosomes are placed separately.

Table 6.5 Classes of chromosome

Group	Chromosome number	Features
A	1 to 3	Large, metacentric
B	4 & 5	Large, submetacentric
C	6 to 12	Medium sized, submetacentric
D	13 to 15	Medium sized acrocentric with satellite
E	16 to 18	Short submetacentric
F	19 & 20	Short metacentric
G	21 & 22	Very short acrocentric

3.   **Karyotyping helps to**

A.   To identify pattern of abnormal chromosome,

B.   Determination of the sex.

Key to memory

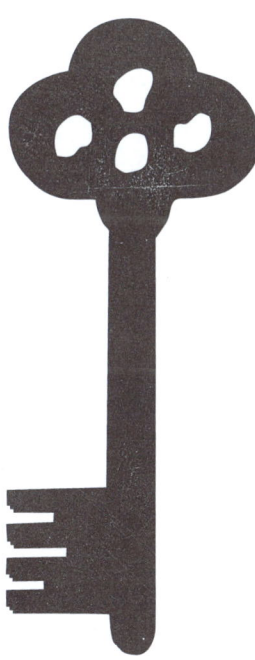

Infex

1. Muscles attached to **linea aspera** (from lateral to medial)
   I love **B**, **Mr B** loves **me**.
   Vastus **i**ntermedius.
   Vastus **l**ateralis.
   Short head of **b**iceps femoris.
   Adductor **m**agnus.
   Adductor **b**revis.
   Adductor **l**ongus.
   Vastus **me**dialis.

2. Course and relations of **great saphenous vein** starts with letter 'M'
   Medial end of the dorsal venous arch.
   It is supplemented by **m**edial marginal vein.
   It runs in front of **m**edial malleous and crosses obliquely on **m**edial surface of lower third of tibia.
   It ascends behind the **m**edial border of tibia to reach knee.
   It runs along the **m**edial side of thigh to drain in saphenous opening present in cribriform fascia.

3. Relations at the base of **femoral triangle** from medial to lateral (VAN)
   Femoral **v**ein,
   Femoral **a**rtery and
   Femoral **n**erve.

4. Branches of **femoral nerve**
   A. The branches of the anterior division can be remembered by Short Cut.
      Muscular: **S**artorius.
      Cutaneous:
      - Medial cutaneous nerve of thigh supplies skin of medial side of thigh.
      - Intermediate cutaneous nerve of thigh.
   B. The branches of posterior division can be remembered by Quadri saph - J
      a. Quadri represents quadreceps femoris. They are
         i. Rectus femoris,
         ii. Vastus lateralis,
         iii. Vastus medialis and
         iv. Vastus intermedius.
      b. Saph represents saphenous nerve.
      c. J represent branches to hip and knee joint.

5. The structures forming the subsartorial plexus of **adductor canal** are remembered by PAS
   A. **P**osterior branch of medial femoral cutaneous nerve.
   B. **A**nterior division of obturator nerve.
   C. **S**aphenous nerve.

6. The gluteus maximus arises from SC ST
   Sacrum
   Coccyx
   Sacro**t**uberous ligament

7. Structure under cover of gluteus maximus can be remembered by grouping the structures i.e. Muscles, nerve, vessels, bones, joints, bursae etc.
   A. Muscles can be remembered by key muscle & other muscles are grouped as ½, 1, 2, 3, 4

    a.   **Key** muscle is piriformis.

    b.   ½ muscle is reflected head of rectus femoris.

    c.   The muscle which is **single**, quadratus femoris.

    d.   The muscles which are in group of **two**:
- I.   Gamelli
  - i.   Superior and
  - ii.   Inferior.
- II.   Obturator
  - i.   Internus &
  - ii.   Externus.

    e.   The muscles which are in group of **three**:
- I.   Gluteus minimus.
- II.   Gluteus medius.

    f.   The muscle which are in group of **four**:
- I.   Semimembranous.
- II.   Semitendinosus.

B.   The key nerve in this region is sciatic nerve. The other nerves under cover of gluteus maximus are recollected by remembering the muscles & their nerve supply.

    a.   Key nerve is sciatic nerve ($L_{4, 5}$, $S_{1, 2, 3}$).

    b.   Nerve to quadratus femoris ($L_{4, 5}$, S_1).

    c.   Nerve to obturator internus (L_5, $S_{1, 2}$).

    d.   Superior gluteal nerve ($L_{4, 5}$, S_1).

    e.   Inferior gluteal nerve (L_5, $S_{1, 2}$).

    f.   Pudendal nerve ($S_{2, 3, 4}$).

    g.   Posterior cutaneous nerve of thigh ($S_{2, 3}$)

    h.   Perforating cutaneous nerve ($S_{2, 3}$) branch of posterior cutaneous nerve of thigh.

C.   Vessels can be remembered by pneumonic 'SIATICA'

    a.   **S**uperior gluteal artery.

    b.   **I**nferior gluteal artery.

    c.   **A**scending branch of medial & lateral circumflex femoral artery (profunda femoris).

    d.   **T**rochanteric anastomosis.

    e.   **I**nternal pudendal vessels.

    f.   **C**ruciate anastomosis.

    g.   **A**scending branch of first perforating artery.

8.   The structures in the **popliteal fossa** at the superior angle, middle and inferior angle are remembered by AVN, AVN & NVA from medial to lateral in the superior and inferior angle and in the middle the structures are from anterior to posterior.

A.   At the superior angle

    a.   Popliteal **a**rtery

    b.   Popliteal **v**ein

    c.   Tibial **n**erve

B.   In middle part

    a.   Popliteal **a**rtery

    b.   Popliteal **v**ein

    c.   Tibial **n**erve

C.   At the inferior angle

    a.   Tibial **n**erve

    b.   Popliteal **v**ein

    c.   Popliteal **a**rtery

9. The action of the **popliteus** is remembered by PPPP
    It pulls the lateral meniscus posteriorly and prevents it from being trapped at the beginning of the flexion.

10. **Layers of the sole** are remembered as follows
    A. First layer contains abductors of great toe and little finger and small tendons of digits.
        a. Abductor hallucis
        b. Abductor digiti minimi
        c. Flexor digitorum brevis
    B. Second layer contains long flexors, their offsprings and their supporters
        a. Flexor hallucis longus
        b. Flexor digitorum longus
        c. Lumbricles
        d. Flexor accessorius
    C. Third layer consist of adductor of great toe, small tendons of the great toe and little finger
        a. Adductor hallucis
        b. Flexor hallucis brevis
        c. Flexor digiti minimi brevis
    D. Fourth layer can be remembered by acronym TIP
        a. **T**ibialis posterior.
        b. **I**nterossei: Three plantar & four dorsal.
        c. Tendon of **p**eroneus longus.

11. The nerve supply of **hip joint** is (**A**ll **s**hould **r**eads **q**uestions **o**ften)
    Accessory obturator nerve
    Sciatic nerve
    Nerve to **r**ectus femoris
    Nerve to **q**uadratus femoris
    Obturator nerve.

12. The functions of the **acetabular labrum** are DMP
    Deepens the acetabular cavity
    Maintains the bony contacts
    Protects the edges.

13. The **intra-articular structures of knee joint** can be remembered as
    A. Key structure is cruciate ligament
    B. All remaining structures can be recollected by recollecting the letters of week days
        a. **M**enisci (**M**on),
        b. **T**endon of popliteus (**T**ue),
        c. **M**enisco femoral ligament (**W**ed),
        d. **T**ransverse ligament (**Th**u),
        e. Haversian pad of **f**at (**F**ri),
        f. **S**ynovial membrane (**S**at) and
        g. **C**oronary ligament (**C**un).

14. The attachment of **cruciate ligament** is remembered by LAMP
    Lateral condyle of femur receives **a**nterior cruciate ligament and **m**edial condyle of femur receives **p**osterior cruciate ligament.

15. The functions of **meniscus** are summerize by 'MENISCUS'
    Maintains the bony contact and potential joint space.
    Escorts the articular surfaces.
    Nourishes the articular surface.
    Increases the concavity of tibial condyle for better adaptation with femoral condyle.
    Serves as a cushion and overcomes the thrust.
    Deepens the joint **c**avity.
    Spreads the synovial fluid **u**niformly.
    Saves from the shock during weight transmission and locomotion between two long bones of the body.

16. **Bursae around knee joint**
    A. SICK - **S**ubcutaneous, **I**nfrapatellar - **C**lergymans **k**nee
    B. PPH - **P**re**p**atellar subcutaneous: **H**ousemaid's knee

17. **Locking of the knee joint** is remembered by the famous tyre company MRF.
    Locking is **m**edial **r**otation of **f**emur on fixed tibia.

18. Relations of **ankle joint** - **T**all **H**imalayas **a**re **n**ever **d**ry **p**laces (From medial to lateral)
    A. Anterior relation
       Tendon of **t**ibialis anterior,
       Extensor **h**allucis longus,
       Anterior tibial vessels,
       Deep peroneal **n**erve,
       Extensor **d**igitorum longus &
       Peroneus tertius.
    B. Posterior relations - **T**alented **D**octors **a**re **n**ever **h**ungry (From anterior to posterior)
       Tendon of **t**ibialis posterior,
       Flexor **d**igitorum longus,
       Posterior tibial **a**rtery,
       Tibial **n**erve &
       Tendon of flexor **h**allucis longus.

19. Posterior boundary of **foramen Winslow** by SIT
    Suprarenal gland (right).
    Inferior vena cava.
    Twelfth thoracic vertebra.

Abdomen

20. The structures forming the **stomach bed** begins with the letters of the days of week
    The **m**ain structure is left crus of diaphragm. (Mon)
    Tortuous splenic artery. (Tue)
    When stomach is distended, gastric surface of spleen also comes in contact. The spleen is separated from the stomach by a recess of greater sac. (Wed)
    Transverse mesocolon. (Thu)
    Left colic **f**lexure. (Fri)
    Anterior **s**urface of the left kidney. (Sat)
    Anterior **s**urface of left suprarenal gland. (Sun)
    Body of the pancreas.

21. External features of **liver** has surfaces, borders, fissures, lobes and peritoneal reflections which are five in number.
   A. **Five** surfaces:
      a. Superior,
      b. Inferior,
      c. Anterior,
      d. Posterior and
      e. Right lateral.
   B. **Five** borders: They are ill defined except inferior border which is well defined.
   C. **Five** fissures:
      a. Fissure for ligamentum teres,
      b. Fissure for ligamentum venosum,
      c. Groove for inferior vena cava,
      d. Fossa for gall bladder and
      e. Porta hepatis.
   D. **Five** lobes:
      a. Anatomical right and left lobes: The liver is divided by a line extending from falciform ligament to the ligamentum teres, which divides into anatomical right and left lobe.
      b. **P**hysiological right and left lobes: It is separated by the **c**holecysto **v**enacaval line into physiological right and left lobe. (PVC)
      c. Caudate lobe.
      d. Quadrate lobe.
      e. Riedel's lobe: Sometimes a tongue like projection arises from the lower border of liver called as Riedel's lobe. It extends below the right costal margin.
   E. **Five** peritoneal ligaments:
      a. Falciform ligament.
      b. Coronary ligament.
      c. Right triangular ligament.
      d. Left triangular ligament.
      e. Lesser omentum.

22. In liver the relations at **porta hepatis** are (from posterior to anterior) as follows: (VAN)
   A. Portal **v**ein,
   B. Hepatic **a**rtery and
   C. Hepatic **d**uct.

23. Interesting about **pancreas**
   The word pancreas has **8** letters.
   It weighs **80** gms
   It measures **8** inch in length.
   It secrets **800** cc of pancreatic juice in 24 hours.
   The pH is **8**.
   It secrets roughly **8** enzymes.

24 Posterior relations of **head of pancreas:**
   IVC, Right renal vein
   Right renal artery, Sympathetic chain,
   Common bile duct, Diaphragm

25. The features of the **kidney** are **1, 2, 3, 4, 5**
   A. Thickness: **1**".
   B. Width: **2**".
   C. Coverings: **3**
   D. Length: **4**".
   E. Weight: **5** ounce i.e.150 gm.

26. The relations of the **posterior surface of the kidney on right and left side** are 1, 2, 3, 4,
   A. On the right side
      a. **1** bone: 12th rib.
      b. **2** vessels:
         i. Subcostal vessels and
         ii. Fourth lumbar artery.
      c. **3** nerves:
         i. Ilio hypogastric,
         ii. Ilio inguinal and
         iii. Subcostal.
      d. **4** muscles:
         i. Psoas major,
         ii. Quadrtus lumborum,
         iii. Transversus abdominis and
         iv. The diaphragm.
   B. The relations of the posterior surface of left kidney are **1, 2, 3, 4,**
      a. **1** Artery: Subcostal.
      b. **2** bones:
         I. Eleventh rib and
         II. Twelfth ribs.
      c. **3** nerves:
         I. Ilio hypogastric,
         II. Ilio inguinal and
         III. Subcostal.
      d. **4** muscles:
         I. Psoas major,
         II. Quadratus lumborum,
         III. Transversus abdominis and
         IV. The diaphragm.

27. The relations of the structures in the **pelvis of kidney** are VAU (from anterior to posterior)
   Renal **v**ein most anteriorly.
   Renal **a**rtery in the middle.
   Ureter most posteriorly.

28. The **ureter** crosses the following structures (VAN from down above)
   Obturator **n**erve,
   Obliterated umbilical **a**rtery,
   Obturator **a**rtery,
   Obturator **v**ein,

29. The hilum of the **left suprarenal gland** is situated on the **l**ower pole of the **l**eft suprarenal gland. (L for the hilum of the left suprarenal gland, l for lower pole of the left suprarenal gland)

30. The lateral part of the right **suprarenal gland** is related to the bare area of the liver (non peritoneal).

31. Origin of the diaphragm is CVS
    Costal
    Vertebral
    Sternal

32. The arterial supply of **diaphragm** is IMP
    Inferior phrenic artery, first branch of the abdominal aorta.
    Musculophrenic, a terminal branch of the internal thoracic artery.
    Lower 5 or 6 **p**osterior intercostal, branches of thoracic aorta.

33. There are three major openings of the **diaphragm.** Each opening contains three important structures
    A. Aortic opening: Main structure is DTA
       Descending **t**horacic **a**orta
       Thoracic duct
       Azygous vein
    B. Oesophageal opening. The word oesophagus contains **ten** letters and it is present at **tenth** thoracic vertebra and contains oesophagus and
       Oesophageal branch of **left gastric artery.**
       Oesophageal vein draining into **left gastric vein.**

34 The development of the diaphragm is from **four** sources which
    Develops at **fourth** cervical vertebra and
    Supplied by phrenic nerve which as root value as C**4**.

35. The hiatus hernia of **diaphragm** is manifested by HARD
    Hiccough
    Anaemia
    Regurgitation
    Dysphagia

36. Th paired muscles of the **perineal body** are formed by BSNL
    Bulbo spongiosus.
    Superficial transverse perinei.
    Deep transverse peri**n**ei.
    Levator ani.

37. Contents of **superficial perineal pouch** of male (SBI)
    Superficial transverse perinei.
    Bulbospongiosus
    Ischiocavernosus.

38. The capacity of **urinary bladder** is 2, 4, 8, 16, 32
    At birth it is **2** ounce (60 ml).
    When the capacity of the bladder reaches **4** ounces (120 ml), one gets sense of filling the bladder.
    When the bladder is filled beyond **8** ounce (240 ml), onegets desire to micturate.
    When the capacity of the bladder reaches **16** ounce (480 ml), it become painful.
    The anatomical capacity of bladder is **32** ounce (960 ml).

39. The anomalies of the **urinary bladder** are A, B, C, D, E, F
    <u>A</u>bsence of the urinary bladder.
    <u>B</u>ladder may be divided into upper & lower compartment by septum (hour glass bladder).
    There may be <u>c</u>ommunication with the rectum - vesicorectal fistula.
    <u>D</u>iverticulum of the urinary bladder. It is usually at the junction of trigone and rest of the bladder.
    <u>E</u>ctopic vesicae: The lower part of the anterior abdominal wall is absent, the bladder is exposed on the surface of the body.
    <u>F</u>istula: Allantosis may remain patent entirely & urine passes through umbilicus.

40. The word **prostate** contains <u>8</u> letters and it weighs <u>8</u> gram.

General Histology
41. Sites of **simple squamous epithelium** are SAHEB
    <u>S</u>erous membrane.
    <u>A</u>lveoli of lung.
    <u>H</u>enles loop.
    <u>E</u>ndothelium of blood vessel.
    <u>B</u>owman's capsule.

42. The word **elastic cartilage** and examples of the elastic cartilage starts with the letter E
    <u>E</u>piglottis,
    Pinna of <u>e</u>ar.
    Lateral part of <u>e</u>xternal acoustic meatus.
    Medial part of <u>E</u>ustachian tube.

General Anatomy
43. The **carpal bones** are (<u>S</u>he <u>l</u>ook <u>t</u>oo <u>p</u>retty, <u>t</u>ry <u>t</u>o <u>c</u>atch <u>h</u>er).
    <u>S</u>caphoid,
    <u>L</u>unate,
    <u>T</u>riquetral,
    <u>P</u>isiform,
    <u>T</u>rapezium,
    <u>T</u>rapezoid,
    <u>C</u>apitate and
    <u>H</u>amate.

44. The exact functions of **sesamoid bone** is not definitely known. However the following functions are attributed which can be remembered by the word SESAMOID
    <u>S</u>erves as a mechanical advantage to the tendon.
    <u>E</u>nsures the prevention of wear and tear of the tendon.
    <u>S</u>tabilises the local circulation.
    <u>A</u>lters the direction of pull of the muscle.
    <u>M</u>aintains the local circulation.
    <u>O</u>vercomes the pressure.
    <u>I</u>nsures the vessels and nerves.
    <u>D</u>iminishes the friction.

45. The examples of the **syndesmoses joints** are IMP
    <u>I</u>nferior tibiofibular joint,
    <u>M</u>iddle radioulnar joint and
    <u>P</u>osterior sacroiliac joint.

46. The examples of the **primary cartilagenous joint** (First, S of second, C & D)
    First condrosternal joint.
    Spheno-occipital.
    Costo-chondral. ('C' third alphabet)
    Diaphysis and epiphysis of long bone. ('D' fourth alphabet)

47. The examples of the **secondary cartilagenous joint** are IMP
    Intervertebral joint.
    Manubrio sternal.
    Pubic symphysis.
    Sacral joint.

Genetics

48. **Lyons hypothesis** - Number of chromosome - One = Number of Barr bodies.

49. Genutype of following syndrome is
    Trisomy 21 (Down's syndrome, Mongolism) 47 XX (+ 21) or 47 XY (+21).
    Cri-du-chat syndrome (5p-)
    Klinefelter's syndrome (47 XXY)
    Turner's syndrome (45 X)

Feed Back

The author humbly request all the students, teachers and well wishers to point out any corrections, which will be rectified in the next edition. Author is very much free for correction and welcomed all sorts of criticism.

Name: .... Designation: ....

Name of the college: ....

Address with phone No. ....

....

....

1. About appearance of the book ....

2. Language ....

3. About text (Grammatical, typographical) ....

4. Content ....

5. Diagram ....

6. Applied anatomy ....

7. Illustration ....

8. Any other comments ....

....

....

....

....

....

....

....

....